P9-CTO-773

W. Nixon Library
Butler Community College
901 South Haverhill Road
El Dorado, Kansas 67042-3280

DISCARD

Injury & Trauma Sourcebook

Learning Disabilities Sourcebook, 4th Edition

Leukemia Sourcebook

Liver Disorders Sourcebook

Medical Tests Sourcebook, 4th Edition

Men's Health Concerns Sourcebook, 4th Edition

Mental Health Disorders Sourcebook, 5th Edition

Mental Retardation Sourcebook

Movement Disorders Sourcebook, 2nd Edition

Multiple Sclerosis Sourcebook

Muscular Dystrophy Sourcebook

Obesity Sourcebook

Osteoporosis Sourcebook

Pain Sourcebook, 4th Edition

Pediatric Cancer Sourcebook

Physical & Mental Issues in Aging Sourcebook

Podiatry Sourcebook, 2nd Edition

Pregnancy & Birth Sourcebook, 3rd Edition

Prostate & Urological Disorders Sourcebook

Prostate Cancer Sourcebook

Rehabilitation Sourcebook

Respiratory Disorders Sourcebook, 3rd Edition

Sexually Transmitted Diseases Sourcebook, 5th Edition

Sleep Disorders Sourcebook, 3rd Edition

Smoking Concerns Sourcebook

Sports Injuries Sourcebook, 4th Edition

Stress-Related Disorders Sourcebook, 3rd Edition

Stroke Sourcebook, 3rd Edition

Surgery Sourcebook, 3rd Edition

Thyroid Disorders Sourcebook

Transplantation Sourcebook

Traveler's Health Sourcebook

Urinary Tract & Kidney Diseases & Disorders Sourcebook, 2nd Edition

Vegetarian Sourcebook

Women's Health Concerns Sourcebook, 4th Edition

Workplace Health & Safety Sourcebook

Worldwide Health Sourcebook

Teen Health Series

Abuse & Violence Information for Teens

Accident & Safety Information for Teens

Alcohol Information for Teens, 3rd Edition

Allergy Information for Teens, 2nd Edition

Asthma Information for Teens, 2nd Edition

Body Information for Teens

Cancer Information for Teens, 3rd Edition

Complementary & Alternative Medicine Information for Teens, 2nd Edition

Diabetes Information for Teens, 2nd Edition

Diet Information for Teens, 3rd Edition

Drug Information for Teens, 3rd Edition

Eating Disorders Information for Teens, 3rd Edition

Fitness Information for Teens, 3rd Edition

Learning Disabilities Information for Teens

Mental Health Information for Teens, 4th Edition

Pregnancy Information for Teens, 2nd Edition

Sexual Health Information for Teens, 3rd Edition

Skin Health Information for Teens, 3rd Edition

Sleep Information for Teens

Sports Injuries Information for Teens, 3rd Edition

Stress Information for Teens, 2nd Edition

Suicide Information for Teens, 2nd Edition

Tobacco Information for Teens, 2nd Edition

Pain

SOURCEBOOK

Fourth Edition

Health Reference Series

Fourth Edition

Pain
SOURCEBOOK

Basic Consumer Health Information about Causes and Types of Acute and Chronic Pain and Disorders and Injuries Characterized by Pain, Including Arthritis, Back Pain, Burns, Carpal Tunnel Syndrome, Headaches, Fibromyalgia, Neuropathy, Neuralgia, Sciatica, Shingles, and More

Along with Facts about Over-the-Counter and Prescription Analgesics, Physical Therapy, and Complementary and Alternative Medicine Therapies, Tips for Managing Pain, a Glossary of Related Terms, and a Directory of Additional Resources

Edited by
Karen Bellenir

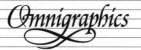

Omnigraphics

155 W. Congress, Suite 200, Detroit, MI 48226

Bibliographic Note

Because this page cannot legibly accommodate all the copyright notices, the Bibliographic Note portion of the Preface constitutes an extension of the copyright notice.

Edited by Karen Bellenir

Health Reference Series
Karen Bellenir, *Managing Editor*
David A. Cooke, MD, FACP, *Medical Consultant*
Elizabeth Collins, *Research and Permissions Coordinator*
EdIndex, Services for Publishers, *Indexers*

* * *

Omnigraphics, Inc.
Matthew P. Barbour, *Senior Vice President*
Kevin M. Hayes, *Operations Manager*

* * *

Peter E. Ruffner, *Publisher*
Copyright © 2013 Omnigraphics, Inc.
ISBN 978-0-7808-1299-4
E-ISBN 978-0-7808-1300-7

Library of Congress Cataloging-in-Publication Data

Pain sourcebook : basic consumer health information about causes and types of acute and chronic pain and disorders and injuries characterized by pain, including arthritis ... / edited by Karen Bellenir. -- Fourth edition.
    pages cm. -- (Health reference series)
Includes bibliographical references and index.
    Summary: "Provides basic consumer health information about the causes and management of various types of acute and chronic pain, along with prevention strategies and coping tips. Includes index, glossary of related terms, and other resources"-- Provided by publisher.
    ISBN 978-0-7808-1299-4 (hardcover : alk. paper) 1. Pain--Popular works. I. Bellenir, Karen.
    RB127.P332123 2013
    616'.0472--dc23
                                                                2013012327

Electronic or mechanical reproduction, including photography, recording, or any other information storage and retrieval system for the purpose of resale is strictly prohibited without permission in writing from the publisher.

The information in this publication was compiled from the sources cited and from other sources considered reliable. While every possible effort has been made to ensure reliability, the publisher will not assume liability for damages caused by inaccuracies in the data, and makes no warranty, express or implied, on the accuracy of the information contained herein.

This book is printed on acid-free paper meeting the ANSI Z39.48 Standard. The infinity symbol that appears above indicates that the paper in this book meets that standard.

Printed in the United States

Table of Contents

Visit www.healthreferenceseries.com to view *A Contents Guide to the Health Reference Series*, a listing of more than 16,000 topics and the volumes in which they are covered.

Preface xiii

Part I—Encountering and Avoiding Pain

Chapter 1—Pain: The Universal Disorder 3

Chapter 2—Facts and Figures on Pain 9

Chapter 3—Pain Perception 19

       Section 3.1—Types of Pain 20

       Section 3.2—The Different Ways People
                   Experience Pain 25

Chapter 4—Chronic Pain Affects Mental Health
             and Sleep 33

       Section 4.1—Depression and Chronic Pain 34

       Section 4.2—Anxiety and Chronic Pain 37

       Section 4.3—Pain and Sleep 40

Chapter 5—Substance Use and Pain 43

       Section 5.1—The Effects of Cigarette
                   Smoke on Pain 44

       Section 5.2—Alcohol and Chronic Pain 46

       Section 5.3—Pain and Illegal Drugs and
                   Marijuana 47

Chapter 6—Coping with Chronic Pain 49

    Section 6.1—Tips for Managing
             Chronic Pain 50

    Section 6.2—Learning to Control Pain 52

    Section 6.3—Quality of Life Scale for
             People with Pain........................ 55

Chapter 7—Stress Management: An Important Tool
    for People with Chronic Pain 57

Chapter 8—Physical Activity Helps Relieve and Avoid
    Spinal Pain.. 65

Chapter 9—Ergonomics to Avoid Workplace Pain 73

Part II: Musculoskeletal Pain

Chapter 10—Arthritis and Rheumatic Diseases........................ 87

    Section 10.1—Questions and Answers
             about Arthritis and Rheumatic
             Diseases 88

    Section 10.2—Rheumatoid Arthritis................. 94

    Section 10.3—Osteoarthritis 98

    Section 10.4—Reactive Arthritis..................... 104

    Section 10.5—Gout... 107

    Section 10.6—Polymyalgia Rheumatica 110

Chapter 11—Back and Spinal Pain 113

    Section 11.1—What You Should Know
             about Back Pain 114

    Section 11.2—Symptoms and Causes of
             Back and Spinal Pain.............. 120

    Section 11.3—Spinal Stenosis........................ 126

Chapter 12—Bone Pain 131

    Section 12.1—Bone Cancer............................. 132

    Section 12.2—Paget's Disease of Bone........... 134

    Section 12.3—Osteonecrosis............................ 136

Chapter 13—Fibromyalgia 139

Chapter 14—Foot Pain 145

Chapter 15—Growing Pains.. 161

Chapter 16—Knee Pain 165

Chapter 17—Muscle Pain.. 175

     Section 17.1—Chronic Myofascial Pain 176

     Section 17.2—Delayed Onset Muscle
               Soreness................................... 179

     Section 17.3—Muscle Cramps........................ 184

Chapter 18—Neck Pain 189

     Section 18.1—What Causes a
               Pain in the Neck? 190

     Section 18.2—Whiplash and
               Whiplash-Associated
               Disorders................................. 193

Chapter 19—Repetitive Motion Disorders 199

     Section 19.1—What Are Repetitive
               Motion Disorders? 200

     Section 19.2—Bursitis and Tendinitis 201

     Section 19.3—Carpal Tunnel Syndrome........ 206

Chapter 20—Shoulder Pain... 213

Chapter 21—Sports Injuries 223

Part III: Other Pain-Related Injuries and Disorders

Chapter 22—Burns 235

     Section 22.1—Facts about Burns 236

     Section 22.2—Burn Pain................................. 238

Chapter 23—Cancer Pain.. 243

Chapter 24—Chest Pain 253

     Section 24.1—Signs and Symptoms of
               a Heart Attack.......................... 254

     Section 24.2—Angina...................................... 256

     Section 24.3—Costochondritis........................ 264

Chapter 25—Dental and Facial Pain 267

    Section 25.1—Tooth Pain 268

    Section 25.2—Temporomandibular
                   Joint Disorders 270

    Section 25.3—Trigeminal Neuralgia 274

Chapter 26—Ear Pain 279

Chapter 27—Gastrointestinal Pain 285

    Section 27.1—Abdominal Adhesions 286

    Section 27.2—Appendicitis 288

    Section 27.3—Crohn Disease 291

    Section 27.4—Diverticulosis and
                   Diverticulitis 294

    Section 27.5—Gallstones 297

    Section 27.6—Gas in the Digestive Tract 299

    Section 27.7—Gastroesophageal Reflux
                   Disease (Heartburn) 302

    Section 27.8—Irritable Bowel Syndrome 305

    Section 27.9—Pancreatitis 309

Chapter 28—Gynecological Pain 313

    Section 28.1—Childbirth and Pain 314

    Section 28.2—Chronic Pelvic Pain 318

    Section 28.3—Dysmenorrhea 321

    Section 28.4—Dyspareunia 324

    Section 28.5—Endometriosis 328

    Section 28.6—Uterine Fibroids 331

    Section 28.7—Vulvodynia 335

Chapter 29—Headaches 339

    Section 29.1—Primary and Secondary
                   Headache Disorders 340

    Section 29.2—Hormones and Migraine 352

    Section 29.3—Analgesic Rebound 354

    Section 29.4—Giant Cell Arteritis 355

Chapter 30—Multiple Sclerosis Pain... 359

Chapter 31—Neuralgia and Neurological Pain........................... 363

    Section 31.1—Understanding Nerve Pain...... 364

    Section 31.2—Arachnoiditis 367

    Section 31.3—Central Pain Syndrome............ 368

    Section 31.4—Complex Regional
                   Pain Syndrome 370

    Section 31.5—Glossopharyngeal Neuralgia ... 371

    Section 31.6—Meralgia Paresthetica.............. 372

    Section 31.7—Paresthesia 373

    Section 31.8—Pinched Nerve 374

    Section 31.9—Piriformis Syndrome................ 375

    Section 31.10–Shingles and
                   Postherpetic Neuralgia 376

    Section 31.11–Tabes Dorsalis 380

    Section 31.12–Tarlov Cysts............................. 381

Chapter 32—Neuropathies... 383

    Section 32.1—Peripheral Neuropathy............ 384

    Section 32.2—Diabetic Neuropathies............. 389

Chapter 33—Phantom and Stump Pain 395

Chapter 34—Sickle Cell Pain 399

Chapter 35—Sinus Pain 405

    Section 35.1—Sinusitis.................................... 406

    Section 35.2—Paranasal Sinus and
                   Nasal Cavity Cancer 411

Chapter 36—Somatoform Pain Disorder 415

Chapter 37—Stroke and Pain 419

Chapter 38—Surgical Pain... 423

    Section 38.1—What You Need to Know
                   about Pain Control after
                   Surgery 424

    Section 38.2—Is Post-Surgery Codeine
                   a Risk for Children? 434

Chapter 39—Urological Pain.. 437

    Section 39.1—Interstitial Cystitis (Painful
               Bladder Syndrome) 438

    Section 39.2—Kidney Stones.......................... 444

Part IV: Medical Management of Pain

Chapter 40—Working with Your Doctor and Pain
    Management Team 449

    Section 40.1—What Is the Specialty
               of Pain Medicine? 450

    Section 40.2—Pain Management Programs ... 451

Chapter 41—Diagnosing and Evaluating Pain 455

    Section 41.1—Getting a Diagnosis
               for Chronic Pain 456

    Section 41.2—X-Rays...................................... 462

    Section 41.3—Magnetic Resonance
               Imaging...................................... 464

    Section 41.4—Electromyograms and Nerve
               Conduction Studies 469

Chapter 42—Conventional and Integrative Approaches
    to Pain Management 473

    Section 42.1—Pain Treatment Plans.............. 474

    Section 42.2—Pain Management
               Therapies 476

    Section 42.3—Rehabilitation Approaches
               to Pain Management 485

Chapter 43—Complementary and Alternative Medicine
    (CAM) Therapies for Pain.................................... 487

    Section 43.1—Chronic Pain and CAM 488

    Section 43.2—Acupuncture 492

    Section 43.3—Dietary Supplements 496

    Section 43.4—Spinal Manipulation 499

    Section 43.5—Massage Therapy 501

    Section 43.6—Relaxation Techniques 504

    Section 43.7—Yoga.. 507

Chapter 44—Over-the-Counter Pain Relievers........................ 509

Chapter 45—Topical Pain Relievers 513

Chapter 46—Non-Opioid Analgesic Pain Relievers 519

Chapter 47—Opioid Pain Relievers 527

    Section 47.1—Commonly Prescribed
                  Opioid Medications.................. 528

    Section 47.2—Opioid Use for Chronic,
                  Non-Terminal Pain Is
                  Controversial........................... 541

Chapter 48—Other Medications Used for Pain
                Management 543

Chapter 49—Corticosteroid Injections for Relieving
                Pain... 559

Chapter 50—Invasive and Implanted Pain Interventions 563

Chapter 51—Surgical Procedures for Pain Relief..................... 571

    Section 51.1—Types of Back Surgery 572

    Section 51.2—Minimally Invasive
                  Spine Surgery 577

    Section 51.3—Nerve Blocks............................ 580

    Section 51.4—Joint Replacement Surgery 583

Chapter 52—Palliative Care 589

Part V: Additional Help and Information

Chapter 53—Terms Related to Pain and
                Pain Management................................ 597

Chapter 54—Resources for More Information about
                Pain Management................................ 609

Index... **623**

Preface

About This Book

According to the National Institutes of Health, pain affects more Americans than diabetes, heart disease, and cancer combined, and chronic pain is the most common cause of long-term disability in the U.S. During the past few decades, medical researchers have learned a great deal about how pain is induced and experienced, but a cure remains elusive. Pain-relieving medications are often insufficient, and many carry the risk of serious side effects, including addiction and death. Other conventional, surgical, and complementary and alternative medicine (CAM) approaches to pain management offer varying degrees of relief, but so far nothing has been discovered that fully addresses the diverse needs of people experiencing pain. Nevertheless, millions of people are able to lessen their suffering and enjoy a better quality of life by taking advantage of medications, therapies, and techniques that can provide some relief.

Pain Sourcebook, Fourth Edition provides updated information about the many ways people encounter pain and the steps they can take to avoid it. It explains the different ways people experience pain and how pain affects mental health, sleep patterns, and everyday tasks. Details about the causes and treatments of the most common types of musculoskeletal pain—including arthritis and back pain—and many other pain-related injuries and disorders, such as burns, headaches, neuropathy, and postoperative pain, are included. A section on pain management offers tips for working with a healthcare provider or pain management team, facts about diagnostic procedures, and information about the most commonly used conventional and CAM therapies for pain relief. The book concludes with a glossary and a directory of resources for additional help and information.

How to Use This Book

This book is divided into parts and chapters. Parts focus on broad areas of interest. Chapters are devoted to single topics within a part.

Part I: Encountering and Avoiding Pain examines the phenomenon of pain, the various ways people experience it, and the differences in pain perception among specific subpopulations. It offers strategies for coping with chronic pain and provides tips for avoiding pain.

Part II: Musculoskeletal Pain describes what is known about disorders and injuries that can cause pain in the joints, tendons, ligaments, bones, and muscles. Individual chapters examine the most common acute and chronic conditions associated with musculoskeletal pain, including arthritis and other rheumatic disorders, back and neck pain, foot pain, and sports injuries.

Part III: Other Pain-Related Injuries and Disorders provides information about conditions of the body's organs, systems, and tissues where pain is the primary symptom or a common complication. These include complaints defined by pain—such as headaches, chronic pelvic pain, and somatoform pain disorder—and a wide variety of diseases associated with pain, such as cancer, heart disease, appendicitis, sickle cell anemia, sinusitis, and kidney stones. Painful injuries and wounds to the body, such as burns, amputations, and surgical incisions, are also discussed.

Part IV: Medical Management of Pain offers tips about effectively communicating pain-related symptoms to a health care provider, and it describes the tools that are used to diagnose the sources of acute and chronic pain. It recounts various approaches to pain management and discusses the benefits and risks associated with some of the most commonly used pain relievers. Invasive, implanted, and surgical interventions are also addressed, and the part concludes with information about palliative care.

Part V: Additional Help and Information includes a glossary of terms related to pain and pain management and a directory of resources for readers seeking more details or assistance.

Bibliographic Note

This volume contains documents and excerpts from publications issued by the following U.S. government agencies: Agency for Healthcare Research and Quality; National Cancer Institute; National Center for Complementary and Alternative Medicine; National Diabetes Information Clearinghouse; National Digestive Diseases Clearinghouse; National Heart Lung and Blood Institute; National Institute of Allergy and Infectious Diseases; National Institute of Arthritis and Musculoskeletal and Skin Diseases; National Institute of Child Health and Human Development; National Institute of Dental and Craniofacial Research; National Institute of Diabetes and Digestive and Kidney Diseases; National Institute of General Medical Sciences; National Institute of Mental Health; National Institute of Neurological Disorders and Stroke; National Institute of Nursing Research; National Institutes of Health; National Kidney and Urologic Diseases Information Clearinghouse; NIH Pain Consortium; Office on Women's Health; U.S. Department of Veterans Affairs; and the U.S. Food and Drug Administration.

In addition, this volume contains copyrighted documents from the following organizations, individuals, and publications: A.D.A.M., Inc.; About.com; American Academy of Orthopaedic Surgeons; American Academy of Pain Medicine; American Association of Endodontists; American Association of Neurological Surgeons; American Board of Pain Medicine; American Chronic Pain Association; American College of Rheumatology; American College of Sports Medicine; American Industrial Hygiene Association; American Psychological Association; Anxiety and Depression Association of America; Beth Israel Medical Center, Department of Pain Medicine and Palliative Care (StopPain.org); Judy Bildner; British Psychological Society; Cleveland Clinic; Jonathan Cluett; Continuum Health Partners, Inc.; Helpguide.org; M.J. Hockenberry; Christian Jarrett; S. Krechel; S. Malviya; S.I. Merkel; Model Systems Knowledge Translation Center; Mosby, Inc./Elsevier; Nemours Foundation; New Zealand Dermatological Society; North American Spine Society; *Paediatric Anaesthesia; The Psychologist;* Regents of the University of California (San Diego); Regents of the University of California (San Francisco); Regents of the University of Michigan; J.R. Shayevitz; Sleep HealthCenters; University of Michigan Health System; T. Voepel-Lewis; and D. Wilson.

Full citation information is provided on the first page of each chapter or section. Every effort has been made to secure all necessary rights to reprint the copyrighted material. If any omissions have been made, please contact Omnigraphics to make corrections for future editions.

Acknowledgements

Thanks go to the many organizations, agencies, and individuals who have contributed materials for this *Sourcebook* and to medical consultant Dr. David Cooke, prepress services provider WhimsyInk, and permissions coordinator Liz Collins for their help and support.

About the Health Reference Series

The *Health Reference Series* is designed to provide basic medical information for patients, families, caregivers, and the general public. Each volume takes a particular topic and provides comprehensive coverage. This is especially important for people who may be dealing with a newly diagnosed disease or a chronic disorder in themselves or in a family member. People looking for preventive guidance, information about disease warning signs, medical statistics, and risk factors for health problems will also find answers to their questions in the *Health Reference Series*. The *Series*, however, is not intended to serve as a tool for diagnosing illness, in prescribing treatments, or as a substitute for the physician/patient relationship. All people concerned about medical symptoms or the possibility of disease are encouraged to seek professional care from an appropriate healthcare provider.

A Note about Spelling and Style

Health Reference Series editors use *Stedman's Medical Dictionary* as an authority for questions related to the spelling of medical terms and the *Chicago Manual of Style* for questions related to grammatical structures, punctuation, and other editorial concerns. Consistent adherence is not always possible, however, because the individual volumes within the *Series* include many documents from a wide variety of different producers and copyright holders, and the editor's primary goal is to present material from each source as accurately as is possible following the terms specified by each document's producer. This sometimes means that information in different chapters or sections may follow other guidelines and alternate spelling authorities. For example, occasionally a copyright holder may require that eponymous terms be shown in possessive forms (Crohn's disease *vs.* Crohn disease) or that British spelling norms be retained (leukaemia *vs.* leukemia).

Locating Information within the Health Reference Series

The *Health Reference Series* contains a wealth of information about a wide variety of medical topics. Ensuring easy access to all the fact sheets, research reports, in-depth discussions, and other material contained within the individual books of the series remains one of our highest priorities. As the *Series* continues to grow in size and scope, however, locating the precise information needed by a reader may become more challenging.

A Contents Guide to the Health Reference Series was developed to direct readers to the specific volumes that address their concerns. It presents an extensive list of diseases, treatments, and other topics of general interest compiled from the Tables of Contents and major index headings. To access *A Contents Guide to the Health Reference Series*, visit www.healthreferenceseries.com.

Medical Consultant

Medical consultation services are provided to the *Health Reference Series* editors by David A. Cooke, MD, FACP. Dr. Cooke is a graduate of Brandeis University, and he received his M.D. degree from the University of Michigan. He completed residency training at the University of Wisconsin Hospital and Clinics. He is board-certified in Internal Medicine. Dr. Cooke currently works as part of the University of Michigan Health System and practices in Ann Arbor, MI. In his free time, he enjoys writing, science fiction, and spending time with his family.

Our Advisory Board

We would like to thank the following board members for providing guidance to the development of this series:

Dr. Lynda Baker, Associate Professor of Library and Information Science, Wayne State University, Detroit, MI

Nancy Bulgarelli, William Beaumont Hospital Library, Royal Oak, MI

Karen Imarisio, Bloomfield Township Public Library, Bloomfield Township, MI

Karen Morgan, Mardigian Library, University of Michigan-Dearborn, Dearborn, MI

Rosemary Orlando, St. Clair Shores Public Library, St. Clair Shores, MI

Health Reference Series *Update Policy*

The inaugural book in the *Health Reference Series* was the first edition of *Cancer Sourcebook* published in 1989. Since then, the *Series* has been enthusiastically received by librarians and in the medical community. In order to maintain the standard of providing high-quality health information for the layperson the editorial staff at Omnigraphics felt it was necessary to implement a policy of updating volumes when warranted.

Medical researchers have been making tremendous strides, and it is the purpose of the *Health Reference Series* to stay current with the most recent advances. Each decision to update a volume is made on an individual basis. Some of the considerations include how much new information is available and the feedback we receive from people who use the books. If there is a topic you would like to see added to the update list, or an area of medical concern you feel has not been adequately addressed, please write to:

Editor
Health Reference Series
Omnigraphics, Inc.
155 W. Congress, Suite 200
Detroit, MI 48226
E-mail: editorial@omnigraphics.com

Part One

Encountering and Avoiding Pain

Chapter 1

Pain: The Universal Disorder

A Brief History of Pain

Ancient civilizations recorded on stone tablets accounts of pain and the treatments used: pressure, heat, water, and sun. Early humans related pain to evil, magic, and demons. Relief of pain was the responsibility of sorcerers, shamans, priests, and priestesses, who used herbs, rites, and ceremonies as their treatments.

The Greeks and Romans were the first to advance a theory of sensation, the idea that the brain and nervous system have a role in producing the perception of pain. But it was not until the Middle Ages and well into the Renaissance—the 1400s and 1500s—that evidence began to accumulate in support of these theories. Leonardo da Vinci and his contemporaries came to believe that the brain was the central organ responsible for sensation. Da Vinci also developed the idea that the spinal cord transmits sensations to the brain.

In the 17th and 18th centuries, the study of the body—and the senses—continued to be a source of wonder for the world's philosophers. In 1664, the French philosopher René Descartes described what is still called a "pain pathway." Descartes illustrated how particles of fire, in contact with the foot, travel to the brain and he compared pain sensation to the ringing of a bell.

Excerpted from "Pain: Hope Through Research," National Institute of Neurological Disorders and Stroke (www.ninds.nih.gov), January 10, 2013.

In the 19th century, pain came to dwell under a new domain—science—paving the way for advances in pain therapy. Physician-scientists discovered that opium, morphine, codeine, and cocaine could be used to treat pain. These drugs led to the development of aspirin, to this day the most commonly used pain reliever. Before long, anesthesia—both general and regional—was refined and applied during surgery.

"It has no future but itself," wrote the 19th century American poet Emily Dickinson, speaking about pain. As the 21st century unfolds, however, advances in pain research are creating a less grim future than that portrayed in Dickinson's verse, a future that includes a better understanding of pain, along with greatly improved treatments to keep it in check.

What We Know about Pain

We may experience pain as a prick, tingle, sting, burn, or ache. Receptors on the skin trigger a series of events, beginning with an electrical impulse that travels from the skin to the spinal cord. The spinal cord acts as a sort of relay center where the pain signal can be blocked, enhanced, or otherwise modified before it is relayed to the brain. One area of the spinal cord in particular, called the dorsal horn, is important in the reception of pain signals.

The most common destination in the brain for pain signals is the thalamus and from there to the cortex, the headquarters for complex thoughts. The thalamus also serves as the brain's storage area for images of the body and plays a key role in relaying messages between the brain and various parts of the body. In people who undergo an amputation, the representation of the amputated limb is stored in the thalamus.

Pain is a complicated process that involves an intricate interplay between a number of important chemicals found naturally in the brain and spinal cord. In general, these chemicals, called neurotransmitters, transmit nerve impulses from one cell to another.

There are many different neurotransmitters in the human body; some play a role in human disease and, in the case of pain, act in various combinations to produce painful sensations in the body. Some chemicals govern mild pain sensations; others control intense or severe pain.

The body's chemicals act in the transmission of pain messages by stimulating neurotransmitter receptors found on the surface of cells; each receptor has a corresponding neurotransmitter. Receptors function much like gates or ports and enable pain messages to pass through and on to neighboring cells. One brain chemical of special interest to neuroscientists is glutamate. During experiments, mice with blocked glutamate receptors show a reduction in their responses to pain. Other important receptors in pain transmission are opiate-like receptors. Morphine and other opioid drugs work by locking on to these opioid receptors, switching on pain-inhibiting pathways or circuits, and thereby blocking pain.

Another type of receptor that responds to painful stimuli is called a nociceptor. Nociceptors are thin nerve fibers in the skin, muscle, and other body tissues, that, when stimulated, carry pain signals to the spinal cord and brain. Normally, nociceptors only respond to strong stimuli such as a pinch. However, when tissues become injured or inflamed, as with a sunburn or infection, they release chemicals that make nociceptors much more sensitive and cause them to transmit pain signals in response to even gentle stimuli such as breeze or a caress. This condition is called allodynia—a state in which pain is produced by innocuous stimuli.

The body's natural painkillers may yet prove to be the most promising pain relievers, pointing to one of the most important new avenues in drug development. The brain may signal the release of painkillers found in the spinal cord, including serotonin, norepinephrine, and opioid-like chemicals. Many pharmaceutical companies are working to synthesize these substances in laboratories as future medications.

Endorphins and enkephalins are other natural painkillers. Endorphins may be responsible for the "feel good" effects experienced by many people after rigorous exercise; they are also implicated in the pleasurable effects of smoking.

Similarly, peptides, compounds that make up proteins in the body, play a role in pain responses. Mice bred experimentally to lack a gene for two peptides called tachykinins-neurokinin A and substance P-have a reduced response to severe pain. When exposed to mild pain, these mice react in the same way as mice that carry the missing gene. But when exposed to more severe pain, the mice exhibit a reduced pain response. This suggests that the two peptides are involved in the production of pain sensations, especially moderate-to-severe pain. Continued research on tachykinins may pave the way for drugs tailored to treat different severities of pain.

Gender and Pain

It is now widely believed that pain affects men and women differently. While the sex hormones estrogen and testosterone certainly play a role in this phenomenon, psychology and culture, too, may account at least in part for differences in how men and women receive pain signals. For example, young children may learn to respond to pain based on how they are treated when they experience pain. Some children may be cuddled and comforted, while others may be encouraged to tough it out and to dismiss their pain.

Many investigators are turning their attention to the study of gender differences and pain. Women, many experts now agree, recover more quickly from pain, seek help more quickly for their pain, and are less likely to allow pain to control their lives. They also are more likely to marshal a variety of resources—coping skills, support, and distraction—with which to deal with their pain.

Research in this area is yielding fascinating results. For example, male experimental animals injected with estrogen, a female sex hormone, appear to have a lower tolerance for pain—that is, the addition of estrogen appears to lower the pain threshold. Similarly, the presence of testosterone, a male hormone, appears to elevate tolerance for pain in female mice: the animals are simply able to withstand pain better. Female mice deprived of estrogen during experiments react to stress similarly to male animals. Estrogen, therefore, may act as a sort of pain switch, turning on the ability to recognize pain.

Investigators know that males and females both have strong natural pain-killing systems, but these systems operate differently. For example, a class of painkillers called kappa-opioids is named after one of several opioid receptors to which they bind, the kappa-opioid receptor, and they include the compounds nalbuphine (Nubain) and butorphanol (Stadol). Research suggests that kappa-opioids provide better pain relief in women.

Though not prescribed widely, kappa-opioids are currently used for relief of labor pain and in general work best for short-term pain. Investigators are not certain why kappa-opioids work better in women than men. Is it because a woman's estrogen makes them work, or because a man's testosterone prevents them from working? Or is there another explanation, such as differences between men and women in their perception of pain? Continued research may result in a better understanding of how pain affects women differently from men, enabling new and better pain medications to be designed with gender in mind.

Pain in Aging and Pediatric Populations

Pain is the number one complaint of older Americans, and one in five older Americans takes a painkiller regularly. In 1998, the American Geriatrics Society (AGS) issued guidelines for the management of pain in older people (*Journal of the American Geriatrics Society.* 1998;

46:635-651). The AGS panel addressed the incorporation of several non-drug approaches in patients' treatment plans, including exercise. AGS panel members recommend that, whenever possible, patients use alternatives to aspirin, ibuprofen, and other nonsteroidal antiinflammatory drugs (NSAIDs) because of the drugs' side effects, including stomach irritation and gastrointestinal bleeding. For older adults, acetaminophen is the first-line treatment for mild-to-moderate pain, according to the guidelines. More serious chronic pain conditions may require opioid drugs (narcotics), including codeine or morphine, for relief of pain.

Pain in younger patients also requires special attention, particularly because young children are not always able to describe the degree of pain they are experiencing. Although treating pain in pediatric patients poses a special challenge to physicians and parents alike, pediatric patients should never be undertreated. Recently, special tools for measuring pain in children have been developed that, when combined with cues used by parents, help physicians select the most effective treatments.

Nonsteroidal agents, and especially acetaminophen, are most often prescribed for control of pain in children. In the case of severe pain or pain following surgery, acetaminophen may be combined with codeine.

Diagnosing Pain

There is no way to tell how much pain a person has. No test can measure the intensity of pain, no imaging device can show pain, and no instrument can locate pain precisely. Sometimes, as in the case of headaches, physicians find that the best aid to diagnosis is the patient's own description of the type, duration, and location of pain. Defining pain as sharp or dull, constant or intermittent, burning or aching may give the best clues to the cause of pain. These descriptions are part of what is called the pain history, taken by the physician during the preliminary examination of a patient with pain.

Physicians, however, do have a number of technologies they use to find the cause of pain. Primarily these include electrodiagnostic procedures, imaging techniques, and neurological examinations.

Electrodiagnostic procedures include electromyography (EMG), nerve conduction studies, and evoked potential (EP) studies. Information from EMG can help physicians tell precisely which muscles or nerves are affected by weakness or pain. Thin needles are inserted in muscles and a physician can see or listen to electrical signals displayed on an EMG machine. With nerve conduction studies the doctor uses two sets of electrodes (similar to those used during an electrocardiogram) that are placed on the skin over the muscles. The first set gives the patient a mild shock that stimulates the nerve that runs to that muscle. The second set of electrodes is used to make a recording of the nerve's electrical signals, and from this information the doctor can determine if there is nerve damage. EP tests also involve two sets of electrodes—one set for stimulating a nerve (these electrodes are attached to a limb) and another set on the scalp for recording the speed of nerve signal transmission to the brain.

X-rays produce pictures of the body's structures, such as bones and joints. Other types of imaging, especially magnetic resonance imaging or MRI, provide physicians with pictures of the body's structures and tissues. MRI uses magnetic fields and radio waves to differentiate between healthy and diseased tissue.

Neurological examinations are inspections in which the physician tests movement, reflexes, sensation, balance, and coordination.

Treating Pain

The goal of pain management is to improve function, enabling individuals to work, attend school, or participate in other day-to-day activities. Patients and their physicians have a number of options for the treatment of pain; some are more effective than others. Sometimes, relaxation and the use of imagery as a distraction provide relief. These methods can be powerful and effective, according to those who advocate their use. Whatever the treatment regime, it is important to remember that pain is treatable.

Surgery, although not always an option, may be required to relieve pain, especially pain caused by back problems or serious musculoskeletal injuries. Surgery may take the form of a nerve block or it may involve an operation to relieve pain from a ruptured disc.

Chapter 2

Facts and Figures on Pain

Overview

Pain is associated with a wide range of injury and disease and is sometimes the disease itself. Some conditions may have pain and associated symptoms arising from a discrete cause, such as postoperative pain or pain associated with a malignancy, or may be conditions in which pain constitutes the primary problem, such as neuropathic pains or headaches.

Millions suffer from acute or chronic pain every year and the effects of pain exact a tremendous cost on our country in health care costs, rehabilitation, and lost worker productivity, as well as the emotional and financial burden it places on patients and their families. The costs of unrelieved pain can result in longer hospital stays, increased rates of rehospitalization, increased outpatient visits, and decreased ability to function fully leading to lost income and insurance coverage. As such, patient's unrelieved chronic pain problems often result in an inability to work and maintain health insurance. According to a recent Institute of Medicine Report, *Relieving Pain in America: A Blueprint for Transforming Prevention, Care, Education, and Research,* pain is a significant public health problem that costs society at least $560–$635

"AAPM Facts and Figures on Pain" is a copyrighted work of the American Academy of Pain Medicine. © 2012 American Academy of Pain Medicine; reprinted with permission. The complete text of this document, including links to references, can be found online at http://www.painmed.org/patientcenter/facts_on_pain.aspx.

billion annually, an amount equal to about $2,000.00 for everyone living in the U.S. This includes the total incremental cost of health care due to pain from ranging between $261 to $300 billion and $297–$336 billion due to lost productivity (based on days of work missed, hours of work lost, and lower wages).

Much more needs to be done to meet these challenges and to increase public awareness of them.

What Is Chronic Pain?

While acute pain is a normal sensation triggered in the nervous system to alert you to possible injury and the need to take care of yourself, chronic pain is different. Chronic pain persists. Pain signals keep firing in the nervous system for weeks, months, even years. There may have been an initial mishap—sprained back, serious infection—or there may be an ongoing cause of pain—arthritis, cancer, ear infection—but some people suffer chronic pain in the absence of any past injury or evidence of body damage. Many chronic pain conditions affect older adults. Common chronic pain complaints include headache, low back pain, cancer pain, arthritis pain, neurogenic pain (pain resulting from damage to the peripheral nerves or to the central nervous system itself).

A recent market research report indicates that more than 1.5 billion people worldwide suffer from chronic pain and that approximately 3–4.5% of the global population suffers from neuropathic pain, with incidence rate increasing in correlation to age.

Incidence of Pain, as Compared to Major Conditions

Pain affects more Americans than diabetes, heart disease, and cancer combined. The information below depicts the number of chronic pain sufferers compared to other major health conditions:

Chronic Pain

- Number of sufferers: 100 million Americans
- Source: Institute of Medicine of the National Academies

Diabetes

- Number of sufferers: 25.8 million Americans (diagnosed and estimated undiagnosed)
- Source: American Diabetes Association

Coronary Heart Disease (Heart Attack and Chest Pain)

- Number of sufferers: 16.3 million Americans
- Source: American Heart Association

Stroke

- Number of sufferers: 7.0 million Americans
- Source: American Heart Association

Cancer

- Number of sufferers: 11.9 million Americans
- Source: American Cancer Society

The Burden of Pain on Every Day Life

The total annual incremental cost of health care due to pain ranges from $560 billion to $635 billion (in 2010 dollars) in the United States, which combines the medical costs of pain care and the economic costs related to disability days and lost wages and productivity.

More than half of all hospitalized patients experienced pain in the last days of their lives, and although therapies are present to alleviate most pain for those dying of cancer, research shows that 50–75% of patients die in moderate to severe pain.

An estimated 20% of American adults (42 million people) report that pain or physical discomfort disrupts their sleep a few nights a week or more.

Commonly Reported Pain Conditions

When asked about four common types of pain, respondents of a National Institute of Health Statistics survey indicated that low back pain was the most common (27%), followed by severe headache or migraine pain (15%), neck pain (15%) and facial ache or pain (4%).

Back pain is the leading cause of disability in Americans under 45 years old. More than 26 million Americans between the ages of 20–64 experience frequent back pain.

Adults with low back pain are often in worse physical and mental health than people who do not have low back pain: 28% of adults with low back pain report limited activity due to a chronic condition, as compared to 10% of adults who do not have low back pain. Also, adults reporting low back pain were three times as likely to be in fair or poor health and more than four times as likely to experience serious psychological distress as people without low back pain.

National Center for Health Statistics

Highlights from the National Center for Health Statistics Report, *Health, United States, 2006, Special Feature on Pain*:

- More than one-quarter of Americans (26%) age 20 years and over—or, an estimated 76.5 million Americans—report that they have had a problem with pain of any sort that persisted for more than 24 hours in duration. [NOTE: This number does not account for acute pain].

- Adults age 45–64 years were the most likely to report pain lasting more than 24 hours (30%). Twenty-five percent (25%) of young adults age 20–44 reported pain, and adults age 65 and over were the least likely to report pain (21%).

Key Findings from the 2006 Voices of Chronic Pain Survey

A 2006 survey conducted for the American Pain Foundation and sponsored by Endo Pharmaceuticals evaluated the impact that chronic pain had on 303 chronic pain sufferers who sought care from their physician and were currently using an opioid to treat their pain.

Control over Chronic Pain

- More than half of respondents (51%) felt they had little or no control over their pain.

- Six out of ten patients (60%) said they experience breakthrough pain one or more times daily, severely impacting their quality of life and overall well-being.

Impact on Quality of Life

- Almost two-thirds (59%) reported an impact on their overall enjoyment of life.

- More than three quarters of patients (77%) reported feeling depressed.

- 70% said they have trouble concentrating.

- 74% said their energy level is impacted by their pain.

- 86% reported an inability to sleep well.

Lost Productive Time and Cost Due to Common Pain Conditions in the United States Workforce

Data from the American Productivity Audit, a computer assisted telephone survey of health and work, of 28,902 working adults between August, 2001 and July 2002, was used to estimate lost productive time due to headache, arthritis, back pain, and other musculoskeletal conditions expressed in hours per worker per week and calculated in US dollars.

- Over half (52.7%) of the workforce surveyed reported having headache, back pain, arthritis, or other musculoskeletal pain in the past two weeks, and 12.7% of all workforce lost productive time in a two-week period due to pain.

- Headache (5.4%) was the most common pain condition prompting lost productive time, followed by back pain (3.2%), arthritis pain (2%) and other musculoskeletal pain (2%).

- Overall, workers lost an average of 4.6 hours per week of productive time due to a pain condition.

- Other musculoskeletal pain (5.5 hours/week) and arthritis or back pain (5.2 hours/week) produced the largest amounts of lost productive time.

- Headache produced, on average, 3.5 hours of lost productive time per week.

- Age did not seem to attenuate the findings.

- Lost productive time from common painful conditions was estimated to be $61.2 billion per year, while 76.6% of lost productive time was explained by reduced work performance, not absenteeism.

America Speaks: Pain in America

[This refers to a] 2003 survey conducted by Peter D. Hart Research Associates as a nationwide survey for Research! America. The purpose of this study was to assess the view of Americans about pain in America. The survey's objectives included gauging Americans' perceptions of how pain sufferers and the medical community deal with the problems of chronic pain.

Dealing with Pain

- Among the major adjustments that chronic pain sufferers have made are such serious steps as taking disability leave from work (20%), changing jobs altogether (17%), getting help with activities of daily living (13%), and moving to a home that is easier to manage (13%).

A Visit to the Doctor

- Most pain sufferers (63%) have seen their family doctor for help.

- Forty percent made an appointment with a specialist, such as an orthopedist.

- Twenty-five percent have visited a chiropractor or a doctor that specializes in pain management (15%).

- While 43% of pain sufferers have been to only one type of doctor for their pain, a large proportion (38%) have consulted more than one practitioner in the medical community.

- Treatments for pain have yielded mixed results. Although 58% of those who took prescription medication say that doing so was very fairly effective for their pain, only 41% of those who took over-the-counter [medications reported the same level of relief].

The Pain Gap

- Seven in ten Americans feel that pain research and management should be one of the medical community's top few priorities (16%) or a high priority (55%).

- Almost six in 10 adults (57%) say they would be willing to pay one dollar more per week in taxes to increase federal funding for the scientific research into the causes and treatment of pain.

Prescription Drug Abuse Facts from the Office of National Drug Control Policy (ONDCP)

- Prescription drugs are the second-most abused category of drugs in the United States, following marijuana.

- Among 12th graders, pharmaceutical drugs used nonmedically are six of the ten most-used substances.

- From 1998 to 2008, the proportion of all substance abuse treatment admissions age 12 or older who reported any pain reliever abuse increased more than fourfold.

- Prescription painkillers are considered a major contributor to the total number of drug deaths. In 2007, for example, nearly 28,000 Americans died from unintentional drug poisoning, and of these, nearly 12,000 involved prescription pain relievers.

- Nearly one-third (29 percent) of people age 12 or older who used illicit drugs for the first time in the past year began by using prescription drugs nonmedically.

- According to a 2008 Department of Defense survey, about one in nine active-duty service members (11 percent) reported past-month prescription drug misuse.

- The estimated number of emergency department visits linked to nonmedical use of prescription pain relievers nearly doubled between 2004 and 2009.

- In 2009, the number of first-time, nonmedical users of psychotherapeutics (prescription opioid pain relievers, tranquilizers, sedatives, and stimulants) was about the same as the number of first-time marijuana users.

- Approximately two million adults age 50 and older (2.1 percent of adults in that age range) used prescription-type drugs nonmedically in the past year.

- Substance abuse treatment admissions for individuals age 50 or older nearly doubled from 1992 to 2008, climbing from 6.6 percent of all admissions to 12.2 percent. The percentage of primary admissions for prescription drug abuse among older individuals increased from 0.7 percent to 3.5 percent over the same time period.

Relieving Pain in America

[The following statistics are from] *Relieving Pain in America: A Blueprint for Transforming Prevention, Care, Education and Research* (Institute of Medicine Report):

- In 2011, at least 100 million adult Americans have common chronic pain conditions, a conservative estimate because it does not include acute pain or children.

- Pain is a significant public health problem that costs society at least $560–$635 billion annually (an amount equal to about $2,000.00 for everyone living in the U.S.).

- In 2008 the cost to federal and state governments of medical expenditures for pain was $99 billion.

- Recent Center for Disease Control and Prevention (CDC) and National Center for Health Statistics (NCHS) data suggest substantial rates of pain from the various causes and that most people in chronic pain have multiple sites of pain. For U.S. adults reporting pain, causes include severe headache or migraine (16.1%), low back pain (28.1%), neck pain (15.1%), knee pain (19.5%), shoulder pain (9.0%), finger pain (7.6%), and hip pain (7.1%).

- According to the National Health and Nutrition Examination Survey (NHANES) data, 17 percent of U.S. children, aged 4–18, experience frequent or severe headaches, including migraine, over the course of a year. Before puberty, boys and girls have headaches at approximately the same rate, but after 12, the rate of recurrent and severe headaches rises among girls.

Summary Health Statistics for U.S. Adults

[These statistics are from the] National Health Interview Survey, 2009 Department of Health and Human Services Report:

- Women were more likely to experience pain (in the form of migraines, neck pain, lower back pain, or face or jaw pain) than men. Women were twice as likely to experience migraines or severe headaches, or pain in the face or jaw, than men.

- The percentage of person experiencing migraines or severe headaches was inversely related to age. Twenty percent adults aged 18–44 years experienced a migraine or severe headache in the three months prior to the interview compared with 15% of adults aged 45–64, 7% of adults aged 65–74, and 6% of adults aged 75 and over.

- Adults aged 18–44 years were less likely to have experienced pain in the lower back during the three months prior to the interview compared with older adults.

- When results are considered by single race without regard to ethnicity, Asian adults were less likely to have pain in the lower back compared to white adults, black adults, and American Indian or Alaska Native (AIAN) adults.

• Adults with a bachelor's degree or higher were less likely to have migraine headaches, neck pain, lower back pain, or pain in the face or jaw, compared to adults who did not graduate from high school.

• Adults in poor and near poor families were more likely to experience migraine headaches, neck pain, lower back pain, or pain in the face or jaw in the three months prior to the interview than were adults in families that were not poor.

• Among adults under age 65, those covered by Medicaid were more likely to have migraine headaches, neck pain, lower back pain, or pain the face or jaw than those with private insurance or those who were uninsured. Among adults aged 65 and over, those covered by Medicaid and Medicare were more likely to have migraine headaches, neck pain, lower back pain, or pain in the face or jaw than those with private insurance or only Medicare health care coverage.

CDC Analysis

[These statistics are from the Centers for Disease Control and Prevention (CDC)'s report] *Vital Signs: Overdoses of Prescription Opioid Pain Relievers—United States, 1999–2008*:

Overdose deaths involving opioid pain relievers (OPR), also known as opioid analgesics, have increased and now exceed deaths involving heroin and cocaine combined.

• Prescription painkiller overdoses killed nearly 15,000 people in the US in 2008. This is more than three times the 4,000 people killed by these drugs in 1999.

• In 2010, about 12 million Americans (age 12 or older) reported nonmedical use of prescription painkillers in the past year.

• One in 20 people in the United States, ages 12 and older, used prescription painkillers nonmedically (without a prescription or just for the "high" they cause) in 2010.

• Nearly half a million emergency department visits in 2009 were due to people misusing or abusing prescription painkillers.

• Sales of opioid pain relievers (OPR) quadrupled between 1999 and 2010. Enough OPR were prescribed last year to medicate every

American adult with a standard pain treatment dose of 5 mg of hydrocodone (Vicodin and others) taken every four hours for a month.

- Nonmedical use of prescription painkillers costs health insurers up to $72.5 billion annually in direct health care costs.

Certain groups are more likely to abuse or overdose on prescription painkillers:

- Many more men than women die of overdoses from prescription painkillers.

- Middle-aged adults have the highest prescription painkiller overdose rates.

- People in rural counties are about two times as likely to overdose on prescription painkillers as people in big cities.

- Whites and American Indian or Alaska Natives are more likely to overdose on prescription painkillers.

- About one in 10 American Indian or Alaska Natives age 12 or older used prescription painkillers for nonmedical reasons in the past year, compared to one in 20 whites and one in 30 blacks.

Some states have a bigger problem with prescription painkillers than others:

- Prescription painkiller sales per person were more than three times higher in Florida (which has the highest rate) than in Illinois (which has the lowest rate).

- In 2008/2009, nonmedical use of painkillers in the past year ranged from one in 12 people (age 12 or older) in Oklahoma to one in 30 in Nebraska.

- States with higher sales per person and more nonmedical use of prescription painkillers tend to have more deaths from drug overdoses.

Chapter 3

Pain Perception

Chapter Contents

Section 3.1—Types of Pain 20
Section 3.2—The Different Ways People
              Experience Pain.. 25

Section 3.1

Types of Pain

Excerpted from "Pain: Hope Through Research," National Institute of Neurological Disorders and Stroke (www.ninds.nih.gov), January 10, 2013.

The Two Faces of Pain: Acute and Chronic

What is pain? The International Association for the Study of Pain defines it as: An unpleasant sensory and emotional experience associated with actual or potential tissue damage or described in terms of such damage.

It is useful to distinguish between two basic types of pain—acute and chronic—and they differ greatly.

Acute pain, for the most part, results from disease, inflammation, or injury to tissues. This type of pain generally comes on suddenly (for example, after trauma or surgery) and may be accompanied by anxiety or emotional distress. The cause of acute pain can usually be diagnosed and treated, and the pain is self-limiting, that is, it is confined to a given period of time and severity. In some rare instances, it can become chronic.

Chronic pain is widely believed to represent disease itself. It can be made much worse by environmental and psychological factors. Chronic pain persists over a longer period of time than acute pain and is resistant to most medical treatments. It can—and often does—cause severe problems for patients. A person may have two or more co-existing chronic pain conditions. Such conditions can include chronic fatigue syndrome, endometriosis, fibromyalgia, inflammatory bowel disease, interstitial cystitis, temporomandibular joint dysfunction, and vulvodynia. It is not known whether these disorders share a common cause.

An A to Z List of Common Types of Pain

Hundreds of pain syndromes or disorders make up the spectrum of pain. There are the most benign, fleeting sensations of pain, such as a pin prick. There is the pain of childbirth, the pain of a heart attack, and the pain that sometimes follows amputation of a limb. There is also pain accompanying cancer and the pain that follows severe trauma, such as that associated with head and spinal cord injuries. A sampling of common pain syndromes follows, listed alphabetically.

Arachnoiditis is a condition in which one of the three membranes covering the brain and spinal cord, called the arachnoid membrane, becomes inflamed. A number of causes, including infection or trauma, can result in inflammation of this membrane. Arachnoiditis can produce disabling, progressive, and even permanent pain.

Arthritis affects millions of Americans. Arthritic conditions include osteoarthritis, rheumatoid arthritis, ankylosing spondylitis, and gout. These disorders are characterized by joint pain in the extremities. Many other inflammatory diseases affect the body's soft tissues, including tendonitis and bursitis.

Back pain has become the high price paid by our modern lifestyle and is a startlingly common cause of disability for many Americans, including both active and inactive people. Back pain that spreads to the leg is called sciatica and is a very common condition (see below). Another common type of back pain is associated with the discs of the spine, the soft, spongy padding between the vertebrae (bones) that form the spine. Discs protect the spine by absorbing shock, but they tend to degenerate over time and may sometimes rupture. Spondylolisthesis is a back condition that occurs when one vertebra extends over another, causing pressure on nerves and therefore pain. Also, damage to nerve roots is a serious condition, called radiculopathy, that can be extremely painful. Treatment for a damaged disc includes drugs such as painkillers, muscle relaxants, and steroids; exercise or rest, depending on the patient's condition; adequate support, such as a brace or better mattress and physical therapy. In some cases, surgery may be required to remove the damaged portion of the disc and return it to its previous condition, especially when it is pressing a nerve root. Surgical procedures include discectomy, laminectomy, or spinal fusion.

Burn pain can be profound and poses an extreme challenge to the medical community. First-degree burns are the least severe; with third-degree burns, the skin is lost. Depending on the injury, pain accompanying burns can be excruciating, and even after the wound has healed patients may have chronic pain at the burn site.

Central pain syndrome results from abnormal signals relayed to and from the brain. See "Trauma" below for more information.

Cancer pain can accompany the growth of a tumor, the treatment of cancer, or chronic problems related to cancer's permanent effects on the body. Fortunately, most cancer pain can be treated to help minimize discomfort and stress to the patient.

Headaches affect millions of Americans. The three most common types of chronic headache are migraines, cluster headaches, and tension headaches. Each comes with its own telltale brand of pain.

- Migraines are characterized by throbbing pain and sometimes by other symptoms, such as nausea and visual disturbances. Migraines are more frequent in women than men. Stress can trigger a migraine headache, and migraines can also put the sufferer at risk for stroke.

- Cluster headaches are characterized by excruciating, piercing pain on one side of the head; they occur more frequently in men than women.

- Tension headaches are often described as a tight band around the head.

Head and facial pain can be agonizing, whether it results from dental problems or from disorders such as cranial neuralgia, in which one of the nerves in the face, head, or neck is inflamed. Another condition, trigeminal neuralgia (also called tic douloureux), affects the largest of the cranial nerves and is characterized by a stabbing, shooting pain.

Muscle pain can range from an aching muscle, spasm, or strain, to the severe spasticity that accompanies paralysis. Another disabling syndrome is fibromyalgia, a disorder characterized by fatigue, stiffness, joint tenderness, and widespread muscle pain. Polymyositis, dermatomyositis, and inclusion body myositis are painful disorders characterized by muscle inflammation. They may be caused by infection or autoimmune dysfunction and are sometimes associated with connective tissue disorders, such as lupus and rheumatoid arthritis.

Myofascial pain syndromes affect sensitive areas known as trigger points, located within the body's muscles. Myofascial pain syndromes are sometimes misdiagnosed and can be debilitating. Fibromyalgia is a type of myofascial pain syndrome.

Neuropathic pain is a type of pain that can result from injury to nerves, either in the peripheral or central nervous system. Neuropathic pain can occur in any part of the body and is frequently described as a hot, burning sensation, which can be devastating to the affected individual. It can result from diseases that affect nerves (such as diabetes) or from trauma, or, because chemotherapy drugs can affect nerves, it can be a consequence of cancer treatment. Among the many neuropathic pain conditions are diabetic neuropathy (which results from nerve damage secondary to vascular problems that occur with diabetes); reflex sympathetic dystrophy syndrome (see below), which can follow injury; phantom limb and post-amputation pain, which can result from the surgical removal of a limb; postherpetic neuralgia, which can occur after an outbreak of shingles; and central pain syndrome, which can result from trauma to the brain or spinal cord.

Reflex sympathetic dystrophy syndrome, or RSDS, is accompanied by burning pain and hypersensitivity to temperature. Often triggered by trauma or nerve damage, RSDS causes the skin of the affected area to become characteristically shiny. In recent years, RSDS has come to be called complex regional pain syndrome (CRPS); in the past it was often called causalgia.

Repetitive stress injuries are muscular conditions that result from repeated motions performed in the course of normal work or other daily activities. They include the following conditions:

- Writer's cramp, which affects musicians and writers and others

- Compression or entrapment neuropathies, including carpal tunnel syndrome caused by chronic overextension of the wrist

- Tendonitis or tenosynovitis, affecting one or more tendons

Sciatica is a painful condition caused by pressure on the sciatic nerve, the main nerve that branches off the spinal cord and continues down into the thighs, legs, ankles, and feet. Sciatica is characterized by pain in the buttocks and can be caused by a number of factors. Exertion, obesity, and poor posture can all cause pressure on the sciatic nerve. One common cause of sciatica is a herniated disc.

Shingles and other painful disorders affect the skin. Pain is a common symptom of many skin disorders, even the most common rashes. One of the most vexing neurological disorders is shingles or herpes zoster, an infection that often causes agonizing pain resistant to treatment. Prompt treatment with antiviral agents is important to arrest the infection, which if prolonged can result in an associated condition known as postherpetic neuralgia. These are some other painful disorders that affect the skin:

- Vasculitis, or inflammation of blood vessels
- Other infections, including herpes simplex
- Skin tumors and cysts
- Tumors associated with neurofibromatosis, a neurogenetic disorder

Sports injuries are common. Sprains, strains, bruises, dislocations, and fractures are all well-known words in the language of sports. Pain is another. In extreme cases, sports injuries can take the form of costly and painful spinal cord and head injuries, which cause severe suffering and disability.

Spinal stenosis refers to a narrowing of the canal surrounding the spinal cord. The condition occurs naturally with aging. Spinal stenosis causes weakness in the legs and leg pain usually felt while the person is standing up and often relieved by sitting down.

Surgical pain may require regional or general anesthesia during the procedure and medications to control discomfort following the operation. Control of pain associated with surgery includes presurgical preparation and careful monitoring of the patient during and after the procedure.

Temporomandibular disorders are conditions in which the temporomandibular joint (the jaw) is damaged and/or the muscles used for chewing and talking become stressed, causing pain. The condition may be the result of a number of factors, such as an injury to the jaw or joint misalignment, and may give rise to a variety of symptoms, most commonly pain in the jaw, face, and/or neck muscles. Physicians reach a diagnosis by listening to the patient's description of the symptoms and by performing a simple examination of the facial muscles and the temporomandibular joint.

Trauma can occur after injuries in the home, at the workplace, during sports activities, or on the road. Any of these injuries can result in severe disability and pain. Some patients who have had an injury to the spinal cord experience intense pain ranging from tingling to burning and, commonly, both. Such patients are sensitive to hot and cold temperatures and touch. For these individuals, a touch can be perceived as intense burning, indicating abnormal signals relayed to and from the brain. This condition is called central pain syndrome or, if the damage is in the thalamus (the brain's center for processing bodily sensations), thalamic pain syndrome. It affects as many as 100,000 Americans with multiple sclerosis, Parkinson disease, amputated limbs, spinal cord injuries, and stroke. Their pain is severe and is extremely difficult to treat effectively. A variety of medications, including analgesics, anti-depressants, anticonvulsants, and electrical stimulation, are options available to central pain patients.

Vascular disease or injury—such as vasculitis or inflammation of blood vessels, coronary artery disease, and circulatory problems—all have the potential to cause pain. Vascular pain affects millions of Americans and occurs when communication between blood vessels and nerves is interrupted. Ruptures, spasms, constriction, or obstruction of blood vessels, as well as a condition called ischemia in which blood supply to organs, tissues, or limbs is cut off, can also result in pain.

Section 3.2

The Different Ways People Experience Pain

"Ouch! The different ways people experience pain," by Christian Jarrett, *The Psychologist*, Vol. 24, Number 6, June 2011. © The British Psychological Society. Reprinted with permission. The complete text of this article, including references, can be found online at http://www.thepsychologist.org.uk/archive/archive_home.cfm?volumeID=24&editionID=202&ArticleID=1860.

Headache, stubbed-toe, injection, broken bone—most of us have suffered pain in one form or another, but our experience of that pain will have varied wildly. In the lab, the same level of stimulation, from extreme cold to electric shock, has been shown to cause a yelp in some but a barely discernible wince in others. Moreover, whereas many people are lucky enough to experience pain as a fleeting encounter, for others pain is a constant companion.

The sensitivity and tolerance people show towards pain varies predictably according to several factors, including gender, ethnicity, personality, and culture, all interacting, overlapping, and playing out in the tissues and synapses of the body. Indeed, the topic of individual differences in pain is like a microcosm of science—it's where biology, psychology, and sociology all meet. So, although the studies that we'll hear about often focus on either psychosocial or biological mechanisms, it's worth remembering that a person's beliefs and cultural upbringing can change the way their body and brain respond to pain. "It's important that we not fight it out as to who's winning—the psychologists or the biomedical folks," says Professor Roger Fillingim, a clinical psychologist at the University of Florida and a leading expert in the field. "We need to integrate all of these factors to better understand how they work together to ultimately create the experience of pain."

Gender

The question of whether men or women have the greater pain threshold is guaranteed to liven up the most soporific of dinner parties. From a lay perspective, evidence exists on both sides. There's no shortage of stories of feminine bravery—for example, in the grip of prolonged labor. On the other hand, it's men who have the greater reputation for a warrior instinct and physical risk-taking. Although some studies turn up negative results, the research points overwhelmingly in one direction. Whether in the lab or in the clinic, men demonstrate greater tolerance of and less sensitivity to pain than women. Women are also far more likely to be diagnosed with chronic pain conditions like fibromyalgia.

Consider a 1998 paper, typical of the field, in which Pamela Paulson and colleagues scanned the brains of 10 women and 10 men while they experienced a heat stimulus applied to their forearm. The participants were told the experiment was testing their ability to discriminate temperatures using a scale from 0 "no heat sensation" to 10 "just barely tolerable pain." Not only did the female participants consistently rate the higher 50° C stimulus as more painful than the male participants, but their brains also showed a greater change in activation in response to it, including in the anterior cingulate cortex (a region known to be associated with the evaluation of painful stimuli) and posterior insula (which regulates internal body states).

These kinds of studies are not without problems. For sociocultural reasons men are less likely to want to admit that they've found a stimulation painful. The sex of the experimenter can play a role here. Several studies have shown that men report lower pain intensity ratings and exhibit greater pain tolerance when the experimenter is a woman. Fredric Levine and Laura Lee De Simone in a 1991 study even chose especially attractive researchers to amplify the effect. At least one study has found that women, too, report higher pain tolerance when tested by the opposite sex.

Other research has shown that the degree to which participants identify with masculinity and femininity influences their response to pain. For example, Cynthia Myers at the University of Florida showed this in relation to the widely used cold-pressor task in which participants are required to hold their hand in icy water for as long as they can. Male and female participants who identified more with masculinity tended to hold their hand in the ice for longer.

Whilst findings like this highlight just how important it is to consider gender-role influences when investigating sex as a factor, this doesn't mean that there aren't also underlying physiological differences in the way the sexes experience pain. Myers, for example, found that sex still predicted pain tolerance even after the influence of gender identity was taken into account.

There's no shortage of potential biological mechanisms that could underlie women's greater sensitivity to pain than men. These include hormonal effects—for example, women's response to pain varies across the menstrual cycle, during and after pregnancy, and with the intake of hormone replacement therapy or the contraceptive pill. Hormones are likely to exert their effects via the inflammatory response, but these pathways are still being worked out. There's also evidence that the body's natural pain killer system—the "endogenous opioids"— works differently in women compared with men. For example, in a 2002 study, Jon-Kar Zubieta and colleagues used positron emission tomography (PET) and a deep-tissue pain stimulation and found less μ-opioid system activation in the brains of female compared with male participants. Men and women respond differently to pain treatments too, with women generally showing more of a response to opioid-based analgesics, although this research is patchy.

There are also cognitive factors that could explain gender differences in pain response. One of these concerns *catastrophizing*—that is perceiving a pain as particularly threatening and believing that it is too severe to cope with. Typical items used to measure this factor include: "it is terrible and I feel it is never going to get any better" and "it is awful, and I feel it overwhelms me." Several studies have shown that women tend to catastrophize about pain more than men. In 2000, for example, when Francis Keefe at the Duke University Medical Centre and his team studied 168 patients with osteoarthritis of the knees, they found that the female patients reported more pain but that this gender difference disappeared once levels of catastrophizing were taken into account.

Ethnicity

Alongside gender, substantial evidence has also accumulated suggesting an association between pain experience and ethnicity. Generally, white

Caucasian people are found to be less sensitive to, and more tolerant of, pain than individuals of African or Asian descent.

Claudia Campbell and colleagues in association with Fillingim's Lab at the University of Florida, for example, reported in 2005 that 62 African American participants were on average less tolerant of heat pain, cold pressor pain, and ischemic pain than white participants. Another study by the same research team found that African American participants exhibited the nociceptive flexion reflex—an automatic withdrawal movement—to an electrical pain stimulus at a lower intensity than did white participants. This paradigm has the advantage of not requiring participants to report the pain they're experiencing, so bypassing some of the sociocultural confounds that that entails.

Although most studies in this field have compared African Americans and white Americans, there are some exceptions. Osamu Komiyama's team at the Nihon University School of Dentistry at Matsudo, for example, compared white Caucasian Belgian and Japanese participants, finding that the latter were more sensitive to needle-like stimuli applied to their cheek, gums, or tongue. Intriguingly, this same study also found that, despite their increased sensitivity, the Japanese participants gave the same stimuli lower pain ratings.

The researchers said this likely reflects the "Japanese cultural emphasis on stoicism and the desirability of concealing pain and emotions." Besides the role played by cultural influences, several physiological and psychological mechanisms underlying ethnic differences have also been identified. One of these is the endogenous pain control mechanism called *diffuse noxious inhibitory controls*. This is the physiological reality behind the folk belief that one way to alleviate an ache is to induce pain somewhere else in the body. Another study by Claudia Campbell and colleagues in 2008 investigated this in relation to an ischemic pain, induced via a tightened arm tourniquet, and a painful electric zap to the leg. In the wake of the arm pain, white participants showed greater reductions in sensitivity to the electric stimulation to their leg than did African American participants.

As regards psychosocial factors, a team led by F. Bridgett Rahim-Williams in Roger Fillingim's lab found that pain sensitivity was greater among African Americans and Hispanics who expressed more identification with their ethnic group—for example, they agreed with statements like "I've spent time trying to find out more about the history and traditions of my ethnic group." Consistent with this, Ben Palmer and colleagues at Manchester University Medical School and the University of Aberdeen found that reports of all-over body pain were four times higher, on average, among a sample of South Asian participants in the United Kingdom (UK) compared with white Europeans, and crucially, that such reports were negatively correlated with participants' degree of assimilation into British culture.

One possible explanation for these effects of ethnic identification and assimilation is that ethnic differences in pain experience are largely cultural and so people who identify more with their ethnic group are more likely to be susceptible to these cultural influences. Again it's important to remember that cultural influences are also likely to have neurobiological correlates, as a person's beliefs and upbringing can affect the way their body responds to pain. "My simplistic assumption is that the only way culture can influence pain is via some psychological mechanism, because for me that's the conduit through which it's manifested in the individual," says Fillingim. "So if I grow up in a culture that believes pain is noble and a sign of a higher power, that would alter my beliefs about pain, would alter my cognitive appraisals of pain, and then those beliefs and appraisals would influence my behavioral, biological, and physiological responses related to pain."

Personality

Another major factor that's associated with the way a person experiences pain is personality. Although research in this area is hampered by the use of varied personality measures, a consistent finding is that people who score higher on neuroticism or a neuroticism-like factor tend to show greater sensitivity to pain and reduced tolerance. Helen Vossen at Maastricht University in a 2006 paper showed this sensitivity is also reflected in an exaggerated cortical response to pain as measured by an electroencephalogram (EEG) in an electrical pain paradigm. Aspects of personality also seem to predict the way a person responds to pain relief. Dorit Pud of the Pain Relief Unit at the Rambam Medical Centre in Israel found that men and women who scored more highly on *harm avoidance* (a trait resembling *neuroticism* that's derived from Robert Cloninger's Tridimensional Personality Questionnaire) showed a larger response to morphine in terms of their subsequent performance on the cold pressor task.

Personality isn't only related to acute pain sensitivity and tolerance, it's also predictive of chronic pain conditions in later life, and people diagnosed with a chronic pain condition tend to exhibit a characteristic personality profile. For instance, Katherine Applegate and colleagues at Duke University Medical Centre caught up with over 2000 university students after a 30-year gap and found that those who'd scored highly in their youth on the Minnesota Multiphasic Personality

Inventory measures of *femininity* (male participants only), *paranoia* (female participants only), *hypochondriasis*, or *hysteria* also tended to be more likely to have a chronic pain condition in middle age.

As for the typical character profile of a chronic pain patient, Rupert Conrad at the University of Bonn in a 2007 paper compared 207 patients with 105 pain-free controls, finding that the patients scored higher on *harm avoidance* and lower on *self-directedness* (a mix of the Big Five factors of Conscientiousness and Extraversion) and *cooperativeness* (akin to the Big Five factor of Agreeableness). The patients also tended to score higher on depression and state anxiety, with 41 percent meeting the psychiatric criteria for a personality disorder (PD)—most frequently paranoid or borderline PD.

It's obviously sensible to take rest, relax, and take precautions after a painful injury. However, Conrad says a person who scores high in harm avoidance will continue to behave in this way even after their injury has healed. He adds that a related personality factor associated with chronic pain is low self-efficacy: "That means a feeling of helplessness and a conviction of not being capable of controlling a situation or being able to overcome obstacles associated with chronic pain."

"As a consequence," he explains, "chronic pain treatment should aim at psychological mechanisms enhancing self-efficacy and lessen avoidance (e.g., cognitive behavioral therapy) and at pharmacologic agents improving supraspinal modulation of pain. It is important to note that psychotherapeutic and pharmacologic approaches should be seen as complementary treatments."

Somewhat paradoxically, whilst the prevalence of borderline PD is elevated among patients diagnosed with a chronic pain condition, the same diagnosis is also associated with reduced pain sensitivity on laboratory measures. In one representative study published in 2004, Christian Schmahl at Johannes Gutenberg-University used an infrared laser as the painful stimulus and found 10 women diagnosed with borderline PD to have higher heat pain thresholds and lower subject pain ratings than 14 nonclinical controls. In 2006 the same researcher and his team linked this reduced pain sensitivity to reduced pain-related activation in the anterior cingulate gyrus and amygdala of patients with borderline PD compared with controls.

Recently attention has turned to identifying the physiological mechanisms, not merely the neural correlates, that might account for the link between personality and pain perception. Two years ago, in an unpleasant-sounding experimental paradigm, Peter Paine and colleagues at Hope Hospital in Manchester identified a link between personality, pain, and autonomic nervous system activity. They used a balloon inflated in the esophagus to simulate visceral pain and found that this triggered an increase in parasympathetic nervous system activity, as identified through heart-rate variability, in participants who scored more highly in neuroticism, whereas repetitions of the same stimulus in those lower in neuroticism led to reduced parasympathetic activity. One possible explanation is that increased parasympathetic nervous system activity corresponds to a *freeze* response in the participants' higher in neuroticism, although how this relates to pain experience remains to be worked out.

Conrad says there's evidence that the personality factors underlying chronic pain may be associated with decreased activation of the prefrontal cortex—a key brain region involved in the top-down modulation of pain. "This neuroanatomical structure can be activated by a cognitive anticipation of the potential controllability of pain," he says. "A personality-based conviction of uncontrollability and helplessness and an avoidance of pain makes activation of these neuroanatomical structures less likely and hampers top-down modulation of pain."

Applications and Controversies

We've seen how factors like ethnicity and personality are related to people's experience of pain. A key challenge now is to use this information to improve people's quality of life. "The goal ultimately," says Fillingim "is to gather all the information we have about an individual—their age, weight, race, sex, genotype data, psychology questionnaire results—put all that into a computer and based on an abundance of evidence that we already have, the computer will tell us, for example, what drug is going to work best for that person." And even more helpful, Fillingim says, is that same information might help predict who's at risk for developing chronic pain. For example, if it's judged that a patient has a high chance of developing a chronic pain condition after surgery, it might be better to pursue alternative treatment options where they exist. "So, it's not just picking the right drug or dose," Fillingim says. "It's really understanding the risk for the development of chronic pain because chronic pain is what we really have trouble helping people with."

Conrad agrees, adding: "Future studies addressing the issue of chronic pain have to give an even deeper insight into the complex interplay of personality factors, psychological mechanisms, and the associated neurobiological mechanisms. The identification of a risk factor such as low self-efficacy by personality questionnaires—for example, temperament and character inventory—may lead to an earlier identification of populations at risk and may lead to an earlier treatment, which may positively affect outcome."

How long until these kind of benefits might be seen? "I'm sure we'll get there one day," Fillingim says, "but I'm not sure how far away that is. The more we get into these individual differences, be it genetic, gender, ethnic group, or whatever, the more complicated everything looks!"

A particularly compelling justification for continuing to study individual differences in pain experience comes from as yet unpublished research looking at genetic influences on pain perception. Fillingim and his colleagues have identified a marker for a particular gene that's associated with increased pain sensitivity in one ethnic group but reduced pain sensitivity in another. This means that if biomedical researchers ignore factors like ethnicity and gender, they risk forming conclusions about genetic influences that are too general. "This just shows that we've got a lot of work to do," says Fillingim, "but hopefully it will be useful in the long run."

Inevitably perhaps, this field has attracted criticism from those who fear the findings will be used to bolster stereotypes. Fillingim and others in the field are sensitive to these concerns and don't want their results to be used in that way. "To me the broader concern is with health disparities such that ethnic groups experience poorer health than white people do—that's obviously driven by many factors including socioeconomic status, but what we're finding may imply that there are individual characteristics of people from different ethnic groups making them more or less prone to experiencing pain or disability associated with pain, and unless we understand what's driving these differences, we're not going to be able to remove the health disparities even if we fix all the system-level problems. So I think the benefits of this kind of research far outweigh the concerns that people have."

Chapter 4

Chronic Pain Affects Mental Health and Sleep

Chapter Contents

Section 4.1—Depression and Chronic Pain 34

Section 4.2—Anxiety and Chronic Pain...................................... 37

Section 4.3—Pain and Sleep.. 40

Section 4.1

Depression and Chronic Pain

Excerpted from "Depression and Chronic Pain,"
National Institute of Mental Health (www.nimh.nih.gov),
NIH Publication No. 11-7744, reviewed January 7, 2013.

Introduction

Depression not only affects your brain and behavior—it affects your entire body. Depression has been linked with other health problems, including chronic pain. Dealing with more than one health problem at a time can be difficult, so proper treatment is important.

Recognizing Depression

Major depressive disorder, or depression, is a serious mental illness. Depression interferes with your daily life and routine and reduces your quality of life. About 6.7 percent of U.S. adults ages 18 and older have depression.

Signs and Symptoms of Depression

- Ongoing sad, anxious, or empty feelings

- Feeling hopeless

- Feeling guilty, worthless, or helpless

- Feeling irritable or restless

- Loss of interest in activities or hobbies once enjoyable, including sex

- Feeling tired all the time

- Difficulty concentrating, remembering details, or making decisions

- Difficulty falling asleep or staying asleep, a condition called insomnia, or sleeping all the time

- Overeating or loss of appetite
- Thoughts of death and suicide or suicide attempts
- Ongoing aches and pains, headaches, cramps, or digestive problems that do not ease with treatment

Chronic Pain

Chronic pain is pain that lasts for weeks, months, or even years. It often does not ease with regular pain medication. Chronic pain can have a distinct cause, such as a temporary injury or infection or a long-term disease. But some chronic pain has no obvious cause. Like depression, chronic pain can cause problems with sleep and daily activities, reducing your quality of life.

The Link between Depression and Chronic Pain

Scientists don't yet know how depression and chronic pain are linked, but the illnesses are known to occur together. Chronic pain can worsen depression symptoms and is a risk factor for suicide in people who are depressed.

Bodily aches and pains are a common symptom of depression. Studies show that people with more severe depression feel more intense pain. According to recent research, people with depression have higher than normal levels of proteins called cytokines. Cytokines send messages to cells that affect how the immune system responds to infection and disease, including the strength and length of the response. In this way, cytokines can trigger pain by promoting inflammation, which is the body's response to infection or injury. Inflammation helps protect the body by destroying, removing, or isolating the infected or injured area. In addition to pain, signs of inflammation include swelling, redness, heat, and sometimes loss of function.

Many studies are finding that inflammation may be a link between depression and illnesses that often occur with depression. Further research may help doctors and scientists better understand this connection and find better ways to diagnose and treat depression and other illnesses.

One disorder that has been shown to occur with depression is fibromyalgia. Fibromyalgia causes chronic, widespread muscle pain, tiredness, and multiple tender points—places on the body that hurt in response to light pressure. People with fibromyalgia are more likely to have depression and other mental illnesses than the general

L.W. Nixon Library
Butler Community College
901 South Haverhill Road
El Dorado, Kansas 67042-3280

population. Studies have shown that depression and fibromyalgia share risk factors and treatments.

Treating Depression in People Who Have Chronic Pain

Depression is diagnosed and treated by a health care provider. Treating depression can help you manage your chronic pain and improve your overall health. Recovery from depression takes time but treatments are effective.

At present, the most common treatments for depression include talk therapy and medication. Cognitive behavioral therapy (CBT) is a type of psychotherapy, or talk therapy, that helps people change negative thinking styles and behaviors that may contribute to their depression. Selective serotonin reuptake inhibitors (SSRIs) are a type of antidepressant medication that includes citalopram (Celexa), sertraline (Zoloft), and fluoxetine (Prozac). Serotonin and norepinephrine reuptake inhibitors (SNRIs) are a type of antidepressant medication similar to SSRIs that includes venlafaxine (Effexor) and duloxetine (Cymbalta).

While currently available depression treatments are generally well tolerated and safe, talk with your health care provider about side effects, possible drug interactions, and other treatment options. For the latest information on medications, visit the U.S. Food and Drug Administration website (www.fda.gov). Not everyone responds to treatment the same way. Medications can take several weeks to work, may need to be combined with ongoing talk therapy, or may need to be changed or adjusted to minimize side effects and achieve the best results.

People living with chronic pain may be able to manage their symptoms through lifestyle changes. For example, regular aerobic exercise may help reduce some symptoms of chronic pain. Exercise may also boost your mood and help treat your depression. Talk therapy may also be helpful in treating your chronic pain.

More information about depression treatments can be found on the National Institute of Mental Health website (www.nimh.nih.gov). If you think you are depressed or know someone who is, don't lose hope. Seek help for depression.

L. W. Nixon Library
Butler Community College
901 South Haverhill Road
El Dorado, Kansas 67042-3280

Section 4.2

Anxiety and Chronic Pain

"Chronic Pain," © 2012 Anxiety and Depression Association of America (www.adaa.org); reprinted with permission.

Muscle tension, body soreness, headaches. For people with anxiety disorders, pain like this may be all too familiar.

Pain can be a common symptom—and sometimes a good indicator— of an anxiety disorder, particularly generalized anxiety disorder (GAD).

Beyond everyday aches and pains, some people will also suffer a diagnosed chronic pain disease such as arthritis or fibromyalgia. And a co-occurring chronic pain disease can make functioning even more difficult for someone with an anxiety disorder.

But people can manage anxiety disorders and chronic pain to lead full and productive lives.

Chronic Pain and Anxiety Disorders

Many chronic pain disorders are common in people with anxiety disorders.

Arthritis: Arthritis is a wide-ranging term that describes a group of more than 100 medical conditions that affect the musculoskeletal system, specifically the joints.

Symptoms include pain, stiffness, inflammation, and damage to joint cartilage and surrounding structures. Damage can lead to joint weakness, instability, and deformities that can interfere with basic daily tasks. Systemic forms of arthritis can affect the whole body and can cause damage to virtually any bodily organ or system.

Anxiety, depression, and other mood disorders are common among people who have arthritis, and very often in younger arthritis sufferers.

Fibromyalgia: Fibromyalgia is a chronic medical condition that causes widespread muscle pain and fatigue.

Migraine: Migraine is severe pain felt on one or both sides of the head, normally occurring around the temples or behind one eye or ear.

Back pain: Back pain is more common in people with anxiety and mood disorders than those without them. Illness, accidents, and infections are among the causes of back pain.

Symptoms include persistent aches or stiffness anywhere along the spine; sharp, localized pain in the neck, upper back, or lower back, especially after lifting heavy objects or engaging in strenuous activity; and chronic ache in the middle or lower back, especially after sitting or standing for extended periods.

Complications

An anxiety disorder along with chronic pain can be difficult to treat. Those who suffer from chronic pain and have an anxiety disorder may have a lower tolerance for pain. People with an anxiety disorder may be more sensitive to medication side effects or more fearful of side effects than, and they may also be more fearful of pain than someone who experiences pain without anxiety.

Treatment

Many treatments for anxiety disorders may also improve chronic pain symptoms. Visit the Anxiety and Depression Association of America's website (www.adaa.org) to find a mental health professional who treats anxiety disorders in your area.

Medication: Some people with an anxiety disorder and chronic pain may be able to take one medication for the symptoms of both conditions, such as treating fibromyalgia with a selective serotonin reuptake inhibitor (SSRI) and some anxiolytics, tricyclic antidepressants, and monoamine oxidase inhibitors (MAOIs) that are effective for headache pain.

Cognitive-behavioral therapy (CBT): CBT is used to treat anxiety disorders as well as chronic pain conditions. It is one type of effective therapy.

Relaxation: Relaxation techniques help people develop the ability to cope more effectively with the stresses that contribute to anxiety and pain. Common techniques include breathing retraining, progressive muscle relaxation, and exercise.

Complementary and alternative treatment: Yoga, acupuncture, and massage are among the complementary and alternative techniques that relieve the symptoms of anxiety disorders as well as chronic pain.

Lifestyle

Many lifestyle changes that improve the symptoms of an anxiety disorder also help the symptoms of chronic pain.

Exercise: Regular exercise strengthens muscles, reduces stiffness, improves flexibility, and boosts mood and self-esteem. Always check with your doctors before beginning an exercise regimen.

Sleep: A good night's sleep is key for anxiety disorders and chronic pain conditions. Symptoms of both types of conditions often become worse without enough sleep.

Consistent sleep and wake times, a good sleep environment (comfortable room temperature, no TV or other distractions), and avoiding caffeine late in the day and at night can help promote restful sleep.

Nutrition: People with anxiety should limit or avoid caffeine and alcohol, which can trigger panic attacks and worsen anxiety symptoms. Some types of food may aggravate some musculoskeletal conditions, including dairy products, gluten (found in wheat, oats, barley, and rye), corn, sugar, and members of the nightshade family (potatoes, tomatoes, eggplant, peppers, and tobacco).

Those who experience pain can reduce their intake of tea, coffee, alcohol, red meat, and acid-forming foods. A health professional can provide more guidance about healthful foods and which to avoid.

Section 4.3

Pain and Sleep

This section includes "What Is Sleep and Why Is It Important?" "Sleep Deprivation," and "Sleep and Pain," © 2012 Sleep HealthCenters. All rights reserved. Reprinted with permission. For additional information, visit www.sleepandyou.com.

What Is Sleep and Why Is It Important?

We spend one third of our lives sleeping; yet, the reason we sleep has long been a scientific mystery. Like humans and other mammals, all animals sleep. Scientists have learned much about the function of sleep from studying the sleep behaviors of different animals from fruit flies to dolphins. What is clear from looking at sleep and sleep-like behaviors in different species is that sleep is a time of restoration and recovery. Sleep serves a variety of possible functions:

- **Energy conservation:** Sleep is a time when our bodies and brains are at rest. Less energy is required compared to when we are awake and active or even awake and at rest, which allows us to conserve energy.

- **Inactivity:** Lack of activity for a period of time makes us less vulnerable to injury and may protect animals from predators.

- **Recovery and growth:** Several important body functions occur during sleep such as release of hormones vital for growth and optimal functioning of various organs in our bodies.

- **Brain function and learning:** The brain reorganizes itself during sleep, which appears to be important for learning and memory.

Sleep Deprivation

Much of the information we know about the function of sleep has come from observing what happens when we don't sleep. The consequences of sleep deprivation highlight why it is worth our while to set aside enough time for sleep, despite a common tendency to "burn the candle at both ends" in our fast-paced world. Studies have shown that sleep deprivation can cause:

Signs of Sleep Deprivation

- Decreased immune function and increased risk of infection
- Changes in hormone levels causing
  - Higher risk of obesity
  - Higher risk of diabetes type 2
- Impaired thinking and attention causing a higher risk of accidents, including motor vehicle accidents
- Decreased ability to learn and form memories
- Increased sensitivity to pain
- Impaired ability to exercise and increased difficulty recovering from exercise
- Higher risk of heart problems
- Increased likelihood of low mood and problems with mood regulation

Sleep and Pain

About Pain

- Pain can be caused by injury or disease, or can be a disease in itself (chronic pain).
- Pain is highly subjective, varying from person to person.
- Pain is the most frequent reason for physician visits.
- Effective management of pain is the key to treating most diseases and injuries.

Pain is usually perceived in one of three ways—through direct stimulation of nerves designed to sense pain, damage to the pain nerves themselves, or damage to the part of the brain responsible for receiving the input from pain nerves.

Pain is an important part of our defenses against injury. Without the ability to sense pain, we would repeat activities that previously caused injury, continue in an activity that will eventually result in injury, or not protect part of the body from further injury (for example, using limping to reduce the weight on a limb).

Treatment of pain depends on whether the pain is chronic (ongoing) or acute (short term). Apart from treating the source of injury, acute pain is treated with drugs (painkillers taken by mouth or applied directly to the site of injury). Chronic pain is much more complicated and difficult to treat and few physicians are expert in the field.

Pain is experienced in many diseases and injuries. Managing pain during the night is important to maintaining sleep quality and quantity. Poor sleep can lead to increased pain.

About Sleep and Pain

- Pain interferes with our ability to sleep.

- A lack of sleep makes you more sensitive to pain.

- Acute pain, for example after surgery, affects sleep length and quality.

- Chronic pain, for example in arthritis, affects all aspects of sleep.

As would be expected, being in pain can affect sleep. Being tired from lack of sleep can also make you more sensitive to pain. Some drugs used to treat acute and chronic pain may cause sleep disorders. Furthermore, it is common for sufferers of some sleep disorders, such as obstructive sleep apnea, to have headache pain upon wakening. The interaction of poor sleep and pain can be a complex problem.

To reduce pain and sleep disorders, you must assess both fully, and treat in a way to minimize both problems. If you visit your physician to discuss pain, it is important to also discuss any problems with your sleep.

Chapter 5

Substance Use and Pain

Chapter Contents

Section 5.1—The Effects of Cigarette Smoke on Pain 44

Section 5.2—Alcohol and Chronic Pain.. 46

Section 5.3—Pain and Illegal Drugs and Marijuana 47

Section 5.1

The Effects of Cigarette Smoke on Pain

Excerpted from "ACPA Resource Guide to Chronic Pain Medication and Treatment," © 2012 American Chronic Pain Association. All rights reserved. Reprinted with permission. For additional information, visit www.theacpa.org.

Smoking causes blood vessels to become constricted, smaller, and narrower; this restricts the amount of oxygen-rich blood flowing to areas of pain. Smoking not only reduces blood flow to your heart but also to other structure such as the skin, bones, and discs. Due to this, you may get accelerated aging leading to degenerative conditions. The lack of blood supply caused by cigarette smoke is also responsible for increased healing time after surgery. After a back fusion surgery, smoking cigarettes can increase the risk of your fusion not healing properly. Cigarette smoke triggers the release of pro-inflammatory cytokines, increasing inflammation and intensifying pain. Smoking makes the bones weak and increases the prevalence of osteoporosis, spinal degenerative disease, and impaired bone and wound healing. Symptoms of depression are more commonly seen among smokers. Below are some tips to help you become smoke free.

Assess your readiness to quit smoking and ask your health care professional or pharmacist for help. They will make recommendations, modifications, and develop a treatment plan to optimize success. Even one less cigarette a day is a step in the right direction. There is nicotine replacement therapy available such as lozenges, gum, or patches. There is also pharmaceutical intervention available to help decrease not only the number of cravings and urges but also the severity.

Keep a smoker's log:

- Cigarettes per day
- Time of each cigarette
- What triggered the craving?
- What were you doing while smoking?
- How did you feel while smoking?

Keeping a log can help you pin point when and why you are smoking. Knowing these triggers can help you replace smoking a cigarette with other less toxic habits.

There are some medications which can help with the craving of cigarettes that many people experience when they are trying to quit. These medications work by affecting dopamine. Dopamine is a neurotransmitter, a chemical messenger, which plays a prominent role in addiction. Dopamine plays a role in movement control, emotional response, and pleasure/pain. It is responsible for the reward pathway and the "feel good" phenomenon experienced when smoking. Nicotine triggers dopamine release in the brain.

Norepinephrine is also a neurotransmitter that sends signal from one neuron to the next. Norepinephrine is similar to adrenaline and is responsible for constricting and narrowing the blood vessels. Norepinephrine can also cause an increase in blood pressure and blood sugar levels. Norepinephrine can affect both mood and behavior.

Varenicline (Chantix) mimics nicotine at the receptors in order to aid in smoking cessation. Varenicline is similar in structure to cytosine, a natural compound that has aided in smoking cessation since the 1960s. Varenicline works via two different mechanisms. First, varenicline is effective because it provides partial nicotine effects to help with nicotine withdrawal symptoms. Second, varenicline also binds to nicotine receptors to block nicotine's effect if one is to relapse. Duration of therapy is normally 12 weeks. Patients who respond to treatment may receive another 12 weeks of therapy to increase their success rate. There is a black box warning for neuropsychiatric symptoms such as change in behavior and mood, agitation, and risk of suicide. Common side effects include the following: nausea, vomiting, insomnia, headache, and abnormal dreams.

Bupropion (Zyban) is an antidepressant; however, it is also used in the smoking cessation process. Bupropion inhibits the reuptake of both dopamine and norepinephrine, increasing their concentrations within the brain. By increasing dopamine the frequency and severity of nicotine cravings and urges are reduced. Norepinephrine plays a role in alleviating symptoms associated with withdrawal. Bupropion effects are not fully seen until one week of treatment is complete. Therefore it is important for patients to start this medication one to two weeks prior to their quit-date. Bupropion is associated with several black box warnings; there is an increased risk of suicide, and neuropsychiatric symptoms may be exhibited. These symptoms include behavior changes, hostility, agitation, and depression. Seizure may occur however they are dose dependent. Less severe, more common side effects include dry mouth, headache, nausea, dizziness, sweating, and insomnia.

Section 5.2

Alcohol and Chronic Pain

Excerpted from "ACPA Resource Guide to Chronic Pain Medication
and Treatment," © 2012 American Chronic Pain Association. All
rights reserved. Reprinted with permission. For additional information, visit www.theacpa.org.

Alcohol is also a drug. The use of alcohol has no place in the treatment of chronic pain, although some individuals turn to alcohol for
relief when they perceive their pain as intolerable.

Alcohol can enhance the effects of certain prescription drugs as well
as markedly increase potential toxic side effects (such as liver damage
when used in conjunction with acetaminophen).

Alcohol affects the nervous system as a depressant, not as a stimulant. It depresses normal mental activity and normal muscle function.
Short-term effects of an average amount of alcohol include relaxation,
breakdown of inhibitions, euphoria, and decreased alertness. Short-
term effects of large amounts of alcohol include nausea, stupor, hang-
over, unconsciousness, and even death. Alcohol increases stomach acid
and impairs liver function. Chronic alcoholism frequently leads to
permanent damage to the liver. Alcohol also affects the heart and
blood vessels by decreasing normal function, leading to heart disease.
Bleeding from the esophagus and stomach frequently accompany liver
disease caused by chronic alcoholism. Many medications cannot be
given to patients with abnormal liver function, thus making it more
difficult to treat chronic pain.

The early signs of alcoholism include the prominent smell of alcohol
on the breath and behavior changes such as aggressiveness, passivity,
lack of sexual inhibition, poor judgment, and outbursts of uncontrolled
emotion such as rage or tearfulness. Intoxication signs of alcoholism
include unsteady gait, slurred speech, poor performance of any brain
or muscle function, stupor or coma in severe alcohol intoxication, with
slow, noisy breathing, cold and clammy skin, and an increased heartbeat.

The long-term effects of alcohol addiction include the compulsive
use of it. When alcohol is unavailable to persons who are severely
addicted, severe withdrawal symptoms are noticed and may be life

threatening if not treated immediately. Even with successful treatment, individuals addicted to alcohol have a high tendency to relapse. Alcohol and chronic pain medications do not mix.

Section 5.3

Pain and Illegal Drugs and Marijuana

Excerpted from "ACPA Resource Guide to Chronic Pain Medication and Treatment," © 2012 American Chronic Pain Association. All rights reserved. Reprinted with permission. For additional information, visit www.theacpa.org.

Health care professionals will not prescribe opioids and other medications to individuals who are known to use illegal "street" drugs (heroin, methamphetamines, etc.) or to be irresponsible with prescription pain medication.

The use of marijuana for pain is controversial. It is allowed by some states for "medicinal" purposes while it is banned by the United States federal government.

Some physicians will prescribe marijuana; others will not prescribe it but not object to its use while prescribing other pain medicines, while some physicians will refuse to prescribe medications (especially opioids) if the patient is using marijuana. Some physicians take a "don't ask, don't tell" philosophy and don't check for marijuana when doing urine drug testing.

The active ingredient found in marijuana (THC) can help pain, but can also lead to dependence and addiction in certain individuals.

Some states allow the legal use of marijuana for health purposes, including pain, although there is no high-level scientific research supporting the long-term use of marijuana for chronic pain. In fact, there is good evidence that excessive smoking of marijuana can be harmful. The use of any substances should be discussed openly between you and your health care professional.

Despite some states allowing medicinal marijuana, it is a federal crime for a health care professional to prescribe a scheduled drug to a patient known to be using illegal drugs, including marijuana. It is also

47

important to remember, if you travel through a state where medicinal marijuana is not allowed, you could be charged with possession of an illegal substance, even if you have the proper documentation from your home state. Additionally, you can be denied employment or fired if your employer or prospective employer conducts drug screenings as a part of the hiring process or has a "no-drug tolerance" policy. Also you can be charged with driving under the influence (DUI) if your driving is impaired and you test positive for marijuana, even in states where medicinal marijuana is allowed.

People who are self-medicating with marijuana for various complaints may not recognize the reality of marijuana withdrawal symptoms. Marijuana withdrawal symptoms, which can start as early as hours after smoking marijuana and last for up to a month, include sleep disturbances, substantial anxiety (which can worsen pain), discomfort, lack of appetite, and commonly trigger marijuana-seeking.

There are risks associated with chronic marijuana use. More frequent marijuana use is associated with increased risk of severe respiratory illnesses, especially chronic bronchitis. Marijuana use leads to reduced workplace productivity, as well as impaired judgment even hours after use. Marijuana intoxication impairs cognitive and psychomotor performance with complex, demanding tasks. Individuals who have used marijuana over long periods of time demonstrate impaired performance on a variety of neuropsychological tests (for example, attention, memory, and processing complex information) even when not acutely intoxicated. A recent review of the existing medical literature concluded the early use of marijuana increased the risk of schizophrenia or a schizophrenia-like psychotic illness by approximately threefold. Emerging evidence suggests a link between more frequent, or severe, marijuana use and anxiety symptoms and disorders.

Chapter 6

Coping with Chronic Pain

Chapter Contents

Section 6.1—Tips for Managing Chronic Pain 50

Section 6.2—Learning to Control Pain 52

Section 6.3—Quality of Life Scale for People
with Pain.. 55

Section 6.1

Tips for Managing Chronic Pain

Copyright © 2012 by the American Psychological Association. Reproduced with permission. American Psychological Association. "Coping with chronic pain." Retrieved from http://www.apa.org/helpcenter/chronic-pain.aspx. No further reproduction or distribution is permitted without written permission from the American Psychological Association.

Chronic pain is physically and psychologically stressful and its constant discomfort can lead to anger and frustration with yourself and your loved ones. By definition, chronic pain is pain that lasts longer than six months and affects how a person lives their daily life. While physicians can provide treatment for the physical dimensions of chronic pain, psychologists are uniquely trained to help you manage the mental and emotional aspects of this often debilitating condition.

Several medical treatments may be used to alleviate chronic pain, including over-the-counter or prescription medication, physical therapy, and less utilized treatments, such as surgery. However, these options are only a few of the pieces necessary to solve the puzzle of chronic pain. Mental and emotional wellness is equally important— psychological techniques and therapy help build resilience and teach the necessary skills for management of chronic pain.

The American Psychological Association (APA) offers the following tips on coping with chronic pain:

Manage your stress: Emotional and physical pain are closely related, and persistent pain can lead to increased levels of stress. Learning how to deal with your stress in healthy ways can position you to cope more effectively with your chronic pain. Eating well, getting plenty of sleep, and engaging in approved physical activity are all positive ways for you to handle your stress and pain.

Talk to yourself constructively: Positive thinking is a powerful tool. By focusing on the improvements you are making, i.e., the pain is less today than yesterday or you feel better than you did a week ago, you can make a difference in your perceived comfort level. For example, instead of considering yourself powerless and thinking that you absolutely cannot deal with the pain, remind yourself that you are uncomfortable, but that you are working toward finding a healthy way to deal with it and living a productive and fulfilling life.

Become active and engaged: Distracting yourself from your pain by engaging in activities you enjoy will help you highlight the positive aspects of your life. Isolating yourself from others fosters a negative attitude and may increase your perception of your pain. Consider finding a hobby or a pastime that makes you feel good and helps you connect with family, friends, or other people via your local community groups or the internet.

Find support: Going through the daily struggle of your pain can be extremely trying, especially if you're doing it alone. Reach out to other people who are in your same position and who can share and understand your highs and lows. Search the internet or your local community for support groups, which can reduce your burden by helping you understand that you're not alone.

Consult a professional: If you continue to feel overwhelmed by chronic pain at a level that keeps you from performing your daily routine, you may want to talk with a mental health professional, such as a psychologist, who can help you handle the physical and psychological repercussions of your condition.

Section 6.2

Learning to Control Pain

"Halt the Hurt! Dealing with Chronic Pain," *NIH News in Health*,
National Institutes of Health, March 2012.

Pain—it's something we've all experienced. From our first skinned knee
to the headaches, back pain, and creaky joints as we age, pain is something
we encounter many times. Most pain is acute and goes away quickly. But
in some cases, when pain develops slowly or persists for months or even
years, then it's called chronic pain, and it can be tricky to treat.

Chronic pain is a huge problem. Over 115 million people nationwide—
about one in three Americans—suffer from some kind of long-term pain.
It's the leading reason that people miss work.

Scientists funded by the National Institutes of Health (NIH) are
working to better understand and treat chronic pain. They're uncovering
the intricate pathways that lead to long-term pain. And they're looking
for approaches beyond medication that might help you control your pain.

Chronic pain differs in many ways from acute pain. Acute pain is
part of the body's response to an injury or short-term illness. Acute
pain can help prevent more serious injury. For instance, it can make
you quickly pull your finger away from a hot stove or keep your weight
off a broken ankle. The causes of acute pain can usually be diagnosed
and treated, and the pain eventually ends.

But the causes of chronic pain aren't always clear. "It's a complex
problem that involves more than just the physical aspects of where the
hurt seems to be," says Dr. John Killen, deputy director of NIH's National Center for Complementary and Alternative Medicine. "There's
a lot of accumulating scientific evidence that chronic pain is partly a
problem of how the brain processes pain."

Chronic pain can come in many forms, and it accompanies several
conditions including low-back pain, arthritis, cancer, migraine, fibromyalgia, endometriosis, and inflammatory bowel disease. These persistent
pains can severely limit your ability to move around and perform day-
to-day tasks. Chronic pain can lead to depression and anxiety. It's hard
to look on the bright side when pain just won't go away. Some experts
say that chronic pain is a disease itself.

The complexities of chronic pain can make it difficult to treat. Many of today's medications for chronic pain target inflammation. These drugs include aspirin, ibuprofen, and COX-2 inhibitors. But if taken at high doses for a long time, these drugs can irritate your stomach and digestive system and possibly harm your kidneys. And they don't work for everyone.

"With hard-to-treat pain, the opioids are also used, sometimes in combination with the other drugs," says Dr. Raymond Dionne, who oversees some of NIH's clinical pain research. Opioids include prescription painkillers such as codeine and morphine and brand-name drugs such as Vicodin, OxyContin, and Percocet. Opioids affect the processes by which the brain perceives pain. If used improperly, though, opioids can be addictive, and increasingly high doses may be needed to keep pain in check.

"As with all drugs, you have to find a balance between effectiveness and side effects," says Dionne. He and other researchers have studied potential new pain medications to learn more about how they work in the body. But for the most part, pain medications are similar to those used five or more decades ago. That's why some researchers are looking for approaches beyond medications.

"One thing we know is that currently available drug therapies don't provide all the answers. Many people find that medications don't fully relieve their chronic pain, and they can experience unpleasant side effects," Killen says. "Evidence on a number of fronts, for several conditions, suggests that mind and body approaches can be helpful additions to conventional medicine for managing chronic pain."

Research has shown that patients with chronic low-back pain might benefit from acupuncture, massage therapy, yoga, or cognitive-behavioral therapy (a type of talk therapy).

NIH-funded scientists have also found that people with fibromyalgia pain might find relief through tai chi. This mind-body technique combines meditation, slow movements, deep breathing, and relaxation.

But how much these approaches truly help is still an open question. Studies of pain relief can be difficult to interpret. Researchers must rely on patients to complete questionnaires and rate their own levels of pain.

One puzzler is that the exposure to the exact same pain-causing thing, or stimulus, can lead to completely different responses in different people. For example, when an identical heat stimulus is applied to different people's arms, one may report feeling uncomfortable, while another might say that the pain is extreme.

"How do we account for these differences? We've now learned that genes play a role," says Dr. Sean Mackey, who heads Stanford

University's neuroscience and pain lab. "Some differences involve our personality and mood states, including anxiety."

Mackey and his team are using brain scans to gain insights into how we process and feel pain. One study found that a painful stimulus can activate different brain regions in people who are anxious than in those who are fearful of pain.

In another study, volunteers were taught strategies that could turn on specific brain regions. One technique involved mentally changing the meaning of the pain and thinking about it in a non-threatening way.

"We found that with repeated training, people can learn how to build up this brain area, almost like a muscle, and make its activity much stronger," says Mackey. "That led to a significant improvement overall in their pain perception." The researchers also found that different types of mental strategies, such as distraction, engaged different brain regions.

Another study found that intense feelings of passionate love can provide surprisingly effective pain relief. "It turns out that the areas of the brain activated by intense love are the same areas that drugs use to reduce pain," says Mackay.

"We can't write a prescription for patients to go home and have a passionate love affair," says Mackey. "But we can suggest that you go out and do things that are rewarding, that are emotionally meaningful. Go for a walk on a moonlit beach. Go listen to some music you never listened to before. Do something that's novel and exciting."

That's a prescription that should be painless to try.

Section 6.3

Quality of Life Scale for People with Pain

"Quality of Life Scale," © 2003 American Chronic Pain Association. All rights reserved. Reprinted with permission. For additional information, visit www.theacpa.org. Reviewed by David A. Cooke, MD, FACP, March 2013.

Pain is a highly personal experience. The degree to which pain interferes with the quality of a person's life is also highly personal.

The American Chronic Pain Association Quality of Life Scale looks at ability to function, rather than at pain alone. It can help people with pain and their health care team to evaluate and communicate the impact of pain on the basic activities of daily life. This information can provide a basis for more effective treatment and help to measure progress over time.

The scale is meant to help individuals measure activity levels. We recognize that homemakers, parents and retirees often don't work outside the home, but activity can still be measured in the amount of time one is able to "work" at fulfilling daily responsibilities be that in a paid job, as a volunteer, or within the home.

With a combination of sound medical treatment, good coping skills, and peer support, people with pain can lead more productive, satisfying lives. The American Chronic Pain Association can help. For more information, contact ACPA:

American Chronic Pain Association
P.O. Box 850
Rocklin, CA 95677
916-632-0922 or 800-533-3231
Fax: 916-632-3208
E-mail: acpa@pacbell.net
Web page: www.theacpa.org

Quality of Life Scale: A Measure of Function for People with Pain

0. Non-functioning; Stay in bed all day; Feel hopeless and helpless about life.

1. Stay in bed at least half the day; Have no contact with outside world.

2. Get out of bed but don't get dressed; Stay at home all day.

3. Get dressed in the morning; Minimal activities at home; Contact with friends via phone, e-mail.

4. Do simple chores around the house; Minimal activities outside of home two days a week.

5. Struggle but fulfill daily home responsibilities; No outside activity; Not able to work/volunteer.

6. Work/volunteer limited hours; Take part in limited social activities on weekends.

7. Work/volunteer for a few hours daily; Can be active at least five hours a day; Can make plans to do simple activities on weekends.

8. Work/volunteer for at least six hours daily; Have energy to make plans for one evening social activity during the week; Active on weekends.

9. Work/volunteer/be active eight hours daily; Take part in family life; Outside social activities limited.

10. Normal quality of life; Go to work/volunteer each day; Normal daily activities each day; Have a social life outside of work; Take an active part in family life.

Chapter 7

Stress Management: An Important Tool for People with Chronic Pain

How to Reduce, Prevent, and Cope with Stress

It may seem that there's nothing you can do about stress. The bills won't stop coming, there will never be more hours in the day, and your career and family responsibilities will always be demanding. But you have more control than you might think. In fact, the simple realization that you're in control of your life is the foundation of stress management. Managing stress is all about taking charge: of your thoughts, emotions, schedule, and the way you deal with problems.

Identify the Sources of Stress in Your Life

Stress management starts with identifying the sources of stress in your life. This isn't as easy as it sounds. Your true sources of stress aren't always obvious, and it's all too easy to overlook your own stress-inducing thoughts, feelings, and behaviors. Sure, you may know that you're constantly worried about work deadlines. But maybe it's your procrastination, rather than the actual job demands, that leads to deadline stress.

"Stress Management," by Melinda Smith, M.A., and Robert Segal, M.A., updated January 2013. © 2013 Helpguide.org. All rights reserved. Reprinted with permission. Helpguide provides a detailed list of references and resources for this article, with links to related Helpguide topics and information from other websites. For a complete list of these resources, go to http://www.helpguide.org/mental/stress_management_relief_coping.htm.

To identify your true sources of stress, look closely at your habits, attitude, and excuses:

- Do you explain away stress as temporary ("I just have a million things going on right now") even though you can't remember the last time you took a breather?

- Do you define stress as an integral part of your work or home life ("Things are always crazy around here") or as a part of your personality ("I have a lot of nervous energy, that's all").

- Do you blame your stress on other people or outside events, or view it as entirely normal and unexceptional?

Until you accept responsibility for the role you play in creating or maintaining it, your stress level will remain outside your control.

Start a Stress Journal

A stress journal can help you identify the regular stressors in your life and the way you deal with them. Each time you feel stressed, keep track of it in your journal. As you keep a daily log, you will begin to see patterns and common themes. Write down:

- What caused your stress (make a guess if you're unsure).
- How you felt, both physically and emotionally.
- How you acted in response.
- What you did to make yourself feel better.

Look at How You Currently Cope with Stress

Think about the ways you currently manage and cope with stress in your life. Your stress journal can help you identify them. Are your coping strategies healthy or unhealthy, helpful or unproductive? Unfortunately, many people cope with stress in ways that compound the problem.

Unhealthy Ways of Coping with Stress

These coping strategies may temporarily reduce stress, but they cause more damage in the long run:

- Smoking
- Drinking too much
- Overeating or undereating

- Zoning out for hours in front of the TV or computer
- Withdrawing from friends, family, and activities
- Using pills or drugs to relax
- Sleeping too much
- Procrastinating
- Filling up every minute of the day to avoid facing problems
- Taking out your stress on others (lashing out, angry outbursts, physical violence)

Learning Healthier Ways to Manage Stress

If your methods of coping with stress aren't contributing to your greater emotional and physical health, it's time to find healthier ones. There are many healthy ways to manage and cope with stress, but they all require change. You can either change the situation or change your reaction. When deciding which option to choose, it's helpful to think of the four As: avoid, alter, adapt, or accept.

Since everyone has a unique response to stress, there is no "one size fits all" solution to managing it. No single method works for everyone or in every situation, so experiment with different techniques and strategies. Focus on what makes you feel calm and in control.

Dealing with Stressful Situations: The Four A's

- Change the situation:
  - Avoid the stressor.
  - Alter the stressor.
- Change your reaction:
  - Adapt to the stressor.
  - Accept the stressor.

Stress Management Strategy #1: Avoid Unnecessary Stress

Not all stress can be avoided, and it's not healthy to avoid a situation that needs to be addressed. You may be surprised, however, by the number of stressors in your life that you can eliminate.

- **Learn how to say "no":** Know your limits and stick to them. Whether in your personal or professional life, refuse to accept added responsibilities when you're close to reaching them. Taking on more than you can handle is a surefire recipe for stress.

- **Avoid people who stress you out:** If someone consistently causes stress in your life and you can't turn the relationship around, limit the amount of time you spend with that person or end the relationship entirely.

- **Take control of your environment:** If the evening news makes you anxious, turn the TV off. If traffic's got you tense, take a longer but less-traveled route. If going to the market is an unpleasant chore, do your grocery shopping online.

- **Avoid hot-button topics:** If you get upset over religion or politics, cross them off your conversation list. If you repeatedly argue about the same subject with the same people, stop bringing it up or excuse yourself when it's the topic of discussion.

- **Pare down your to-do list:** Analyze your schedule, responsibilities, and daily tasks. If you've got too much on your plate, distinguish between the "shoulds" and the "musts." Drop tasks that aren't truly necessary to the bottom of the list or eliminate them entirely.

Stress Management Strategy #2: Alter the Situation

If you can't avoid a stressful situation, try to alter it. Figure out what you can do to change things so the problem doesn't present itself in the future. Often, this involves changing the way you communicate and operate in your daily life.

- **Express your feelings instead of bottling them up:** If something or someone is bothering you, communicate your concerns in an open and respectful way. If you don't voice your feelings, resentment will build and the situation will likely remain the same.

- **Be willing to compromise:** When you ask someone to change their behavior, be willing to do the same. If you both are willing to bend at least a little, you'll have a good chance of finding a happy middle ground.

- **Be more assertive:** Don't take a backseat in your own life. Deal with problems head on, doing your best to anticipate and prevent them. If you've got an exam to study for and your chatty roommate just got home, say up front that you only have five minutes to talk.

- **Manage your time better:** Poor time management can cause a lot of stress. When you're stretched too thin and running behind, it's hard to stay calm and focused. But if you plan ahead and make sure you don't overextend yourself, you can alter the amount of stress you're under.

Stress Management Strategy #3: Adapt to the Stressor

If you can't change the stressor, change yourself. You can adapt to stressful situations and regain your sense of control by changing your expectations and attitude.

- **Reframe problems:** Try to view stressful situations from a more positive perspective. Rather than fuming about a traffic jam, look at it as an opportunity to pause and regroup, listen to your favorite radio station, or enjoy some alone time.

- **Look at the big picture:** Take perspective of the stressful situation. Ask yourself how important it will be in the long run. Will it matter in a month? A year? Is it really worth getting upset over? If the answer is no, focus your time and energy elsewhere.

- **Adjust your standards:** Perfectionism is a major source of avoidable stress. Stop setting yourself up for failure by demanding perfection. Set reasonable standards for yourself and others, and learn to be okay with "good enough."

- **Focus on the positive:** When stress is getting you down, take a moment to reflect on all the things you appreciate in your life, including your own positive qualities and gifts. This simple strategy can help you keep things in perspective.

Adjusting Your Attitude

How you think can have a profound effect on your emotional and physical well-being. Each time you think a negative thought about yourself, your body reacts as if it were in the throes of a tension-filled situation. If you see good things about yourself, you are more likely to feel good; the reverse is also true. Eliminate words such as "always," "never," "should," and "must." These are telltale marks of self-defeating thoughts.

Stress Management Strategy #4: Accept the Things You Can't Change

Some sources of stress are unavoidable. You can't prevent or change stressors such as the death of a loved one, a serious illness, or a national recession. In such cases, the best way to cope with stress is to accept things as they are. Acceptance may be difficult, but in the long run, it's easier than railing against a situation you can't change.

- **Don't try to control the uncontrollable:** Many things in life are beyond our control— particularly the behavior of other people. Rather than stressing out over them, focus on the things you can control such as the way you choose to react to problems.

- **Look for the upside:** As the saying goes, "What doesn't kill us makes us stronger." When facing major challenges, try to look at them as opportunities for personal growth. If your own poor choices contributed to a stressful situation, reflect on them and learn from your mistakes.

- **Share your feelings:** Talk to a trusted friend or make an appointment with a therapist. Expressing what you're going through can be very cathartic, even if there's nothing you can do to alter the stressful situation.

- **Learn to forgive:** Accept the fact that we live in an imperfect world and that people make mistakes. Let go of anger and re-sentments. Free yourself from negative energy by forgiving and moving on.

Stress Management Strategy #5: Make Time for Fun and Relaxation

Beyond a take-charge approach and a positive attitude, you can reduce stress in your life by nurturing yourself. If you regularly make time for fun and relaxation, you'll be in a better place to handle life's stressors when they inevitably come.

Healthy Ways to Relax and Recharge

- Go for a walk.
- Spend time in nature.
- Call a good friend.
- Sweat out tension with a good workout.
- Write in your journal.
- Take a long bath.
- Light scented candles.

- Savor a warm cup of coffee or tea.
- Play with a pet.
- Work in your garden.
- Get a massage.
- Curl up with a good book.
- Listen to music.
- Watch a comedy.

Don't get so caught up in the hustle and bustle of life that you forget to take care of your own needs. Nurturing yourself is a necessity, not a luxury.

- **Set aside relaxation time:** Include rest and relaxation in your daily schedule. Don't allow other obligations to encroach. This is your time to take a break from all responsibilities and recharge your batteries.

- **Connect with others:** Spend time with positive people who enhance your life. A strong support system will buffer you from the negative effects of stress.

- **Do something you enjoy every day:** Make time for leisure activities that bring you joy, whether it be stargazing, playing the piano, or working on your bike.

- **Keep your sense of humor:** This includes the ability to laugh at yourself. The act of laughing helps your body fight stress in a number of ways.

Stress Management Strategy #6: Adopt a Healthy Lifestyle

You can increase your resistance to stress by strengthening your physical health.

- **Exercise regularly:** Physical activity plays a key role in reducing and preventing the effects of stress. Make time for at least 30 minutes of exercise, three times per week. Nothing beats aerobic exercise for releasing pent-up stress and tension.

- **Eat a healthy diet:** Well-nourished bodies are better prepared to cope with stress, so be mindful of what you eat. Start your day right with breakfast, and keep your energy up and your mind clear with balanced, nutritious meals throughout the day.

- **Reduce caffeine and sugar:** The temporary "highs" caffeine and sugar provide often end in with a crash in mood and energy. By reducing the amount of coffee, soft drinks, chocolate, and sugar snacks in your diet, you'll feel more relaxed and you'll sleep better.

- **Avoid alcohol, cigarettes, and drugs:** Self-medicating with alcohol or drugs may provide an easy escape from stress, but the relief is only temporary. Don't avoid or mask the issue at hand; deal with problems head on and with a clear mind.

- **Get enough sleep:** Adequate sleep fuels your mind, as well as your body. Feeling tired will increase your stress because it may cause you to think irrationally.

Chapter 8

Physical Activity Helps Relieve and Avoid Spinal Pain

The Importance of Exercise

Spine experts agree that physical activity is important for people with low back pain. This chapter will show you how to stay active while controlling your pain, and how proper activity may help protect against recurring back pain.

Your health care provider's goals in treating your low back pain include:

- communicate well;

- explain and reassure you about your condition;

- reduce your fears;

- promote physical activity;

- teach proper exercise;

- improve body mechanics; and

- avoid prolonged use of passive therapies.

Printed with permission from: NASS Patient Education Committee. *Exercise: The Backbone of Spine Treatment.* © 2006–2012 North American Spine Society. Available at: http://www.knowyourback.org.

What Kind of Exercise Should Be Done?

So how do you stay physically active without making your pain worse? Many people are surprised to learn that carefully selected exercises can *reduce* pain. Some of the exercises in this chapter can provide quick and significant relief, speeding recovery.

Once pain lessens or disappears, other exercises can help restore back movement and core muscle strength. These will help you reach full recovery and protect against recurring pain. Many doctors think an increase in pain during activity is okay as long as that increase doesn't continue after completing the activity. So try to stay active.

Remember, this is only a guide. Not all exercises are appropriate for everyone. If you experience substantially more pain while exercising, discontinue and let your health care provider know.

Monitoring Your Pain while Selecting Your Exercise

It is important to choose exercises carefully to avoid making your back pain worse. One way to know if your back is getting worse is when symptoms spread:

- away from the center of your low back;

- into your buttock; or

- down into, or further down, your leg(s).

This can happen during exercise and activity or even in certain positions.

The good news is that the opposite is also true! Symptoms can move out of your leg(s) or buttock so they are felt closer to *the center* of your low back (called "pain centralization"). This usually means that you are improving and moving toward recovery. You may find exercises and positions to make that happen. Once all symptoms have returned to the center of your low back, they will often improve and disappear with continued exercise.

Four exercises that most commonly centralize and reduce symptoms are:

- walking on level ground (*Figure 8.1*);

- standing backbends (*Figure 8.2*);

- face-down on elbows (*Figure 8.3*); and

- press-ups (*Figure 8.4*).

When doing these exercises, as well as other activities, monitor your pain. Make sure it is centralizing, going away or at least remaining the same—not getting worse.

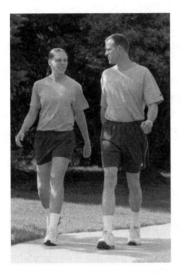

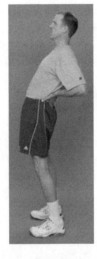

Figure 8.1. Walking: Begin with 10 minutes and increase to 30 minutes or more. Increase distance and pace as tolerated.

Figure 8.2. *Standing Extension: Place hands with fingers in the small of back. Bend backward as far as tolerated, pressing inward with fingers. Hold for 1–2 seconds. Repeat 10 times, trying to bend further each time. Unless pain gets worse, repeat every two hours.*

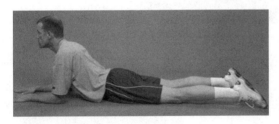

Figure 8.3. *Face Down on Elbows: Raise up on elbows, letting the low back sag. Hold for 10 seconds. Repeat three times. Unless pain gets worse, repeat every two hours.*

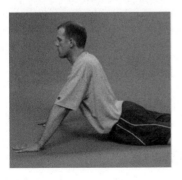

Figure 8.4. *Press-up: Push upward with arms, letting the low back sag. Hold for 1–2 seconds. Return to lying position. Repeat 10 times with a deeper sag each time. Unless pain gets worse, repeat every two hours.*

Posture Is Important, Too

Along with proper exercise, good posture is essential, whether standing (*Figure 8.5*) or sitting (*Figure 8.6*). When seated, avoid sitting for longer than necessary and avoid slouching.

If your symptoms get worse when sitting (and may even move toward or into the buttock or down your leg), check your posture. For many people, sitting erect may help centralize and lessen pain. It helps to think of sitting erect as an exercise to build muscle stamina and develop better sitting habits. Once pain-free, sitting erect often keeps symptoms from returning. When you must sit for a long time, it can be very helpful to put a firm support behind your low back to deepen its natural inward curve and keep your hips slightly higher than your knees.

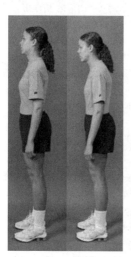

Figure 8.5. Standing Posture: Draw the head backward, tucking your chin; ears and shoulders should be vertically aligned with the hips and balanced above the legs (good posture on left; poor posture on right).

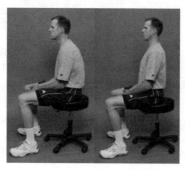

Figure 8.6. Seated Posture: Ears and shoulders should be aligned over the hips, reproducing the same hollow in the low back as when standing (poor posture on left; good posture on right).

Exercising Once Pain Has Lessened

In many cases, it may take only one or two days to control or eliminate symptoms. Once your pain is much better or gone, gradually and carefully increase your range of motion, starting with some simple forward-bending exercises (*Figures 8.7 and 8.8*). *Continue as long as your symptoms do not return, get worse or move away from the center of the back.*

For most people, continuing to sit erect is very helpful.

Figure 8.7. Single Knee-to-Chest: Pull one knee up to the chest and gently pull for 10 seconds. Repeat three times. Do this for each leg.

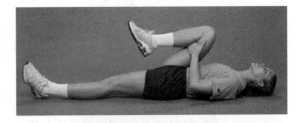

Figure 8.8. Double Knee-to-Chest: Pull both knees up to the chest and gently pull for 10 seconds. Repeat three times. Be sure pain is not getting worse. Unless pain is getting worse, perform 2–3 times per day.

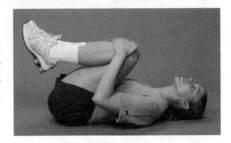

Strengthening Can Help

Many people with low back pain have weak core muscles. Strengthening exercises (*Figures 8.9–16*) protect you from future problems. All body movements and posture (including sitting erect) need adequate muscle strength and flexibility that require some strength training as well as stretching. Moderate strength training is one of the most valuable things you can do for your overall health and is especially important if you have low back pain.

Low back strengthening is helpful in two ways: (1) it helps repair injury by increasing blood flow; and (2) improves function in daily life by increasing strength and stamina.

To heal and repair injuries, nutrients must be delivered to the injured area by good blood flow. Strength training for low back muscles (*Figures 8.9–11*) increases blood flow to the muscles exercised and to nearby tissues. This is also true for aerobic exercise (for example, walking, swimming, bicycling) but is especially true for strength training.

Building strong muscles also increases your ability to function throughout the day. In addition to strengthening the low back, the trunk (*Figures 8.12–14*) and large muscles of the upper and lower legs (*Figures 8.15–16*) deserve attention, too. These muscles provide important stability to the back and trunk by improving balance and gait. It allows you to do daily activities with greater ease and reduces the chance of falling.

Special equipment and gyms can be helpful but there are good, low-tech and inexpensive ways to strengthen low back muscles at home.

In *Figure 8.9*, simply placing a pillow or two beneath your waist adds more resistance. Two simple pieces of equipment often used and very helpful include the popular Swiss balls (*Figures 8.10, 8.14 and 8.16*) or a basic Roman chair (*Figure 8.11*).

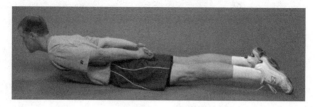

Figure 8.9. *Face-Down Extension: Place hands behind the back and lift head and shoulders from the floor. Hold for 5-10 seconds. Repeat three times.*

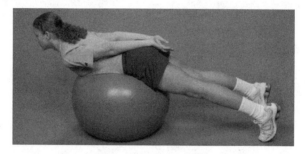

Figure 8.10. *Face-Down Ball Extension: Place hands behind the back and lift head and shoulders upward. Hold for 5-10 seconds. Repeat three times.*

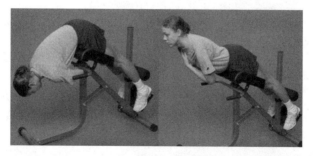

Figure 8.11. *Roman Chair Extension: This is a more advanced exercise and may not be appropriate for everyone. Hip pad is placed at the crest of the hips. Bend forward as far as possible and lift the trunk using your low back muscles. Perform exercise slowly (three count up and four count down). Repeat 5-10 times.*

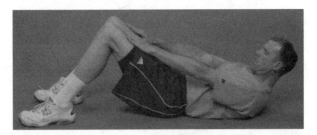

Figure 8.12. Curl Up: Place arms out toward the knees, tilt pelvis to flatten back. Raise head and shoulders from the floor. Hold for 5-10 seconds. Repeat three times.

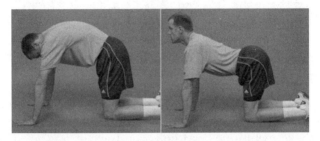

Figure 8.13. Cat/Camel: Place hands under the shoulders and knees under the hips. (1) Raise and round back by contracting the stomach muscles. Hold for 5-10 seconds. (2) Release and let the back sag.

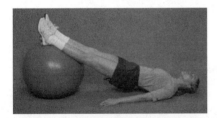

Figure 8.14. Supine Ball Extension: Place hands on the floor and raise hips from the floor. Hold for 5-10 seconds. Repeat three times.

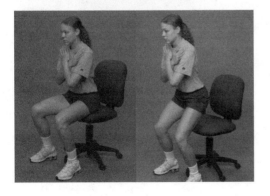

Figure 8.15. Chair Stand: Sit with arms across the chest; stand slowly and slowly return to seated position (count to three up and three down). Repeat 5-10 times.

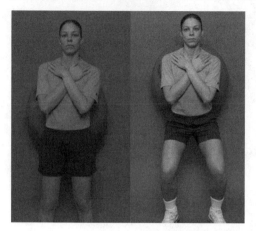

Figure 8.16. Ball/Wall Stand: Stand with straight knees and ball at your back. Bend knees slowly (three second count) to three quarters position and hold for five seconds. Return to standing position slowly (three second count). Repeat 5-10 times.

Summary

Good low back care includes pain-relieving exercises and proper stretching, followed by moderate strengthening. Taking care of yourself using these techniques can help you recover and provide a good defense for preventing future symptoms.

Chapter 9

Ergonomics to Avoid Workplace Pain

Oh, My Aching Back! (and Burning Eyes and Sore Wrists)

Working Americans spend about 2,000 hours a year in the workplace. Not surprisingly, all of these hours can take a toll—on your eyes, your back, your arms, and your neck.

Exposure to adverse working conditions can result in momentary pain or long-term injury. Moreover, poorly designed working environments contribute to reduced efficiency, decreased production, loss of income, increased medical claims, and permanent disability. Fortunately, professionals like the members of the American Industrial Hygiene Association use a science called *ergonomics* to help remedy the conditions that cause occupational disorders and injuries.

The ultimate goal of ergonomics is to design the workplace so that it accommodates the variety of human capabilities and limitations to prevent musculoskeletal disorders. While designing ergonomic hazards out of the workplace is ideal, other measures such as administrative controls (including training or employee rotation) and changes to work practices are often more feasible initially. We will examine several of the risk factors that affect employees, as well as solutions that you and your employer can use to eliminate or lessen these conditions.

"An Ergonomics Approach to Avoiding Workplace Injury," © 2009 American Industrial Hygiene Association (www.aiha.org); reprinted with permission.

Naturally, there are additional problems specific to certain industries, but the following pages will give you an overview of many of today's most common occupational disorders, which often affect muscles, tendons, and nerves of the body.

Let Your Fingers Do the Walking ...

Perhaps the most commonly discussed workplace injuries of the last decade have been carpal tunnel syndrome and related maladies of the wrist and hand. Although typewriters have been in use for more than 100 years in American offices, the popularity of the computer—with intensive keyboard use for data entry and word processing—has given rise to a generation at risk for such injuries. Carpal tunnel syndrome and related disorders (including tendonitis, trigger finger, hand-arm vibration disease, de Quervain disease, and myalgia) are part of a group of illnesses known as cumulative trauma disorders (CTDs). CTDs are a family of muscle, tendon, and nerve disorders that are caused, accelerated, or aggravated by repeated movements of the body, particularly when awkward postures, high forces, contact stresses, vibration, and/or exposure to cold are evident. The elbow, shoulders, neck, and back are also subject to CTDs.

Despite the connection between CTDs and computer-related office jobs, many non-office workers who perform repetitive work may be at risk for these injuries. In particular, employees in the fields of aerospace, agriculture, automotive, clerical, electronics, fabric cutting, food processing, glassware, health care, manufacturing, postal services, metal forming, plastics molding, and the performing arts (particularly music and dance) are susceptible to CTDs.

What CTDs Are Not

First of all, cumulative trauma disorders are not fatigue. Though it is a potential contributing factor, fatigue is classified as tiredness, physical stress, and discomfort that subsides a few minutes or hours after you stop the activity. Repeated and sustained activities that might potentially cause long-term problems usually cause fatigue as well. Although being weary after performing certain job tasks certainly has an effect on work performance and daily living, and may even cause pain, fatigue is not considered a serious medical problem.

As a general rule, symptoms that persist after a night of rest or interfere significantly with work or daily activities indicate something more serious than fatigue. At this point, you should see a physician; if the problem is indeed work-related, report the problem to the appropriate company representative. Finally, you should speak to your employer about adjusting your work environment or equipment to help alleviate the problem.

How CTDs Occur

The hands, wrists, arms, shoulders, neck, and back are comprised of a complex network of nerves, bones, tendons, and fluid. Irritation of these tissues during certain work activities can, over time, result in elevated fluid pressure around nerves. This can cause compression and may eventually cause nerve damage. Nerves can also be damaged by inflamed tendons pressing on them. Carpal tunnel syndrome is a common example of this: The median nerve in the wrist becomes compressed and ultimately damaged as tendon structures swell. A chief cause of this is repeated or sustained work involving high force or using a bent or extended wrist. Even truck drivers who grip a vibrating steering wheel all day may fall prey to this painful disorder.

Unfortunately, since repetition is one of the key factors in causing CTDs, non-work related activities, such as needlework, gardening, fly-casting, and bowling, can also affect the progress of the illness and recovery. These activities may aggravate CTDs. This can make it difficult at times to identify the main cause of a person's CTD.

Risk factors for CTDs, as noted above, can occur in a variety of occupations. In order to properly analyze and correct these factors, job-related tasks must be evaluated for each of the risk factors. For instance, how many minutes or hours does a utility worker run a drill (vibration) or how long does a butcher handle refrigerated meat (cold temperature)?

Some occupations have combinations of stresses, such as prolonged contact stresses and posture (a fabric cutter using poorly designed scissors at a low workbench, for instance).

Cumulative trauma disorders are a major cause of lost time in many labor-intensive industries. If you notice repeated pain or injury related to your work, your specific environment may need to be analyzed, equipment adjusted or added, and procedures modified. Applying ergonomics to the workplace will help you and your employer strike a proper balance between production requirements and staff capabilities, lessening the likelihood of CTDs arising.

How Ergonomics Can Help

Specialists in the science of ergonomics offer numerous solutions to make the workplace a more hospitable environment for employees. Cumulative trauma disorders and lower back injuries in particular have received considerable attention. There are six major CTD risk factors; those risk factors and several possible corrections or solutions to each are offered below.

Repeated Actions and Sustained Postures

- Use mechanical aids. These might include arm or wrist rests for keyboard use or substituting power tools for manual tools. This is the most practical solution.
- Adjust the work standard. Modify the amount of work due in the allotted time to allow you to pace yourself.
- Use task rotation. Move through different tasks during the day to avoid undue stress and repetition of any one kind.
- Use work enlargement. Combine jobs of different motion patterns. (This may require redesigning the work setting.)

Forceful Actions (Lifting, Carrying, Hoisting, Pushing, Etc.)

- Select gloves that improve your grip on an object.
- Avoid thick gloves that interfere with closing your hand around the work object.
- Pick up fewer objects at a time to reduce weight.
- Select tools to reduce weight.
- Attach balancers and handles to steady tools.
- Use reaction bars and articulating arms to reduce powerful "bounce-back" recoils or counteractions.
- Use hoists to raise and support work objects and materials.
- Use rollers and powered belt conveyors to move materials.
- Use gravity to make materials handling easier.
- Use jigs and fixtures to hold parts.
- Use handles to make gripping easier.
- Enlarge grip size.
- Push rather than pull.

Prolonged Contact Stresses from Tools, Equipment, Etc.

- Use elongated handles on tools, such as scissors and pliers.
- Use rounded edges on handles and on work benches.

- Use materials that yield to pressure on handle grips, such as rubber, instead of using hard surfaces, such as metal.

- Use tools, rather than your hands, for pounding parts.

- Pad your hand or wear gloves.

- Avoid compression of leaning on wrists, elbows, and abdomen.

Posture

- Adjust the location of work and the angle of the work piece in such a way that your body can maintain an unstrained, comfortable position with your arms, forearms, and shoulders relaxed.

- Select or design a tool size and shape to maintain a comfortable body position and a straight wrist when gripping the tool.

Vibration

Depending on the job, isolating the hand and wrist entirely from vibration may be impossible. If you begin to show symptoms of a CTD, however, you may need to discuss with your employer the possibility of minimizing exposure to vibration. This can be done through tool selection, gloves, or limiting your time of exposure.

Cold Temperature

- Use insulated gloves.

- Use handles and grips that do not conduct cold easily.

- For pneumatic tools, direct exhaust air away from yourself and not through the tool handle.

- Wear additional clothes on your upper body to retain heat.

Making Your Computer Truly "User-Friendly"

Computer workstations, including the components of monitors, keyboards, and chairs, present a whole set of problems in addition to the cumulative trauma disorders discussed above. The explosive growth in the use of computers over the last 25 years has led to a special group of ergonomic dilemmas unique to their use. For instance, the screen introduces new lighting and vision considerations. Many computer jobs offer few opportunities for alternate activities or postures, and, thanks to the fluidity of computer keyboards compared to typewriters, workers can key faster and for longer uninterrupted stretches than ever before.

In addition, some people who use computers are concerned about the effects of heat and electrostatic and electromagnetic fields in the immediate vicinity of their terminals. And working at computers is sometimes associated with psychological stress, either because of the technology itself or because of job conditions (such as monitoring) associated with the work.

As computers spread from the office to the factory to the fast food restaurant, workers and their employers need to be aware of these problems in order to avoid them. By following the recommendations below, computers can be time-saving and labor-enhancing devices and not potential "pains in the neck."

The Eyes Have It (Soreness, That Is)

The most frequent physical complaint by people who spend a lot of time in front of a monitor is eyestrain. Specialists in ergonomics have identified several problem areas and possible corrections for eyestrain, including glare:

- Move or shield the light source.

- Move the monitor.

- Change the monitor's angle.

- Apply a good quality glare filter to the monitor, preferably one made of glass or plastic instead of mesh, which tends to collect dust.

- When correcting for glare, don't create other problems. For instance, if you move your monitor, don't put it in a place that will produce neck strain. The monitor should be directly in front of you.

- When possible, place your monitor at a right angle with the window.

Light Brightness Ratio (Between the Screen and Surrounding Environment)

- Set the background lighting or source document so that it's no more than 10 times brighter than the screen. Some experts recommend that it be no more than three times brighter.

- Adjust the screen brightness to match the surrounding room.

- Work with a light screen background (dark type or images on white or pale background)—you'll find it is easier on your eyes.

Lighting Levels

- Following the preceding recommendations, adjust your screen position and lighting sources (lamps, etc.) to achieve best results.

- In almost all cases, avoid high levels of lighting.

Viewing Distance and Document Height

- Place the monitor and source documents so that they are about the same distance from your eyes. Use a document holder to place the document immediately next to the monitor.

- Rest the muscles of your eyes by focusing on a distant object occasionally.

- When using a laptop, look into the distance more frequently. A laptop monitor will probably not have the best placement, since it is usually attached to the keyboard.

Readability of Screen and Document

- Place monitors and documents so they are perpendicular to the line of sight to avoid character distortion.

- Upgrade or replace monitors with poor resolution or flicker.

- Adjust your monitor's refresh rate.

Vision Correction

- If you wear glasses, consider getting full-frame reading glasses prescribed for a working distance of 20 to 30 inches. These will allow you to place the monitor correctly and see well without stressing your posture.

- Place the monitor so that the top of the screen is below your line of sight.

- Don't skip visits to the eye doctor! Eye strain could indicate a problem with your vision beyond the use of a computer monitor.

Mom Was Right ... Posture IS Important

In addition to cumulative trauma disorders and vision difficulties, back problems are another common complaint during the prolonged use of computer terminals. Poor posture (held for long periods), poorly designed work areas and poorly adjusted chairs, and sustained activity without breaks can all contribute to varying amounts of back, shoulder, and neck pain.

Posture

Although your own work habits can contribute to back and shoulder pain, using good posture is not a simple matter of finding the "right" position in which to sit. Even "poor" postures (feet up on chair rungs, slumping, twisting your body into odd positions) can prove comfortable if you don't remain in them for extended periods of time. In fact, shifting about periodically actually proves useful for many people.

Ergonomic specialists recommend the following changes to your behavior and work environment to avoid back, neck, and shoulder pain:

- Change your body position periodically throughout the day.

- Use a document stand to reduce the amount of neck twisting or bending forward if typing from a source document.

- Position your keyboard directly in front of you and at approximately elbow height. This should enable you to type with straight wrists. If this is not possible with the keyboard atop the work surface, use an adjustable-height keyboard tray.

- Center your monitor with your keyboard and chair.

- Avoid ear-to-shoulder neck positioning while on the phone.

- Rearrange the work area to avoid excess bending, stooping, and reaching.

- Try to relax. Many injuries and painful episodes arise from continuously tensing your neck and shoulder muscles while working.

- Consider increasing the amount of exercise you get, since there seems to be a strong relationship between poor physical condition and workplace injury. Overall attention to all aspects of your health such as diet, stress management, and weight control is recommended.

Seating

Not surprisingly, a good chair can contribute significantly to reducing the risk of lower back pain or injury. A good ergonomic chair includes all or most of the following characteristics, not just one or two:

- Adjustable lumbar support;

- Angle between the backrest and seat that allows you to sit without leaning forward uncomfortably;

- Adjustable armrests;

- Slightly inclined backrest;

- Allows for a variety of seated postures;

- Seat height adjustability;

- Seat pan adjustability;

- Soft, rounded edges;

- Size that fits you;

- High backrest or headrest for deeply reclining postures; and

- Comfortable but slip-resistant fabric.

If your feet don't reach the floor, consider using a footrest. In addition, if you have an older chair without lumbar support, try using a small pillow or towel roll to relieve pressure on your lower back. Don't get too large a pillow, however, or you may find it forces you to lean forward too much, creating even more strain.

Also, remember that ergonomic features won't help you if the chair doesn't suit your body or sitting habits, so adjustability is important. Be sure to have the adjustable features of your chair explained to you to ensure the best fit.

Repetition

As with cumulative trauma disorders, one of the best ways to avoid back, neck, and shoulder injuries is to minimize sustained exertions. The following tips should help you:

- Alternate tasks. If possible, get up from your workstation periodically to use the phone, make copies, file paperwork, etc.

- Take several rest breaks. For many people, "microbreaks" that allow you to pause frequently are more effective than the traditional 15-minute break every two hours.

- Consider installing software that reminds you to take periodic breaks throughout the workday.

- Take short breaks that involve active exercise (walking, stretching); they are often the most effective in relieving stress on the back, neck, and shoulders.

Other Risks in the Workplace from Computers

Other problems posed by continued use of computers and possible solutions include:

Heat: Since computers, monitors, and printers create heat, employers should be sure that the work environment is properly cooled and ventilated. Panels, walls, and furniture should be placed in such a way that they do not block air circulation. The American Society of Heating, Refrigerating, and Air-Conditioning Engineers (ASHRAE) has established guidelines for providing adequate ventilation in various types of workplaces and can offer more information for your specific work situation.

Electrostatic fields: Besides causing annoying jolts of low-level electricity, constant exposure to static can cause dermatitis (skin inflammation) in some users. Use a grounded keyboard pad or grounded glare screen to reduce static electricity.

Electromagnetic radiation and magnetic fields: Though this is an area of continuing debate, many workers have expressed worries about continuing exposure to electromagnetic radiation from their computers. The focus of research has been on extremely low frequencies (ELFs), the type of emission from all types of appliances and lighting, not just computers. Although research has not proven that work exposure is harmful in the long run-and some studies indicate that computer users are exposed to as many ELFs in the home as at work—it is recommended that you should sit at least an arm's length from the back or side of any terminal. Very few emissions come from the front of your monitor. Another area of concern is the relationship between ELFs and pregnancy. Most experts believe that standard exposure to ELFs in the home and office has no impact on pregnant women or their unborn children.

Psychological Stresses

Stress may be factored into work injuries in two interconnected ways:

- How stress contributes to physical ergonomic problems.
- How using a computer contributes to stress.

For instance, a stressful work environment may cause you to remain tense for long periods of time, use repetitive motions, take fewer breaks, or fail to report work-related medical problems when they arise. In addition, the use of computers, especially by new users, can contribute to this overall feeling of stress. Obviously, these two factors create a cycle that can contribute to pain and injury.

Although workers may not have extensive input into stressful elements of a job (such as the number of staff available to handle the workload), one way to reduce stress is to give personnel awareness of, and control over, ergonomic conditions. Understanding your work environment is essential; so is gaining control over certain aspects of your surroundings, such as user-adjustable chairs and lighting levels. Information and control go a long way to reducing stress levels.

A Productive Partnership

It is in everyone's best interest to apply modern ergonomic science to the workplace. As we stated at the outset, poor working conditions are bad news for both employees and employers—resulting in physical suffering and adverse economic impact. Although the checklists and suggestions offered here should help, many employers may wish to take the extra step of consulting directly with a professional in the field of ergonomics to analyze specific working conditions and make recommendations. A partnership among staff, employers, and ergonomics specialists can help redesign the workplace to meet the capabilities and potential of every employee.

For More Information

American Industrial Hygiene Association
2700 Prosperity Ave., Suite 250
Fairfax, VA 22031
Phone: 703-849-8888
Fax: 703-207-3561
Website: www.aiha.org
E-mail: infonet@aiha.org

Human Factors and Ergonomics Society
P.O. Box 1369
Santa Monica, CA 90406
Phone: 213-394-1811
Website: www.hfes.org
E-mail: info@hfes.org

National Institute for Occupational Safety and Health
Toll-Free: (800) 356-4674 (Information Inquiry Service)
Website: www.cdc.gov/niosh/topics/ergonomics

Occupational Safety and Health Administration
U.S. Department of Labor—OSHA
200 Constitution Avenue, NW
Washington, D.C. 20210
Website: www.osha.gov/SLTC/ergonomics/index.html

Part Two

Musculoskeletal Pain

Chapter 10

Arthritis and Rheumatic Diseases

Chapter Contents

Section 10.1—Questions and Answers about Arthritis
and Rheumatic Diseases.................................... 88

Section 10.2—Rheumatoid Arthritis............................ 94

Section 10.3—Osteoarthritis 98

Section 10.4—Reactive Arthritis............................... 104

Section 10.5—Gout.. 107

Section 10.6—Polymyalgia Rheumatica 110

Section 10.1

Questions and Answers about Arthritis and Rheumatic Diseases

Excerpted from "Questions and Answers about Arthritis and Rheumatic Diseases," National Institute of Arthritis and Musculoskeletal and Skin Diseases (www.niams.nih.gov), NIH Publication No. 12-4999, April 2012.

What is arthritis and what are rheumatic diseases?

Arthritis literally means joint inflammation. Although joint inflammation describes a symptom or sign rather than a specific diagnosis, the term *arthritis* is often used to refer to any disorder that affects the joints. These disorders fall within the broader category of rheumatic diseases. These are diseases characterized by inflammation (signs include redness or heat, swelling, and symptoms such as pain) and loss of function of one or more connecting or supporting structures of the body. These diseases especially affect joints, tendons, ligaments, bones, and muscles. Common signs and symptoms are pain, swelling, and stiffness. Some rheumatic diseases also can involve internal organs.

There are more than 100 rheumatic diseases. Some are described as connective tissue diseases because they affect the supporting framework of the body and its internal organs. Others are known as autoimmune diseases because they occur when the immune system, which normally protects the body from infection and disease, harms the body's own healthy tissues. Throughout this chapter, the terms *arthritis* and *rheumatic diseases* are used interchangeably.

The burden of arthritis in the United States is enormous. More than 46 million people in the United States have arthritis or other rheumatic conditions.

What are some examples of rheumatic diseases?

Osteoarthritis: Osteoarthritis affects both the cartilage, which is the tissue that cushions the ends of bones within the joint, as well as the underlying bone. Osteoarthritis can cause joint pain and stiffness.

Disability results most often when the disease affects the spine and the weight-bearing joints (the knees and hips).

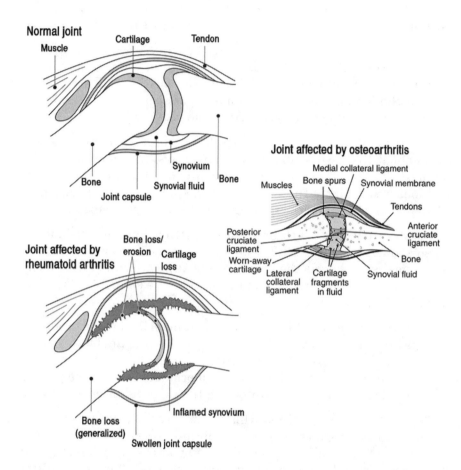

Figure 10.1. *In a healthy joint, the ends of bones are encased in smooth cartilage. Together, they are protected by a joint capsule lined with a synovial membrane that produces synovial fluid. The capsule and fluid protect the cartilage, muscles, and connective tissues. With osteoarthritis, the cartilage becomes worn away. Spurs grow out from the edge of the bone, and synovial fluid increases. The joint feels stiff and sore. In rheumatoid arthritis, the synovium becomes inflamed, causing warmth, redness, swelling, and pain. As the disease progresses, the inflamed synovium invades and damages the cartilage and bone of the joint. (Source: National Institute of Arthritis and Musculoskeletal and Skin Diseases)*

Rheumatoid arthritis: This inflammatory disease of the immune system targets first the synovium, or lining of the joint, resulting in pain, stiffness, swelling, joint damage, and loss of function of the joints. Inflammation most often affects joints of the hands and feet and tends to be symmetrical (occurring equally on both sides of the body). This symmetry helps distinguish rheumatoid arthritis from other forms of the disease.

Juvenile arthritis: This disease is the most common form of arthritis in childhood, causing pain, stiffness, swelling, and loss of function of the joints. This condition may be associated with rashes or fevers and may affect various parts of the body.

Fibromyalgia: Fibromyalgia is a chronic disorder that causes pain throughout the tissues that support and move the bones and joints. Pain, stiffness, and localized tender points occur in the muscles and tendons, particularly those of the neck, spine, shoulders, and hips. Patients also may experience fatigue and sleep disturbances.

Systemic lupus erythematosus: Systemic lupus erythematosus (also known as lupus or SLE) is an autoimmune disease in which the immune system harms the body's own healthy cells and tissues. This can result in inflammation of and damage to the joints, skin, kidneys, heart, lungs, blood vessels, and brain.

Scleroderma: Also known as systemic sclerosis, scleroderma means literally *hard skin*. The disease affects the skin, blood vessels, and joints. It may also affect internal organs, such as the lungs and kidneys. In scleroderma, there is an abnormal and excessive production of collagen (a fiber-like protein) in the skin and internal organs.

Spondyloarthropathies: This group of rheumatic diseases principally affects the spine. One common form—ankylosing spondylitis—also may affect the hips, shoulders, and knees. The tendons and ligaments around the bones and joints become inflamed, resulting in pain and stiffness. Ankylosing spondylitis tends to affect people in late adolescence or early adulthood. Reactive arthritis is another spondyloarthropathy. It develops after an infection involving the lower urinary tract, bowel, or other organ. It is commonly associated with eye problems, skin rashes, and mouth sores.

Infectious arthritis: This is a general term used to describe forms of arthritis that are caused by infectious agents, such as bacteria or viruses. Parvovirus arthritis and gonococcal arthritis are examples of infectious arthritis. Arthritis symptoms also may occur in Lyme disease, which is caused by a bacterial infection following the bite of certain ticks. In those cases of arthritis caused by bacteria, early diagnosis and treatment with antibiotics are crucial to removing the infection and minimizing damage to the joints.

Gout: This type of arthritis results from deposits of needle-like crystals of uric acid in the joints. The crystals cause episodic inflammation, swelling, and pain in the affected joint, which is often the big toe.

Polymyalgia rheumatica: Because this disease involves tendons, muscles, ligaments, and tissues around the joint, symptoms often include pain, aching, and morning stiffness in the shoulders, hips, neck, and lower back. It is sometimes the first sign of giant cell arteritis, a disease of the arteries characterized by headaches, inflammation, weakness, weight loss, and fever.

Polymyositis: This rheumatic disease causes inflammation and weakness in the muscles. The disease may affect the whole body and cause disability.

Psoriatic arthritis: This form of arthritis occurs in some patients with psoriasis, a scaling skin disorder. Psoriatic arthritis often affects the joints at the ends of the fingers and toes and is accompanied by changes in the fingernails and toenails. Back pain may occur if the spine is involved.

Bursitis: This condition involves inflammation of the bursae, small, fluid-filled sacs that help reduce friction between bones and other moving structures in the joints. The inflammation may result from arthritis in the joint or injury or infection of the bursae. Bursitis produces pain and tenderness and may limit the movement of nearby joints.

Tendinitis (tendonitis): This condition refers to inflammation of tendons (tough cords of tissue that connect muscle to bone) caused by overuse, injury, or a rheumatic condition. Tendinitis produces pain and tenderness and may restrict movement of nearby joints.

How are rheumatic diseases diagnosed?

Diagnosing rheumatic diseases can be difficult because some symptoms and signs are common to many different diseases. Common signs and symptoms of arthritis include swelling in one or more joints, stiffness around the joints that lasts for at least one hour in the early morning, constant or recurring pain or tenderness in a joint, difficulty using or moving a joint normally, and warmth and redness in a joint.

A general practitioner or family doctor may be able to evaluate a patient or refer him or her to a rheumatologist (a doctor who specializes in treating arthritis and other rheumatic diseases). The doctor will review the patient's medical history, conduct a physical examination, and obtain laboratory tests and x-rays or other imaging tests. The doctor may need to see the patient more than once and possibly a number of times to make an accurate diagnosis.

It is vital for people with joint pain to give the doctor a complete medical history. It may be helpful for people to keep a daily journal that describes the pain. Patients should write down what the affected joint looks like, how it feels, how long the pain lasts, and what they were doing when the pain started.

The doctor will examine the patient's joints for redness, warmth, damage, ease of movement, and tenderness. Because some forms of arthritis, such as lupus, may affect internal organs, a complete physical examination that includes the heart, lungs, abdomen, nervous system, eyes, ears, mouth, and throat may be necessary.

To see what the joint looks like inside, the doctor may order x-rays or other imaging procedures. X-rays provide an image of the bones, but they do not show cartilage, muscles, and ligaments. Other noninvasive imaging methods such as computed tomography (CT or CAT scan), magnetic resonance imaging (MRI), and arthrography show the whole joint. The doctor also may look for damage to a joint by using an arthroscope, a small, flexible tube that is inserted through a small incision at the joint. The arthroscope transmits the image from inside the joint to a video screen.

What laboratory tests are used to help identify rheumatic diseases?

The doctor may order some laboratory tests to help confirm a diagnosis. Samples of blood, urine, or synovial fluid (lubricating fluid found in the joint) may be needed for the tests. Many of these same tests may be useful later for monitoring the disease or the effectiveness of treatments. Common laboratory tests and procedures include the following:

- **Antinuclear antibody (ANA):** This test checks blood levels of antibodies that are often present in people who have connective tissue diseases or other autoimmune disorders, such as lupus.

- **CCP (or anti-CCP):** This test checks blood levels of antibodies to citrulline, a protein that can be detected in up to 70 percent of people in the early stages of rheumatoid arthritis.

- **C-reactive protein test:** This nonspecific test is used to detect generalized inflammation.

- **Complement:** This test measures the level of complement, a group of proteins in the blood. Complement helps destroy germs and other foreign substances that enter the body. A low blood level of complement is common in people who have active lupus.

- **Complete blood count (CBC):** This test determines the number of white blood cells, red blood cells, and platelets present in a sample of blood. Some rheumatic conditions or drugs used to treat arthritis are associated with a low white blood count (leukopenia), low red blood count (anemia), or low platelet count (thrombocytopenia).

- **Creatinine:** This blood test measures the level of creatinine, a breakdown product of creatine, which is an important component of muscle. This test is commonly used to diagnose and monitor kidney disease in patients who have a rheumatic condition such as lupus.

- **Erythrocyte sedimentation rate (sed rate or ESR):** This blood test is used to detect inflammation in the body.

- **Hematocrit (PCV or packed cell volume):** This test and the test for hemoglobin (a substance in the red blood cells that carries oxygen throughout the body) measure the number of red blood cells present in a sample of blood.

- **Rheumatoid factor:** This test detects the presence of rheumatoid factor, an antibody found in the blood of most (but not all) people who have rheumatoid arthritis.

- **Synovial fluid examination:** Synovial fluid may be examined for white blood cells (found in patients with rheumatoid arthritis and infections), bacteria or viruses (found in patients with infectious arthritis), or crystals in the joint (found in patients with gout or other types of crystal-induced arthritis). To obtain a specimen, the doctor injects a local anesthetic, then inserts a needle into the joint to withdraw the synovial fluid into a syringe. The procedure is called arthrocentesis or joint aspiration.

- **Urinalysis:** In this test, a urine sample is studied for protein, red blood cells, white blood cells, and bacteria.

Can arthritis be cured?

At this time, the only type of arthritis that can be cured is that caused by infections. Although symptoms of other types of arthritis can be effectively managed with rest, exercise, and medication, there are no cures. Some people claim to have been cured by treatment with herbs, oils, chemicals, special diets, radiation, or other products. However, there is no scientific evidence that such treatments cure arthritis. Moreover, some may lead to serious side effects. Patients should talk to their doctor before using any therapy that has not been prescribed or recommended by their health care team.

Section 10.2

Rheumatoid Arthritis

Excerpted from "Handout on Health: Rheumatoid Arthritis,"
National Institute of Arthritis and Musculoskeletal and Skin Diseases
(www.niams.nih.gov), NIH Publication No. 09-4179, April 2009.

What is rheumatoid arthritis?

Rheumatoid arthritis (RA) is an inflammatory disease that causes pain, swelling, stiffness, and loss of function in the joints. It occurs when the immune system, which normally defends the body from invading organisms, turns its attack against the membrane lining the joints.

Rheumatoid arthritis has several features that make it different from other kinds of arthritis. For example, rheumatoid arthritis generally occurs in a symmetrical pattern, meaning that if one knee or hand is involved, the other one also is. The disease often affects the wrist joints and the finger joints closest to the hand. It can also affect other parts of the body besides the joints. In addition, people with rheumatoid arthritis may have fatigue, occasional fevers, and a general sense of not feeling well.

The course of rheumatoid arthritis can range from mild to severe. In most cases it is chronic, meaning it lasts a long time—often a lifetime. For many people, periods of relatively mild disease activity are punctuated by flares, or times of heightened disease activity. In others, symptoms are constant.

What happens in rheumatoid arthritis?

Like many other rheumatic diseases, rheumatoid arthritis is an autoimmune disease (*auto* means self), so-called because a person's immune system, which normally helps protect the body from infection and disease, attacks joint tissues for unknown reasons. White blood cells, the agents of the immune system, travel to the synovium and cause inflammation (synovitis), characterized by warmth, redness, swelling, and pain—typical symptoms of rheumatoid arthritis. During the inflammation process, the normally thin synovium becomes thick and makes the joint swollen and puffy to the touch.

As rheumatoid arthritis progresses, the inflamed synovium invades and destroys the cartilage and bone within the joint. The surrounding muscles, ligaments, and tendons that support and stabilize the joint become weak and unable to work normally. These effects lead to the pain and joint damage often seen in rheumatoid arthritis. Researchers studying rheumatoid arthritis now believe that it begins to damage bones during the first year or two that a person has the disease, one reason why early diagnosis and treatment are so important.

Some people with rheumatoid arthritis also have symptoms in places other than their joints. Many people with rheumatoid arthritis develop anemia, or a decrease in the production of red blood cells. Other effects that occur less often include neck pain and dry eyes and mouth. Very rarely, people may have inflammation of the blood vessels (vasculitis), the lining of the lungs (pleurisy), or the sac enclosing the heart (pericarditis).

How is rheumatoid arthritis treated?

Doctors use a variety of approaches to treat rheumatoid arthritis. These are used in different combinations and at different times during the course of the disease and are chosen according to the patient's individual situation. No matter what treatment the doctor and patient choose, however, the goals are the same: to relieve pain, reduce inflammation, slow down or stop joint damage, and improve the person's sense of well-being and ability to function.

Good communication between the patient and doctor is necessary for effective treatment. Talking to the doctor can help ensure that exercise and pain management programs are provided as needed, and that drugs are prescribed appropriately. Talking to the doctor can also help people who are making decisions about surgery.

Health behavior changes: Certain activities can help improve a person's ability to function independently and maintain a positive outlook.

- *Rest and exercise:* People with rheumatoid arthritis need a good balance between rest and exercise, with more rest when the disease is active and more exercise when it is not. Exercise is important for maintaining healthy and strong muscles, preserving joint mobility, and maintaining flexibility.

- *Joint care:* Some people find using a splint for a short time around a painful joint reduces pain and swelling by supporting the joint and letting it rest. Other ways to reduce stress on joints include self-help devices, devices to help with standing, and changes in the ways that a person carries out daily activities.

- *Stress reduction:* Although there is no evidence that stress plays a role in causing rheumatoid arthritis, it can make living with the disease difficult at times. Stress also may affect the amount of pain a person feels.

- *Healthful diet:* An overall nutritious diet with enough—but not an excess of—calories, protein, and calcium is important. Some people may need to be careful about drinking alcoholic beverages because of the medications they take.

- *Climate:* Moving to a new place with a different climate usually does not make a long-term difference in a person's rheumatoid arthritis.

Medications: Most people who have rheumatoid arthritis take medications. Some medications (analgesics) are used only for pain relief; others (corticosteroids and nonsteroidal anti-inflammatory drugs, which are called NSAIDs) are used to reduce inflammation. Still others, often called disease-modifying antirheumatic drugs (DMARDs), are used to try to slow the course of the disease. The newest and perhaps most promising class of arthritis medications are the biologic response modifiers. These are genetically engineered medications that help reduce inflammation and structural damage to the joints by interrupting the cascade of events that drive inflammation.

For many years, doctors initially prescribed aspirin or other pain-relieving drugs for rheumatoid arthritis, and waited to prescribe more powerful drugs only if the disease worsened. In recent decades this approach to treatment has changed as studies have shown that early treatment with more powerful drugs—and the use of drug combinations instead of one medication alone—may be more effective in reducing or preventing joint damage. Someone with persistent rheumatoid arthritis symptoms should see a doctor familiar with the disease and its treatment to reduce the risk of damage.

Many of the new drugs that help reduce disease in rheumatoid arthritis do so by reducing the inflammation that can cause pain and joint damage. However, in some instances, inflammation is one mechanism the body normally uses to maintain health, such as to fight infection and possibly to stop tumors from growing. The magnitude of the risk from the treatment is hard to judge because infections and cancer can occur in patients with rheumatoid arthritis who are not on treatment, and probably more commonly than in healthy individuals. Nevertheless, appropriate caution and vigilance are justified.

Surgery: Several types of surgery are available to patients with severe joint damage. The primary purpose of these procedures is to reduce pain, improve the affected joint's function, and improve the patient's ability to perform daily activities. Surgery is not for everyone, however, and the decision should be made only after careful consideration by the patient and doctor. Together they should discuss the patient's overall health, the condition of the joint or tendon that will be operated on, and the reason for, as well as the risks and benefits of, the surgical procedure. Cost may be another factor.

Following are some of the more common surgeries performed for rheumatoid arthritis:

- *Joint replacement:* Joint replacement involves removing all or part of a damaged joint and replacing it with synthetic components.
- *Arthrodesis (fusion):* Arthrodesis is a surgical procedure that involves removing the joint and fusing the bones into one immobile unit.
- *Tendon reconstruction:* This surgery, which is used most frequently on the hands, reconstructs the damaged tendon by attaching an intact tendon to it.
- *Synovectomy:* In this surgery, the doctor actually removes the inflamed synovial tissue. Synovectomy is done as part of reconstructive surgery, especially tendon reconstruction.

Routine monitoring and ongoing care: Regular medical care is important to monitor the course of the disease, determine the effectiveness and any negative effects of medications, and change therapies as needed. Monitoring typically includes regular visits to the doctor. It also may include blood, urine, and other laboratory tests and x-rays.

Alternative and complementary therapies: Special diets, vitamin supplements, and other alternative approaches have been suggested for treating rheumatoid arthritis. Research shows that some of these, for example, fish oil supplements, may help reduce arthritis inflammation. For most, however, controlled scientific studies either have not been conducted on them or have found no definite benefit to these therapies.

What can you do?

Patient education and arthritis self-management programs, as well as support groups, help people to become better informed and to participate in their own care. Self-management programs teach about rheumatoid arthritis and its treatments, exercise and relaxation approaches, communication between patients and health care providers, and problem solving. Research on these programs has shown that they help people understand the disease and reduce their pain while remaining active. They also help people cope physically, emotionally, and mentally and feel greater control over the disease and build a sense of confidence in the ability to function and lead full, active, and independent lives.

Section 10.3

Osteoarthritis

Excerpted from "Handout on Health: Osteoarthritis,"
National Institute of Arthritis and Musculoskeletal and Skin Diseases
(www.niams.nih.gov), NIH Publication No. 10-4617, July 2010.

What is osteoarthritis?

Osteoarthritis is the most common type of arthritis and is seen especially among older people. Sometimes it is called degenerative joint disease or osteoarthrosis.

Osteoarthritis mostly affects cartilage, the hard but slippery tissue that covers the ends of bones where they meet to form a joint. Healthy cartilage allows bones to glide over one another. It also absorbs energy from the shock of physical movement. In osteoarthritis, the surface layer of cartilage breaks and wears away. This allows bones under the cartilage to rub together, causing pain, swelling, and loss of motion of the joint. Over time, the joint may lose its normal shape. Also, small deposits of bone—called osteophytes or bone spurs—may grow on the edges of the joint. Bits of bone or cartilage can break off and float inside the joint space. This causes more pain and damage.

How does osteoarthritis affect people?

People with osteoarthritis usually have joint pain and stiffness. Unlike some other forms of arthritis, such as rheumatoid arthritis, osteoarthritis affects only joint function. It does not affect skin tissue, the lungs, the eyes, or the blood vessels. The most commonly affected joints are those at the ends of the fingers (closest to the nail), thumbs, neck, lower back, knees, and hips.

Osteoarthritis affects different people differently. It may progress quickly, but for most people, joint damage develops gradually over years. In some people, osteoarthritis is relatively mild and interferes little with day-to-day life; in others, it causes significant pain and disability.

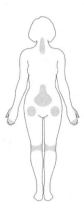

Figure 10.2. Osteoarthritis most often occurs in the hands (at the ends of the fingers and thumbs), spine (neck and lower back), knees, and hips. (Source: National Institute of Arthritis and Musculoskeletal and Skin Diseases)

How is osteoarthritis treated?

Most successful treatment programs include ways to manage pain and improve function. These can involve exercise, weight control, rest and relief from stress on joints, pain relief techniques, medications, surgery, and complementary and alternative therapies.

Exercise: Research shows that exercise is one of the best treatments for osteoarthritis. Exercise can improve mood and outlook, decrease pain, increase flexibility, strengthen the heart and improve blood flow, maintain weight, and promote general physical fitness.

You can use exercises to keep strong and limber, improve cardiovascular fitness, extend your joints' range of motion, and reduce your weight. The following types of exercise are part of a well-rounded arthritis treatment plan.

- **Strengthening exercises:** These exercises strengthen muscles that support joints affected by arthritis. They can be performed with weights or with exercise bands, inexpensive devices that add resistance.

- **Aerobic activities:** These are exercises, such as brisk walking or low-impact aerobics, that get your heart pumping and can keep your lungs and circulatory system in shape.

- **Range-of-motion activities:** These keep your joints limber.

- **Balance and agility exercises:** These help you maintain daily living skills.

Ask your doctor or physical therapist what exercises are best for you. Ask for guidelines on exercising when a joint is sore or if swelling is present. Also, check if you should (1) use pain-relieving drugs, such as analgesics or anti-inflammatories (also called NSAIDs or nonsteroidal anti-inflammatory drugs) to make exercising easier, or (2) use ice afterward.

Weight control: Osteoarthritis patients who are overweight or obese should try to lose weight. Weight loss can reduce stress on weight-bearing joints, limit further injury, and increase mobility. A dietitian can help you develop healthy eating habits. A healthy diet and regular exercise help reduce weight.

Rest and relief from stress on joints: Treatment plans include regularly scheduled rest. Patients must learn to recognize the body's signals, and know when to stop or slow down. If joint pain interferes with your ability to sleep or rest, consult your doctor.

Some people find relief from special footwear and insoles that can reduce pain and improve walking or from using canes to take pressure off painful joints. They may use splints or braces to provide extra support for joints and/or keep them in proper position during sleep or activity. Splints should be used only for limited periods of time because joints and muscles need to be exercised to prevent stiffness and weakness. If you need a splint, an occupational therapist or a doctor can help you get a properly fitted one.

Nondrug pain relief and alternative therapies: People with osteoarthritis may find many nondrug ways to relieve pain. Below are some examples:

- **Heat and cold:** Heat can be applied in a number of different ways—with warm towels, hot packs, or a warm bath or shower—to increase blood flow and ease pain and stiffness. In some cases, cold packs (bags of ice or frozen vegetables wrapped in a towel), which reduce inflammation, can relieve pain or numb the sore area. (Check with a doctor or physical therapist to find out if heat or cold is the best treatment.)

- **Transcutaneous electrical nerve stimulation (TENS):** TENS is a technique that uses a small electronic device to direct mild electric pulses to nerve endings that lie beneath the skin in the painful area.

- **Massage:** This may increase blood flow and bring warmth to a stressed area. However, arthritis-stressed joints are sensitive, so the therapist must be familiar with the problems of the disease.

- **Complementary and alternative therapies:** A study reported in 2004 revealed that acupuncture relieves pain and improves function in knee osteoarthritis, and it serves as an effective complement to standard care. Nutritional supplements such as glucosamine and chondroitin sulfate have been reported to improve the symptoms of people with osteoarthritis, as have certain vitamins. No scientific research to date shows that some popular folk remedies—such as the wearing of copper bracelets, following special diets, and rubbing WD-40 on joints to "lubricate" them—are helpful in treating osteoarthritis. Although these practices may or may not be harmful, they can be expensive, and using them may cause people to delay or even abandon useful medical treatment.

Medications to control pain: Doctors prescribe medicines to eliminate or reduce pain and to improve functioning. By working together, you and your doctor can find the medication that best relieves your pain with the least risk of side effects. The following types of medicines are commonly used in treating osteoarthritis:

- **Acetaminophen:** Acetaminophen, is available without a prescription. It is often the first medication doctors recommend for osteoarthritis patients because of its safety relative to some other drugs and its effectiveness against pain.

- **NSAIDs (nonsteroidal anti-inflammatory drugs):** NSAIDs are staples in arthritis treatment. Aspirin, ibuprofen, naproxen, and naproxen sodium are examples of NSAIDs. They are often the first type of medication used. All NSAIDs work similarly: by blocking substances called prostaglandins that contribute to inflammation and pain. However, each NSAID is a different chemical, and each has a slightly different effect on the body. Some NSAIDs are available over the counter, while others are available only with a prescription. All NSAIDs can have significant side effects, and some people seem to respond better to one NSAID than another. Any person taking NSAIDs regularly should be monitored by a doctor.

- **Narcotic or central acting agents:** Tramadol is a prescription pain reliever and synthetic opioid. Tramadol carries risks that don't exist with acetaminophen and NSAIDs, including the potential for addiction. Mild narcotic painkillers containing analgesics such as codeine or hydrocodone are often effective against osteoarthritis pain. But because of concerns about the potential dependence, doctors generally reserve them for short-term use.

- **Injections:** Corticosteroids are powerful anti-inflammatory hormones. They may be injected into the affected joints to temporarily relieve pain.

- **Hyaluronic acid substitutes:** Sometimes called viscosupplements, hyaluronic acid substitutes are designed to replace a normal component of the joint involved in joint lubrication and nutrition. Depending on the particular product your doctor prescribes, it will be given in a series of three to five injections. These products are approved only for osteoarthritis of the knee.

- **Other medications:** Doctors may prescribe several other medicines for osteoarthritis. They include topical pain-relieving creams, rubs, and sprays, which are applied directly to the skin over painful joints.

Because most medicines used to treat osteoarthritis have side effects, it's important to learn as much as possible about the medications you take, even the ones available without a prescription. Certain health problems and lifestyle habits can increase the risk of side effects from NSAIDs. These include a history of peptic ulcers or digestive tract bleeding, use of oral corticosteroids or anticoagulants (blood thinners), smoking, and alcohol use.

There are measures you can take to help reduce the risk of side effects associated with NSAIDs. These include taking medications with food and avoiding stomach irritants such as alcohol, tobacco, and caffeine. In some cases, it may help to take another medication along with an NSAID to coat the stomach or block stomach acids. Although these measures may help, they are not always completely effective.

Surgery: For many people, surgery helps relieve the pain and disability of osteoarthritis. Surgery may be performed to achieve one or more of the following:

- Removal of loose pieces of bone and cartilage from the joint if they are causing symptoms of buckling or locking (arthroscopy)

- Repositioning of bones (osteotomy)

- Resurfacing (smoothing out) bones (joint resurfacing)

- Replacing affected joints with artificial joints called prostheses

The decision to use surgery depends on several factors, including the patient's age, occupation, level of disability, pain intensity, and the degree to which arthritis interferes with his or her lifestyle. After surgery and rehabilitation, the patient usually feels less pain and swelling and can move more easily.

What can you do?

Although health care professionals can prescribe or recommend treatments to help you manage your arthritis, the real key to living well with the disease is you. Research shows that people with osteoarthritis who take part in their own care report less pain and make fewer doctor visits. They also enjoy a better quality of life.

Living well and enjoying good health despite arthritis requires an everyday lifelong commitment. The following six habits are worth committing to:

1. Get educated.

2. Stay active.

3. Eat well.

4. Get plenty of sleep.

5. Have fun.

6. Keep a positive attitude.

Section 10.4

Reactive Arthritis

Excerpted from "Questions and Answers about Reactive Arthritis,"
National Institute of Arthritis and Musculoskeletal and Skin Diseases
(www.niams.nih.gov), NIH Publication No. 09-5039, updated October 2012.

What is reactive arthritis?

Reactive arthritis is a form of arthritis, or joint inflammation that occurs as a reaction to an infection elsewhere in the body. Inflammation is a characteristic reaction of tissues to injury or disease and is marked by swelling, redness, heat, and pain. Besides this joint inflammation, reactive arthritis is associated with two other symptoms: redness and inflammation of the eyes (conjunctivitis) and inflammation of the urinary tract (urethritis). These symptoms may occur alone, together, or not at all.

Reactive arthritis is also known as a seronegative spondyloarthropathy. The seronegative spondyloarthropathies are a group of disorders that can cause inflammation throughout the body, especially in the spine. (Examples of other disorders in this group include psoriatic arthritis, ankylosing spondylitis, and the kind of arthritis that sometimes accompanies inflammatory bowel disease.)

In many patients, reactive arthritis is triggered by a venereal infection in the bladder, the urethra, or, in women, the vagina (the urogenital tract) that is often transmitted through sexual contact. This form of the disorder is sometimes called genitourinary or urogenital reactive arthritis. Another form of reactive arthritis is caused by an infection in the intestinal tract from eating food or handling substances that are contaminated with bacteria. This form of arthritis is sometimes called enteric or gastrointestinal reactive arthritis.

The symptoms of reactive arthritis usually last several months, although symptoms can return or develop into a long-term disease in a small percentage of people.

What are the symptoms of reactive arthritis?

Reactive arthritis most typically results in inflammation of the urogenital tract, the joints, and the eyes. Less common symptoms are mouth ulcers and skin rashes. Any of these symptoms may be so mild that patients do not notice them. They usually come and go over a period of several weeks to several months.

Joint symptoms: Reactive arthritis typically involves pain and swelling in the knees, ankles, and feet. Wrists, fingers, and other joints are affected less often. People with reactive arthritis commonly develop inflammation of the tendons (tendinitis) or at places where tendons attach to the bone. In many people with reactive arthritis, this results in heel pain or irritation of the Achilles tendon at the back of the ankle. Some people with reactive arthritis also develop heel spurs, which are bony growths in the heel that may cause chronic (long-lasting) foot pain. Approximately half of people with reactive arthritis report low-back and buttock pain.

Reactive arthritis also can cause spondylitis (inflammation of the vertebrae in the spinal column) or sacroiliitis (inflammation of the joints in the lower back that connect the spine to the pelvis). People with reactive arthritis who have the HLA-B27 gene are even more likely to develop spondylitis and/or sacroiliitis.

Eye involvement: Conjunctivitis, an inflammation of the mucous membrane that covers the eyeball and eyelid, develops in approximately half of people with reactive arthritis. Some people may develop uveitis, which is an inflammation of the inner eye. Conjunctivitis and uveitis can cause redness of the eyes, eye pain and irritation, and blurred vision. Eye involvement typically occurs early in the course of reactive arthritis, and symptoms may come and go.

How is reactive arthritis treated?

Although there is no cure for reactive arthritis, some treatments relieve symptoms of the disorder. The doctor is likely to use one or more of the following treatments:

Nonsteroidal anti-inflammatory drugs (NSAIDs): Aspirin, ibuprofen, naproxen, and naproxen sodium are examples of NSAIDs. They are often the first type of medication used. Some NSAIDs are available over the counter, while more than a dozen others, including a subclass called COX-2 inhibitors, are available only with a prescription. All NSAIDs can have significant side effects.

Corticosteroid injections: For people with severe joint inflammation, injections of corticosteroids directly into the affected joint may reduce inflammation. Doctors usually prescribe these injections only after trying unsuccessfully to control arthritis with NSAIDs.

Topical corticosteroids: These corticosteroids come in a cream or lotion and can be applied directly on the skin lesions, such as ulcers, associated with reactive arthritis. Topical corticosteroids reduce inflammation and promote healing.

Antibiotics: The doctor may prescribe antibiotics to eliminate the bacterial infection that triggered reactive arthritis. The specific antibiotic prescribed depends on the type of bacterial infection present. It is important to follow instructions about how much medicine to take and for how long; otherwise the infection may persist.

Immunosuppressive medicines: A small percentage of patients with reactive arthritis have severe symptoms that cannot be controlled with any of the above treatments. For these people, medicine that suppresses the immune system, may be effective.

TNF inhibitors: Several relatively new treatments that suppress tumor necrosis factor (TNF), a protein involved in the body's inflammatory response, may be effective for reactive arthritis and other spondyloarthropathies. These treatments, also sometimes called *biologics*, were first used to treat rheumatoid arthritis.

Exercise: Exercise, when introduced gradually, may help improve joint function. In particular, strengthening and range-of-motion exercises will maintain or improve joint function. Strengthening exercises build up the muscles around the joint to better support it. Muscle-tightening exercises that do not move any joints can be done even when a person has inflammation and pain. Range-of-motion exercises improve movement and flexibility and reduce stiffness in the affected joint. For patients with spine pain or inflammation, exercises to stretch and extend the back can be particularly helpful in preventing long-term disability. Aquatic exercise also may be helpful. Before beginning an exercise program, patients should talk to a health professional who can recommend appropriate exercises.

What is the prognosis for people who have reactive arthritis?

Most people with reactive arthritis recover fully from the initial flare of symptoms and are able to return to regular activities a few months after the first symptoms appear. In such cases, the symptoms of arthritis may last up to a year, although these are usually very mild and do not interfere with daily activities. Some people with reactive arthritis will have chronic (long-term) arthritis, which usually is mild. Studies show that between 15 and 50 percent of patients will develop symptoms again sometime after the initial flare has disappeared. It is possible that such relapses may be caused by reinfection. Back pain and arthritis are the symptoms that most commonly reappear. A few patients will have chronic, severe arthritis that is difficult to control with treatment and may cause joint damage.

Section 10.5

Gout

Excerpted from "Questions and Answers about Gout,"
National Institute of Arthritis and Musculoskeletal and Skin Diseases
(www.niams.nih.gov), NIH Publication No. 12-5027, April 2012.

What is gout?

Gout is a painful condition that occurs when the bodily waste product uric acid is deposited as needle-like crystals in the joints and/or soft tissues. In the joints, these uric acid crystals cause inflammatory arthritis, which in turn leads to intermittent swelling, redness, heat, pain, and stiffness in the joints.

In many people, gout initially affects the joints of the big toe (a condition called podagra). But many other joints and areas around the joints can be affected in addition to or instead of the big toe. These include the insteps, ankles, heels, knees, wrists, fingers, and elbows. Chalky deposits of uric acid, also known as tophi, can appear as lumps under the skin that surrounds the joints and covers the rim of the ear. Uric acid crystals can also collect in the kidneys and cause kidney stones.

Gout can progress through four stages:

- **Asymptomatic (without symptoms) hyperuricemia:** In this stage, a person has elevated levels of uric acid in the blood (hyperuricemia), but no other symptoms. Treatment is usually not required.

- **Acute gout, or acute gouty arthritis:** In this stage, hyperuricemia has caused the deposit of uric acid crystals in joint spaces. This leads to a sudden onset of intense pain and swelling in the joints, which also may be warm and very tender. An acute attack commonly occurs at night and can be triggered by stressful events, alcohol, or drugs, or the presence of another illness. Attacks usually subside within 3–10 days, even without treatment, and the next attack may not occur for months or even years. Over time, however, attacks can last longer and occur more frequently.

- **Interval or intercritical gout:** This is the period between acute attacks. In this stage, a person does not have any symptoms.

- **Chronic tophaceous gout:** This is the most disabling stage of gout. It usually develops over a long period, such as 10 years. In this stage, the disease may have caused permanent damage to the affected joints and sometimes to the kidneys. With proper treatment, most people with gout do not progress to this advanced stage.

What causes gout?

A number of risk factors are associated with hyperuricemia and gout. They include genetics, male gender, adult age, being overweight, drinking too much alcohol, eating too many foods that are rich in purines, and exposure to lead in the environment. Other health problems associated with increased risk of gout include renal insufficiency, high blood pressure, hypothyroidism (underactive thyroid gland), and conditions that cause an excessively rapid turnover of cells, such as psoriasis, hemolytic anemia, or some cancers. Kelley-Seegmiller syndrome and Lesch-Nyhan syndrome are two rare conditions in which the enzyme that helps control uric acid levels either is not present or is found in insufficient quantities.

Additionally, a number of medications may put people at risk for developing hyperuricemia and gout. They include diuretics, salicylate-containing drugs (such as aspirin), niacin, cyclosporine, and levodopa.

How is gout treated?

The most common treatments for an acute attack of gout are non-steroidal anti-inflammatory drugs (NSAIDs) taken orally (by mouth), or corticosteroids, which are taken orally or injected into the affected joint. NSAIDs reduce the inflammation caused by deposits of uric acid crystals, but have no effect on the amount of uric acid in the body. The longer a person uses NSAIDs, the more likely he or she is to have side effects, ranging from mild to serious. Check with your health care provider or pharmacist before you take NSAIDs.

Corticosteroids are strong anti-inflammatory hormones. The most commonly prescribed corticosteroid is prednisone. Patients often begin to improve within a few hours of treatment with a corticosteroid, and the attack usually goes away completely within a week or so.

When NSAIDs or corticosteroids do not control symptoms, the doctor may consider using colchicine. This drug is most effective when taken within the first 12 hours of an acute attack.

For some patients, the doctor may prescribe either NSAIDs or oral colchicine in small daily doses to prevent future attacks. The doctor also may consider prescribing other medicines to treat hyperuricemia and reduce the frequency of sudden attacks and the development of tophi.

People who have other medical problems, such as high blood pressure or high blood triglycerides (fats), may find that the drugs they take for those conditions can also be useful for gout.

The doctor may also recommend losing weight, for those who are overweight; limiting alcohol consumption; and avoiding or limiting high-purine foods, which can increase uric acid levels.

What can people with gout do to stay healthy?

People with gout can decrease the severity of attacks and reduce their risk of future attacks by taking their medications as prescribed. Acute gout is best controlled if medications are taken at the first sign of pain or inflammation.

Tell your doctor about all the medicines and vitamins you take. He or she can tell you if any of them increase your risk of hyperuricemia. Plan followup visits with your doctor to evaluate your progress. Drink plenty of nonalcoholic fluids, especially water. Nonalcoholic fluids help remove uric acid from the body. Alcohol, on the other hand, can raise the levels of uric acid in your blood.

Exercise regularly and maintain a healthy body weight. Lose weight if you are overweight, but avoid low-carbohydrate diets that are designed for quick weight loss. When carbohydrate intake is insufficient, your body can't completely burn its own fat. As a consequence, substances called ketones form and are released into the bloodstream, resulting in a condition called ketosis. After a short time, ketosis can increase the level of uric acid in your blood.

Avoid foods that are high in purines:

- Anchovies
- Asparagus
- Beef kidneys
- Brains
- Fried beans and peas
- Game meats
- Gravy
- Herring
- Liver
- Mackerel
- Mushrooms
- Sardines
- Scallops
- Sweetbreads

Section 10.6

Polymyalgia Rheumatica

"Polymyalgia Rheumatica," © 2012 American College of Rheumatology (www.rheumatology.org). All rights reserved. Reprinted with permission.

Polymyalgia rheumatica (sometimes referred to as PMR) is a common cause of widespread aching and stiffness in older adults. Because PMR does not often cause swollen joints, it may be hard to recognize. PMR may occur with another health problem, giant cell arteritis.

Fast Facts

- PMR affects adults over the age of 50.

- Aching and stiffness in PMR affect the upper arms, neck, buttocks, and thighs, and are most severe in the morning.

- These symptoms respond quickly and completely to low doses of corticosteroids.

What Is Polymyalgia Rheumatica?

The typical symptoms (what you feel) of PMR are aching and stiffness about the upper arms, neck, lower back, and thighs. Symptoms tend to come on quickly, over a few days or weeks, and sometimes even overnight. Both sides of the body are equally affected. Involvement of the upper arms, with trouble raising them above the shoulders, is most common. Sometimes, aching occurs at joints such as the hands and wrists.

Achiness is always worse in the morning and improves as the day goes by. Yet inactivity, such as a long car ride or sitting too long in one position, may cause stiffness to return. Stiffness may be so severe that it causes any of these problems:

- Disturbed sleep

- Trouble getting dressed in the morning (for instance, putting on a jacket or bending over to pull on socks and shoes)

- Problems getting up from a sofa or in and out of a car

What Causes Polymyalgia Rheumatica

The cause of PMR is unknown. PMR does not result from side effects of medications. The abrupt onset of symptoms suggests the possibility of an infection but, so far, none has been found. *Myalgia* comes from the Greek word for *muscle pain*. However, specific tests of the muscles, such as a blood test for muscle enzymes or a muscle biopsy (surgical removal of a small piece of muscle for inspection under a microscope), are all normal.

Recent research suggests that inflammation in PMR involves the shoulder and hip joints themselves, and the bursae (or sacs) around these joints. So pains at the upper arms and thighs, in fact, start at the nearby shoulder and hip joints. This is what doctors call *referred pain*.

PMR should not be confused with fibromyalgia, a poorly understood health problem that affects mainly younger adults.

Who Gets Polymyalgia Rheumatica?

PMR affects older adults over the age of 50. The average age at onset (start) of symptoms is 70, so people who have PMR may be in their 80s or even older. The disease affects women somewhat more often than men. It is more frequent in whites than nonwhites, but all races can get PMR.

How Is Polymyalgia Rheumatica Diagnosed?

In PMR, results of blood tests to detect inflammation are most often abnormally high. One such test is the erythrocyte sedimentation rate, also called "sed rate." Another test is the C-reactive protein, or CRP. Both tests may be very elevated in PMR but, in some patients, these tests may have normal or only slightly high results.

PMR can be hard to diagnose. Your health care providers should rule out other health problems, such as cancer and rheumatoid arthritis.

How Is Polymyalgia Rheumatica Treated?

If your doctor strongly suspects PMR, you will receive a trial of low-dose corticosteroids. Often, the dose is 10–15 milligrams (shortened as mg) per day of prednisone (Deltasone, Orasone, etc.). If PMR is present, the medicine quickly relieves stiffness. The response to corticosteroids can be dramatic. Sometimes patients are better after only one dose. Improvement can be slower, though. But, if symptoms do not go away after two or three weeks of treatment, the diagnosis of PMR is not likely, and your doctor will consider other causes of your illness.

Nonsteroidal anti-inflammatory drugs (commonly called NSAIDs), such as ibuprofen (Advil, Motrin, etc.) and naproxen (Naprosyn, Aleve), are not effective in treating PMR.

When your symptoms are under control, your doctor will slowly decrease (*taper*) the dose of corticosteroid medicine. The goal is to find the lowest dose that keeps you comfortable. Some people can stop taking corticosteroids within a year. Others, though, will need a small amount of this medicine for 2–3 years, to keep aching and stiffness under control. Symptoms can recur. Because the symptoms of PMR are sensitive to even small changes in the dose of corticosteroids, your doctor should direct the gradual decrease of this medicine.

Living with Polymyalgia Rheumatica

Once stiffness has gone away, you can resume all normal activities, including exercise.

Even low doses of corticosteroids can cause side effects. These include higher blood sugar, weight gain, sleeplessness, osteoporosis (bone loss), cataracts, thinning of the skin, and bruising. Checking for these problems, including bone density testing, is an important part of follow-up visits with your doctor. Older patients may need medicine to prevent osteoporosis.

PMR can occur with a more serious condition, giant cell arteritis. Thus, see your doctor right away if you have PMR and you get symptoms of headache, changes in vision or fever.

Points to Remember

- Aching and stiffness develop quickly in PMR and are most common about the shoulders and upper arms.

- Symptoms are worse in the morning.

- Symptoms respond promptly to low doses of corticosteroids, but may recur as the dose is lowered.

The Rheumatologist's Role in the Treatment of Polymyalgia Rheumatica

PMR may be hard to diagnose. Rheumatologists are experts in diagnosing and treating diseases of the joints, muscles, and bones. Therefore, they are more likely to make a proper diagnosis and expertly manage medications to minimize side effects.

Chapter 11

Back and Spinal Pain

Chapter Contents

Section 11.1—What You Should Know about
Back Pain.. 114

Section 11.2—Symptoms and Causes of Back and
Spinal Pain 120

Section 11.3—Spinal Stenosis 126

Section 11.1

What You Should Know about Back Pain

Excerpted from "Handout on Health: Back Pain," National Institute of
Arthritis and Musculoskeletal and Skin Diseases (www.niams.nih.gov),
NIH Publication No. 09-5282, updated April 2012.

What is back pain?

Back pain is an all-too-familiar problem that can range from a dull,
constant ache to a sudden, sharp pain that leaves you incapacitated.
It can come on suddenly—from an accident, a fall, or lifting something
heavy—or it can develop slowly, perhaps as the result of age-related
changes to the spine.

Regardless of how back pain happens or how it feels, you know it
when you have it. And chances are, if you don't have back pain now,
you will eventually. In a three-month period, about one-fourth of U.S.
adults experience at least one day of back pain. It is one of our society's
most common medical problems.

Should I see a doctor for back pain?

In most cases, it is not necessary to see a doctor for back pain because pain usually goes away with or without treatment. However,
a trip to the doctor is probably a good idea if you have numbness or
tingling, if your pain is severe and doesn't improve with medication
and rest, or if you have pain after a fall or an injury. It is also important to see your doctor if you have pain along with any of the following problems: trouble urinating; weakness, pain, or numbness in your
legs; fever; or unintentional weight loss. Such symptoms could signal
a serious problem that requires treatment soon.

Many different types of doctors treat back pain, from family physicians to doctors who specialize in disorders of the nerves and musculoskeletal system. In most cases, it is best to see your primary care
doctor first. In many cases, he or she can treat the problem. In other
cases, your doctor may refer you to an appropriate specialist.

How is back pain diagnosed?

Often a doctor can find the cause of your pain with a physical and medical history alone. However, depending on what the history and exam show, your doctor may order medical tests to help find the cause. Many times, the precise cause of back pain is never known. In these cases, it may be comforting to know that most back pain gets better whether or not you find out what is causing it.

Following are some tests your doctor may order:

X-rays: Traditional x-rays use low levels of radiation to project a picture onto a piece of film (some newer x rays use electronic imaging techniques). They are often used to view the bones and bony structures in the body. Your doctor may order an x-ray if he or she suspects that you have a fracture or osteoarthritis or that your spine is not aligned properly.

Magnetic resonance imaging (MRI): MRI uses a strong magnetic force instead of radiation to create an image. Unlike an x-ray, which shows only bony structures, an MRI scan produces clear pictures of soft tissues, too, such as ligaments, tendons, and blood vessels. Your doctor may order an MRI scan if he or she suspects a problem such as an infection, tumor, inflammation, or pressure on a nerve. An MRI scan, in most instances, is not necessary during the early phases of low back pain unless your doctor identifies certain "red flags" in your history and physical exam. An MRI scan is needed if the pain persists for longer than three to six weeks or if your doctor feels there may be a need for surgical consultation. Because most low back pain goes away on its own, getting an MRI scan too early may sometimes create confusion for the patient and the doctor.

Computed tomography (CT) scan: A CT scan allows your doctor to see spinal structures that cannot be seen on traditional x-rays. A computer creates a three-dimensional image from a series of two-dimensional pictures that it takes of your back. Your doctor may order a CT scan to look for problems including herniated disks, tumors, or spinal stenosis.

Blood tests: Although blood tests are not used generally in diagnosing the cause of back pain, your doctor may order them in some cases.

How is back pain treated?

Treatment for back pain generally depends on what kind of pain you experience: acute or chronic. Acute pain comes on quickly and often leaves just as quickly. To be classified as acute, pain should last no longer than six weeks. Chronic pain, on the other hand, may come on either quickly or slowly, and it lingers a long time. In general, pain that lasts longer than three months is considered chronic.

- **Acute back pain:** Acute back pain usually gets better on its own and without treatment, although you may want to try acetaminophen, aspirin, or ibuprofen to help ease the pain. Perhaps the best advice is to go about your usual activities as much as you can with the assurance that the problem will clear up. Getting up and moving around can help ease stiffness, relieve pain, and have you back doing your regular activities sooner. Exercises or surgery are not usually advisable for acute back pain.

- **Chronic back pain:** Treatment for chronic back pain falls into two basic categories: the kind that requires an operation and the kind that does not. In the vast majority of cases, back pain does not require surgery. Doctors will nearly always try nonsurgical treatments before recommending surgery. In a very small percentage of cases—when back pain is caused by a tumor, an infection, or a nerve root problem called cauda equina syndrome, for example—prompt surgery is necessary to ease the pain and prevent further problems.

Following are some of the more commonly used nonsurgical treatments for chronic back pain.

Hot or cold: Hot or cold packs—or sometimes a combination of the two—can be soothing to chronically sore, stiff backs. Heat dilates the blood vessels, both improving the supply of oxygen that the blood takes to the back and reducing muscle spasms. Heat also alters the sensation of pain. Cold may reduce inflammation by decreasing the size of blood vessels and the flow of blood to the area. Although cold may feel painful against the skin, it numbs deep pain. Applying heat or cold may relieve pain, but it does not cure the cause of chronic back pain.

Exercise: Although exercise is usually not advisable for acute back pain, proper exercise can help ease chronic pain and perhaps reduce the risk of it returning. Flexion, extension, stretching, and aerobic types of exercise are important to general physical fitness and may be helpful for certain specific causes of back pain:

The purposes of *flexion exercises*, which are exercises in which you bend forward, are to (1) widen the spaces between the vertebrae, thereby reducing pressure on the nerves; (2) stretch muscles of the back and hips; and (3) strengthen abdominal and buttock muscles. Many doctors think that strengthening the muscles of the abdomen will reduce the load on the spine. One word of caution: If your back pain is caused by a herniated disk, check with your doctor before performing flexion exercises because they may increase pressure within the disk, making the problem worse.

With *extension exercises*, you bend backward. They may minimize radiating pain, which is pain you can feel in other parts of the body besides where it originates. Examples of extension exercises are leg lifting and raising the trunk, each exercise performed while lying prone. The theory behind these exercises is that they open up the spinal canal in places and develop muscles that support the spine.

The goal of *stretching exercises*, as their name suggests, is to stretch and improve the extension of muscles and other soft tissues of the back. This can reduce back stiffness and improve range of motion.

Aerobic exercise is the type that gets your heart pumping faster and keeps your heart rate elevated for a while. For fitness, it is important to get at least 30 minutes of aerobic (also called cardiovascular) exercise three times a week. Aerobic exercises work the large muscles of the body and include brisk walking, jogging, and swimming. For back problems, you should avoid exercise that requires twisting or vigorous forward flexion, such as aerobic dancing and rowing, because these actions may raise pressure in the disks and actually do more harm than good. In addition, avoid high-impact activities if you have disk disease. If back pain or your fitness level make it impossible to exercise 30 minutes at a time, try three 10-minute sessions to start with and work up to your goal. But first, speak with your doctor or physical therapist about the safest aerobic exercise for you.

Medications: A wide range of medications are used to treat chronic back pain. Some are available over the counter. Others require a doctor's prescription.

Analgesic medications are those designed specifically to relieve pain. They include over-the-counter acetaminophen (for example, Tylenol [Brand names included in this book are provided as examples only, and their inclusion does not mean that these products are endorsed by the National Institutes of Health or any other agency. Also, if a particular brand name is not mentioned, this does not mean or imply that the product is unsatisfactory.]) and aspirin, as well as prescription narcotics, such as oxycodone with acetaminophen (Percocet) or hydrocodone with acetaminophen (Vicodin). Aspirin and acetaminophen are the most commonly used analgesics; narcotics should only be used for a short time for severe pain or pain after surgery. People with muscular back pain or arthritis pain that is not relieved by medications may find topical analgesics helpful. These creams, ointments, and salves are rubbed directly onto the skin over the site of pain. They use one or more of a variety of ingredients to ease pain.

Nonsteroidal anti-inflammatory drugs (NSAIDs) are drugs that relieve pain and inflammation, both of which may play a role in some cases of back pain. NSAIDs include the nonprescription products ibuprofen

117

(Motrin, Advil), ketoprofen (Actron, Orudis KT), and naproxen sodium (Aleve). More than a dozen others, including a subclass of NSAIDs called COX-2 inhibitors, are available only with a prescription. All NSAIDs work similarly by blocking substances called prostaglandins that contribute to inflammation and pain. However, each NSAID is a different chemical, and each has a slightly different effect on the body. The longer a person uses NSAIDs, the more likely he or she is to have side effects, ranging from mild to serious. Check with your health care provider or pharmacist before you take NSAIDs. It's important to work with your doctor to choose the one that's safest and most effective for you.

Muscle relaxants and certain *antidepressants* have also been prescribed for chronic back pain, but their usefulness is questionable. If the cause of back pain is an inflammatory form of arthritis, medications used to treat that specific form of arthritis may be helpful against the pain.

Traction: Traction involves using pulleys and weights to stretch the back. The rationale behind traction is to pull the vertebrae apart to allow a bulging disk to slip back into place. Some people experience pain relief while in traction, but that relief is usually temporary. Once traction is released, the stretch is not sustained and back pain is likely to return. There is no scientific evidence that traction provides any long-term benefits for people with back pain.

Corsets and braces: Corsets and braces include a number of devices, such as elastic bands and stiff supports with metal stays, that are designed to limit the motion of the lumbar spine, provide abdominal support, and correct posture. Although these may be appropriate after certain kinds of surgery, there is little, if any, evidence that corsets and braces help treat chronic low back pain. In fact, by keeping you from using your back muscles, they may actually cause more problems than they solve by causing lower back muscles to weaken from lack of use.

Behavioral modification: Developing a healthy attitude and learning to move your body properly while you do daily activities, particularly those involving heavy lifting, pushing, or pulling, are sometimes part of the treatment plan for people with back pain. Other behavior changes that might help pain include adopting healthy habits, such as exercise, relaxation, and regular sleep, and dropping bad habits, such as smoking and eating poorly.

Injections: When medications and other nonsurgical treatments fail to relieve chronic back pain, doctors may recommend injections for pain relief. Following are some of the most commonly used injections, although some are of questionable value:

If a nerve is inflamed or compressed as it passes from the spinal column between the vertebrae, an injection called a *nerve root block* may be used to help ease the resulting back and leg pain. The injection contains a steroid medication or anesthetic and is administered to the affected part of the nerve. Whether the procedure helps or not depends on finding and injecting precisely the right nerve.

The *facet joints* are those where the vertebrae connect to one another, keeping the spine aligned. Although arthritis in the facet joints themselves is rarely the source of back pain, the injection of anesthetics or steroid medications into facet joints is sometimes tried as a way to relieve pain. The effectiveness of these injections is questionable. One study suggests that this treatment is overused and ineffective.

In *trigger point injections*, an anesthetic is injected into specific areas in the back that are painful when the doctor applies pressure to them. Some doctors add a steroid medication to the injection. Although the injections are commonly used, researchers have found that injecting anesthetics or steroids into trigger points provides no more relief than "dry needling" (inserting a needle and not injecting a medication).

Complementary and alternative treatments: When back pain becomes chronic or when medications and other conventional therapies do not relieve it, many people try complementary and alternative treatments. Although such therapies won't cure diseases or repair the injuries that cause pain, some people find them useful for managing or relieving pain.

Spinal manipulation refers to procedures in which professionals use their hands to mobilize, adjust, massage, or stimulate the spine or surrounding tissues. This type of therapy is often performed by osteopathic doctors and chiropractors. It tends to be most effective in people with uncomplicated pain and when used with other therapies. Spinal manipulation is not appropriate if you have a medical problem such as osteoporosis, spinal cord compression, or inflammatory arthritis (such as rheumatoid arthritis), or if you are taking blood-thinning medications such as warfarin (Coumadin) or heparin (Calciparine, Liquaemin).

Transcutaneous electrical nerve stimulation (TENS) involves wearing a small box over the painful area that directs mild electrical impulses to nerves there. The theory is that stimulating the nervous system can modify the perception of pain. Early studies of TENS suggested it could elevate the levels of endorphins, the body's natural pain-numbing chemicals, in the spinal fluid. But subsequent studies of its effectiveness against pain have produced mixed results.

The ancient Chinese practice of *acupuncture* has been gaining increasing acceptance and popularity in the United States. Acupuncture is based on the theory that a life force called Qi (pronounced *chee*) flows through the body along certain channels, which if blocked can cause illness. According to the theory, the insertion of thin needles at precise locations along these channels by practitioners can unblock the flow of Qi, relieving pain and restoring health.

Although few Western-trained doctors would agree with the concept of blocked Qi, some believe that inserting and then stimulating needles (by twisting or passing a low-voltage electrical current through them) may foster the production of the body's natural pain-numbing chemicals, such as endorphins, serotonin, and acetylcholine.

As with acupuncture, the theory behind *acupressure* is that it unblocks the flow of Qi. The difference between acupuncture and acupressure is that no needles are used in acupressure. Instead, a therapist applies pressure to points along the channels with his or her hands, elbows, or even feet. (In some cases, patients are taught to do their own acupressure.) Acupressure has not been well studied for back pain.

A type of massage called *Rolfing* involves using strong pressure on deep tissues in the back to relieve tightness of the fascia, a sheath of tissue that covers the muscles, that can cause or contribute to back pain. The theory behind Rolfing is that releasing muscles and tissues from the fascia enables the back to align itself properly. So far, the usefulness of Rolfing for back pain has not been scientifically proven.

Section 11.2

Symptoms and Causes of Back and Spinal Pain

Excerpted from "Back Pain and Sciatica,"
© 2013 A.D.A.M., Inc. Reprinted with permission.

The origin of the pain is often unknown, and imaging studies may fail to determine its cause. Disk disease, spinal arthritis, and muscle spasms are the most common diagnoses. Other problems can also cause back pain, however.

Muscle and Ligament Injuries and Lumbar Strain

Strain and injury to the muscles and ligaments supporting the back are the major causes of low back pain. The pain is typically more spread out in the muscles next to the spine, and may be associated with spasms in those muscles. The pain may move to the buttocks but rarely any farther down the leg.

Sciatica

The sciatic nerve is a large nerve that starts in the lower back.

- It forms near the spine and is made up from branches of the roots of the lumbar spinal nerves.

- It travels through the pelvis and then deep into each buttock.

- It then travels down each leg. It is the longest and widest single nerve in the body.

Sciatica is not a diagnosis but a description of symptoms. Anything that places pressure on one or more of the lumbar nerve roots can cause pain in parts or all of the sciatic nerve. A herniated disk, spinal stenosis, degenerative disc disease, spondylolisthesis, or other abnormalities of vertebrae can all cause pressure on the sciatic nerve.

Some cases of sciatica pain may occur when a muscle located deep in the buttocks pinches the sciatic nerve. This muscle is called the piriformis. The resulting condition is called piriformis syndrome. Piriformis syndrome usually develops after an injury. It is sometimes difficult to diagnose.

Pain or numbness due to sciatica can vary widely. It may feel like a mild tingling, dull ache, or a burning sensation. In some cases, the pain is severe enough to cause immobility.

The pain most often occurs on one side and may radiate to the buttocks, legs, and feet. Some people have sharp pain in one part of the leg or hip and numbness in other parts. The affected leg may feel weak or cold.

The pain often starts slowly. Sciatica pain may get worse:

- At night

- After standing or sitting for long periods of time

- When sneezing, coughing, or laughing

- After bending backwards or walking more than 50–100 yards (particularly if it is caused by spinal stenosis)

Sciatica pain usually goes away within six weeks, unless there are serious underlying conditions. Pain that lasts longer than 30 days, or gets worse with sitting, coughing, sneezing, or straining may indicated a longer recovery. Depending on the cause of the sciatica, symptoms may come and go.

Herniated Disk

A herniated disk, sometimes (incorrectly) called a slipped disk, is a common cause of severe back pain and sciatica. A disk in the lumbar area becomes herniated when it ruptures or thins out, and degenerates to the point that the gel within the disk (the nucleus pulposus) pushes outward. The damaged disk can take on many forms:

- **A bulge:** The gel has been pushed out slightly from the disk and is evenly distributed around the circumference.

- **Protrusion:** The gel has pushed out slightly and asymmetrically in different places.

- **Extrusion:** The gel balloons extensively into the area outside the vertebrae or breaks off from the disk.

Pain in the leg may be worse than the back pain in cases of herniated disks. There is also some debate about how pain develops from a herniated disk and how frequently it causes low back pain. Many people have disks that bulge or protrude and do not suffer back pain. Extrusion (which is less common than the other two conditions) is much more likely to cause back pain, since the gel extends out far enough to press against the nerve root, most often the sciatic nerve. Extrusion is very uncommon, however, while sciatic and low back pain are very common. But there may be other causes of low back pain.

Abnormalities in the Annular Ring

The annular ring, the fibrous band that surrounds and protects the disk, contains a dense nerve network and high levels of peptides that heighten perception of pain. Tears in the annular ring are a frequent finding in patients with degenerative disk disease.

Cauda Equina Syndrome

Cauda equina syndrome is the impingement of the cauda equina (the four strands of nerves leading through the lowest part of the spine). The cause is usually massive extrusion of the disk material. Cauda equina syndrome is an emergency condition that can cause severe complications to bowel or bladder function. It can cause permanent incontinence if not promptly treated with surgery. Symptoms of the cauda equina syndrome include:

- Dull back pain

- Weakness or numbness in the buttocks—in the area between the legs, or in the inner thigh, backs of legs, or feet—may cause stumbling or difficulty in standing

- An inability to control urination and defecation

- Pain accompanied by fever (can indicate an infection)

Lumbar Degenerative Joint Disease

Osteoarthritis occurs in joints of the spine, usually as a result of aging, but also in response to previous back injuries, excessive wear and tear, previously herniated discs, prior surgeries, and fractures. Cartilage between the joints of the spine is destroyed and extra bone growth or bone spurs develop. Spinal discs dry out and become thinner and more brittle. The rate at which these changes develop varies between people.

The end result of these changes is a gradual loss of mobility of the spine and narrowing of the spaces for spinal nerves and spinal cord, eventually leading to spinal stenosis. Symptoms may be similar to that of a herniated disc or spinal stenosis (narrowing of the spinal canal).

Spinal Stenosis

Spinal stenosis is the narrowing of the spinal canal, or narrowing of the openings (called neural foramina) where spinal nerves leave the spinal column. This condition typically develops as a person ages and the disks become drier and start to shrink. At the same time, the bones and ligaments of the spine swell or grow larger due to arthritis and chronic inflammation. However, other problems, including infection and birth defects, can sometimes cause spinal stenosis.

Most patients will report the presence of gradually worsening history of back pain over time. For others, there may be minimal history of back pain, but at some point in this process any disruption, such as a minor injury that results in disk inflammation, can cause impingement on the nerve root and trigger pain.

Patients may experience pain or numbness, which can occur in both legs, or on just one side. Other symptoms include a feeling of weakness or heaviness in the buttocks or legs. Symptoms are usually present or will worsen only when the person is standing or walking upright. Often the symptoms will ease or disappear when sitting down or leaning forward. These positions may create more space in the spinal canal, thus relieving pressure on the spinal cord or the spinal nerves. Patients with spinal stenosis are not usually able to walk for long periods of time, but they may be able to ride a bicycle with little pain.

Spondylolisthesis

Spondylolisthesis occurs when one of the lumbar vertebrae slips over another, or over the sacrum.

In children, spondylolisthesis usually occurs between the fifth bone in the lower back (lumbar vertebra) and the first bone in the sacrum area. It is often due to a birth defect in that area of the spine. In adults, the most common cause is degenerative disease (such as arthritis). The slip usually occurs between the fourth and fifth lumbar vertebrae. It is more common in adults over 65 and women.

Other causes of spondylolisthesis include stress fractures (typically seen in gymnasts) and traumatic fractures. Spondylolisthesis may occasionally be associated with bone diseases.

Spondylolisthesis may vary from mild to severe. It can produce increased lordosis (swayback), but in later stages may result in kyphosis (roundback) as the upper spine falls off the lower spine.

Symptoms may include:

- Lower back pain
- Stiffness
- Tenderness in the slipped area
- Pain in the thighs and buttocks
- Muscle tightness

Pain generally occurs with activity and is better with rest. Neurological damage (leg weakness or changes in sensation) may result from pressure on nerve roots, and may cause pain radiating down the legs.

Inflammatory Conditions and Arthritis

Inflammatory disorders and arthritis syndromes can produce inflammation in the spine. Rheumatoid arthritis can involve the cervical spine (neck). A group of disorders called seronegative spondyloarthropathies may cause back pain. These include:

- *Ankylosing spondylitis* is a chronic inflammation of the spine that may gradually result in a fusion of vertebrae. The back is usually stiff and painful in the morning; pain improves with movement or exercise. In most cases, symptoms develop slowly over time. In severe cases, symptoms become much worse over a short period of time, and the patient develops a stooped over posture. It occurs mostly in young Caucasian men in their mid-20s, and in most cases the cause is believed to be hereditary.

- *Reactive arthritis* or *Reiter syndrome* is a group of inflammatory conditions that involve certain joints, the lower back, urethra, and eyes. There may also be sores (lesions) on the skin and mucus membranes.

- *Psoriatic arthritis* is found in about 20% of people with psoriasis who develop arthritis involving the spine, as well as many other joints.

- *Enteropathic arthritis* is a type of arthritis associated with inflammatory bowel disease, the most common forms being ulcerative colitis and Crohn disease. About 20% of people with inflammatory bowel disease develop symptoms in the spine.

There are multiple medical treatments for these potentially disabling diseases, and in most cases surgery is not beneficial.

Osteoporosis and Compression Fractures

Osteoporosis is a disease of the skeleton in which the amount of calcium present in the bones slowly decreases to the point where the bones become fragile and prone to fractures. It usually does not cause pain unless the vertebrae collapse suddenly, in which case the pain is often severe. More than one vertebra may be affected.

In a compression fracture of the vertebrae, the bone tissue of the vertebra collapses. More than one vertebra may collapse as a result. When the fracture is the result of osteoporosis, the vertebrae in the thoracic (chest) and lower spine are usually affected, and symptoms may be worse with walking.

With multiple fractures, kyphosis (a forward hump-like curvature of the spine) may result. In addition, compression fractures are often responsible for loss of height. Pressure on the spinal cord may also occur, producing symptoms of numbness, tingling, or weakness. Symptoms depend upon the area of the back that is affected. However, most fractures are stable and do not produce neurological symptoms.

Back Pain Emergencies

Several serious conditions can also cause back pain. Often, these symptoms develop over a short period of time, become more severe, and may have other findings that go along with them. Some of these conditions include:

- Infection in the bone (osteomyelitis) or the disk (diskitis).

- Cancer that has spread to the spine from another part of the body (most commonly lung cancer, colon cancer, prostate cancer, and breast cancer).

- Cancer that begins in the bones (the most common diagnosis in adults is probably multiple myeloma, seen in middle age or older adults). Benign tumors such as osteoblastoma or neurofibroma and cancers, including leukemia, can also cause back pain in children.

- Trauma

Miscellaneous Abnormalities and Diagnoses

Other causes of back pain include:

- Fibromyalgia and other myofascial pain syndromes.

- Other medical conditions that cause referred back pain, occurring in conjunction with problems in organs unrelated to the spine (although usually located near it); such conditions include ulcers, kidney disease (including kidney stones), ovarian cysts, and pancreatitis.

- Chronic uterine or pelvic infections can cause low back pain in women.

Section 11.3

Spinal Stenosis

Excerpted from "Questions and Answers about Spinal Stenosis,"
National Institute of Arthritis and Musculoskeletal and Skin Disease
(www.niams.nih.gov), NIH Publication No. 09-5327, updated October 2012.

What is spinal stenosis?

Spinal stenosis is a narrowing of spaces in the spine (backbone) that results in pressure on the spinal cord and/or nerve roots. This disorder usually involves the narrowing of one or more of three areas of the spine: (1) the canal in the center of the column of bones (vertebral or spinal column) through which the spinal cord and nerve roots run, (2) the canals at the base or roots of nerves branching out from the spinal cord, or (3) the openings between vertebrae (bones of the spine) through which nerves leave the spine and go to other parts of the body. The narrowing may involve a small or large area of the spine. Pressure on the lower part of the spinal cord or on nerve roots branching out from that area may give rise to pain or numbness in the legs. Pressure on the upper part of the spinal cord (that is, the neck area) may produce similar symptoms in the shoulders, or even the legs.

This disorder is most common in men and women over 50 years of age. However, it may occur in younger people who are born with a narrowing of the spinal canal or who suffer an injury to the spine.

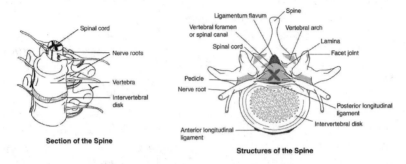

Figure 11.1. *The vertebral column provides the main support for the upper body, allowing humans to stand upright or bend and twist. Many of its structures can be involved in spinal stenosis. (Source: National Institute of Arthritis and Musculoskeletal and Skin Diseases)*

What are the symptoms of spinal stenosis?

The space within the spinal canal may narrow without producing any symptoms. However, if narrowing places pressure on the spinal cord, cauda equina, or nerve roots, there may be a slow onset and progression of symptoms. The neck or back may or may not hurt. More often, people experience numbness, weakness, cramping, or general pain in the arms or legs. If the narrowed space within the spine is pushing on a nerve root, people may feel pain radiating down the leg (sciatica). Sitting or flexing the lower back should relieve symptoms. (The flexed position "opens up" the spinal column, enlarging the spaces between vertebrae at the back of the spine.) Flexing exercises are often advised, along with stretching and strengthening exercises.

People with more severe stenosis may have problems with bowel and bladder function and foot disorders. For example, cauda equina syndrome is a severe, and very rare, form of spinal stenosis. It occurs because of compression of the cauda equina, and symptoms may include loss of control of the bowel, bladder, or sexual function and/or pain, weakness, or loss of feeling in one or both legs. Cauda equina syndrome is a serious condition requiring urgent medical attention.

127

Who treats spinal stenosis?

Nonsurgical treatment of spinal stenosis may be provided by internists or general practitioners. The disorder is also treated by specialists such as rheumatologists, who treat arthritis and related disorders; and neurologists, who treat nerve diseases. Orthopaedic surgeons and neurosurgeons also provide nonsurgical treatment and perform spinal surgery if it is required. Allied health professionals such as physical therapists may also help treat patients.

What are some nonsurgical treatments for spinal stenosis?

In the absence of severe or progressive nerve involvement, a doctor may prescribe one or more of the following conservative treatments:

- Nonsteroidal anti-inflammatory drugs (NSAIDs), such as aspirin, naproxen, ibuprofen, or indomethacin, to reduce inflammation and relieve pain. Warning: NSAIDs can cause stomach irritation or, less often, they can affect kidney function. The longer a person uses NSAIDs, the more likely he or she is to have side effects, ranging from mild to serious. Many other drugs cannot be taken when a patient is being treated with NSAIDs because NSAIDs alter the way the body uses or eliminates these other drugs. Check with your health care provider or pharmacist before you take NSAIDs. Also, NSAIDs sometimes are associated with serious gastrointestinal problems, including ulcers, bleeding, and perforation of the stomach or intestine. People age 65 and older, as well as those with any history of ulcers or gastrointestinal bleeding, should use NSAIDs with caution.

- Analgesics, such as acetaminophen, to relieve pain.

- Corticosteroid injections into the outermost of the membranes covering the spinal cord and nerve roots to reduce inflammation and treat acute pain that radiates to the hips or down a leg.

- Anesthetic injections, known as nerve blocks, near the affected nerve to temporarily relieve pain.

- Restricted activity (varies depending on extent of nerve involvement).

- Prescribed exercises and/or physical therapy to maintain motion of the spine, strengthen abdominal and back muscles, and build endurance, all of which help stabilize the spine. Some patients may be encouraged to try slowly progressive aerobic activity such as swimming or using exercise bicycles.

- A lumbar brace or corset to provide some support and help the patient regain mobility. This approach is sometimes used for patients with weak abdominal muscles or older patients with degeneration at several levels of the spine.

What are some alternative therapies for spinal stenosis?

Alternative (or complementary) therapies are diverse medical and health care systems, practices, and products that are not presently considered to be part of conventional medicine. Some examples of these therapies used to treat spinal stenosis follow:

- **Chiropractic treatment:** This treatment is based on the philosophy that restricted movement in the spine reduces proper function and may cause pain. Chiropractors may manipulate (adjust) the spine to restore normal spinal movement. They may also employ traction, a pulling force, to help increase space between the vertebrae and reduce pressure on affected nerves. Some people report that they benefit from chiropractic care. Research thus far has shown that chiropractic treatment is about as effective as conventional, nonoperative treatments for acute back pain.

- **Acupuncture:** This treatment involves stimulating certain places on the skin by a variety of techniques, in most cases by manipulating thin, solid, metallic needles that penetrate the skin. Research has shown that low back pain is one area in which acupuncture has benefited some people.

More research is needed before the effectiveness of these or other possible alternative therapies can be definitively stated. Health care providers may suggest these therapies in addition to more conventional treatments.

When should surgery be considered and what is involved?

In many cases, the conditions causing spinal stenosis cannot be permanently altered by nonsurgical treatment, even though these measures may relieve pain for a period of time. To determine how much nonsurgical treatment will help, a doctor may recommend such treatment first. However, surgery might be considered immediately if a patient has numbness or weakness that interferes with walking, impaired bowel or bladder function, or other neurological involvement. The effectiveness of nonsurgical treatments, the extent of the patient's pain, and the patient's preferences may all factor into whether or not to have surgery.

The purpose of surgery is to relieve pressure on the spinal cord or nerves and restore and maintain alignment and strength of the spine. This can be done by removing, trimming, or adjusting diseased parts that are causing the pressure or loss of alignment. The most common surgery is called decompressive laminectomy: removal of the lamina (roof) of one or more vertebrae to create more space for the nerves. A surgeon may perform a laminectomy with or without fusing vertebrae or removing part of a disk. Various devices may be used to enhance fusion and strengthen unstable segments of the spine following decompression surgery.

Patients with spinal stenosis caused by spinal trauma or achondroplasia may need surgery at a young age. When surgery is required in patients with achondroplasia, laminectomy (removal of the roof) without fusion is usually sufficient.

What are the major risks of surgery?

All surgery, particularly that involving general anesthesia and older patients, carries risks. The most common complications of surgery for spinal stenosis are a tear in the membrane covering the spinal cord at the site of the operation, infection, or a blood clot that forms in the veins. These conditions can be treated but may prolong recovery. The presence of other diseases and the physical condition of the patient are also significant factors to consider when making decisions about surgery.

What are the long-term outcomes of surgical treatment for spinal stenosis?

Removal of the obstruction that has caused the symptoms usually gives patients some relief; most patients have less leg pain and are able to walk better following surgery. However, if nerves were badly damaged before surgery, there may be some remaining pain or numbness or no improvement. Also, the degenerative process will likely continue, and pain or limitation of activity may reappear after surgery.

Researchers supported by the National Institute of Arthritis and Musculoskeletal and Skin Diseases (NIAMS) have published results from the Spine Patient Outcomes Research Trial (SPORT), the largest trial to date comparing surgical and non-surgical interventions for the treatment of low back and associated leg pain caused by spinal stenosis. The study found that for patients with spinal stenosis, surgical treatment was more effective than non-surgical treatment in relieving symptoms and improving function. However, the functional status of patients who received non-surgical therapies also improved somewhat during the study.

Chapter 12

Bone Pain

Chapter Contents

Section 12.1—Bone Cancer.. 132

Section 12.2—Paget's Disease of Bone................................... 134

Section 12.3—Osteonecrosis... 136

Section 12.1

Bone Cancer

Excerpted from "Bone Cancer," National Cancer Institute (www.cancer.gov),
March 13, 2008. Reviewed by David A. Cooke, MD, FACP, March 2013.

What is bone cancer?

Bone cancer is a malignant (cancerous) tumor of the bone that destroys normal bone tissue. Not all bone tumors are malignant. In fact, benign (noncancerous) bone tumors are more common than malignant ones. Both malignant and benign bone tumors may grow and compress healthy bone tissue, but benign tumors do not spread, do not destroy bone tissue, and are rarely a threat to life.

Malignant tumors that begin in bone tissue are called primary bone cancer. Cancer that metastasizes (spreads) to the bones from other parts of the body, such as the breast, lung, or prostate, is called metastatic cancer, and is named for the organ or tissue in which it began. Primary bone cancer is far less common than cancer that spreads to the bones.

There are different types of primary bone cancer. Cancer can begin in any type of bone tissue. Bones are made up of osteoid (hard or compact), cartilaginous (tough, flexible), and fibrous (threadlike) tissue, as well as elements of bone marrow (soft, spongy tissue in the center of most bones). Common types of primary bone cancer include the following:

- Osteosarcoma, which arises from osteoid tissue in the bone. This tumor occurs most often in the knee and upper arm.

- Chondrosarcoma, which begins in cartilaginous tissue. Cartilage pads the ends of bones and lines the joints. Chondrosarcoma occurs most often in the pelvis (located between the hip bones), upper leg, and shoulder. Sometimes a chondrosarcoma contains cancerous bone cells. In that case, doctors classify the tumor as an osteosarcoma.

- The Ewing sarcoma family of tumors (ESFTs), which usually occur in bone but may also arise in soft tissue (muscle, fat, fibrous tissue, blood vessels, or other supporting tissue). Scientists think that ESFTs arise from elements of primitive nerve tissue in the bone or soft tissue. ESFTs occur most commonly along the backbone and pelvis and in the legs and arms.

Other types of cancer that arise in soft tissue are called soft tissue sarcomas. They are not bone cancer.

What are the symptoms of bone cancer?

Pain is the most common symptom of bone cancer, but not all bone cancers cause pain. Persistent or unusual pain or swelling in or near a bone can be caused by cancer or by other conditions. It is important to see a doctor to determine the cause.

What are the treatment options for bone cancer?

Treatment options depend on the type, size, location, and stage of the cancer, as well as the person's age and general health. Treatment options for bone cancer include surgery, chemotherapy, radiation therapy, and cryosurgery.

Surgery is the usual treatment for bone cancer. The surgeon removes the entire tumor with negative margins (no cancer cells are found at the edge or border of the tissue removed during surgery). The surgeon may also use special surgical techniques to minimize the amount of healthy tissue removed with the tumor.

Dramatic improvements in surgical techniques and preoperative tumor treatment have made it possible for most patients with bone cancer in an arm or leg to avoid radical surgical procedures (removal of the entire limb). However, most patients who undergo limb-sparing surgery need reconstructive surgery to maximize limb function.

Chemotherapy is the use of anticancer drugs to kill cancer cells. Patients who have bone cancer usually receive a combination of anticancer drugs. However, chemotherapy is not currently used to treat chondrosarcoma.

Radiation therapy, also called radiotherapy, involves the use of high-energy x-rays to kill cancer cells. This treatment may be used in combination with surgery. It is often used to treat chondrosarcoma, which cannot be treated with chemotherapy, as well as ESFTs. It may also be used for patients who refuse surgery.

Cryosurgery is the use of liquid nitrogen to freeze and kill cancer cells. This technique can sometimes be used instead of conventional surgery to destroy the tumor.

What does follow-up treatment involve?

Bone cancer sometimes metastasizes, particularly to the lungs, or can recur (come back), either at the same location or in other bones in the body. People who have had bone cancer should see their doctor regularly and should report any unusual symptoms right away. Follow-up varies for different types and stages of bone cancer. Generally, patients are checked frequently by their doctor and have regular blood tests and x-rays. People who have had bone cancer, particularly children and adolescents, have an increased likelihood of developing another type of cancer, such as leukemia, later in life. Regular follow-up care ensures that changes in health are discussed and that problems are treated as soon as possible.

Section 12.2

Paget's Disease of Bone

Excerpted from "Pain and Paget's Disease of Bone," National Institute of Arthritis and Musculoskeletal and Skin Diseases (www.niams.nih.gov), January 2012.

Types of Pain Associated with Paget's Disease

Paget's disease can cause several different kinds of pain, as described below.

- **Bone pain:** Small breaks called microfractures can occur in pagetic bone. These breaks can cause pain, especially in weight-bearing bone such as the spine, pelvis, or leg.

- **Joint pain:** Cartilage (a hard but slippery tissue that cushions the joints) can be damaged when Paget's disease reaches the end of a long bone or changes the shape of bones located near joints. This can result in osteoarthritis and joint pain.

- **Muscle pain:** When bone is changed by Paget's disease, the muscles that support the bone may have to work harder and at different angles, causing muscle pain.

- **Nervous system pain:** Bones enlarged by Paget's disease can put pressure on the brain, spinal cord, or nerves. This can cause headache; pain in the neck, back, and legs; and sciatica, a "shooting" pain that travels down the sciatic nerve from the lower back to the leg.

Available Treatments

It is important for most people with Paget's disease to receive medical treatment as soon as possible. Today's treatments can help reduce pain and possibly prevent the development of further complications.

Several types of medicines are used to address the pain caused by Paget's disease. A doctor may recommend drugs designed to control the Paget's disease or to relieve pain. The doctor also may recommend drugs to address painful complications of Paget's disease, such as arthritis.

When severe pain cannot be controlled with medicine, surgery on the affected bone or joint may be needed.

An appropriate program of regular exercise also can help people with Paget's disease reduce or eliminate pain.

Medicines used to treat Paget's disease help slow the rate at which affected bone is changed, thereby reducing pain. The U.S. Food and Drug Administration (FDA) has approved several bisphosphonates and calcitonin for the treatment of Paget's disease.

Several over-the-counter (nonprescription) drugs can be used to reduce the pain associated with Paget's disease. Each of these medicines is taken orally (by mouth), usually in tablet form. Although there are many brand names for these drugs, they can be purchased on the basis of their key ingredient, which is ibuprofen, naproxen, aspirin, or acetaminophen. In some cases physicians will recommend the use of pain-relieving medicine that requires a prescription.

Surgery to Manage Pain

Although surgery is rarely required for Paget's disease, it should be considered in certain circumstances. Hip or knee replacement surgery may help people with severe pain from Paget's disease-related arthritis. Surgery can also realign affected leg bones to reduce the stress and pain at knee and ankle joints or help broken bones heal in a better position.

The Value of Exercise

Physical exercise is an important tool for persons with Paget's disease. Regular exercise can help patients maintain bone strength, avoid weight gain (and the pressure added weight puts on weakened bone), and keep weight-bearing joints mobile and free of pain. To make sure that pagetic bone is not harmed, patients should discuss their plans with a doctor before beginning any exercise program.

There Is No Need to Be in Pain

Although there is no cure for Paget's disease, people with the disorder do not have to live with constant pain. Available therapies—especially when started early—can greatly reduce or, in some cases, eliminate the pain associated with the disease.

Section 12.3

Osteonecrosis

Excerpted from "Questions and Answers about Osteonecrosis (Avascular Necrosis)," National Institute of Arthritis and Musculoskeletal and Skin Diseases (www.niams.nih.gov), NIH Publication No. 09-4857, updated October 2012.

What is osteonecrosis?

Osteonecrosis is a disease resulting from the temporary or permanent loss of blood supply to the bones. Without blood, the bone tissue dies, and ultimately the bone may collapse. If the process involves the bones near a joint, it often leads to collapse of the joint surface. Osteonecrosis is also known as avascular necrosis, aseptic necrosis, and ischemic necrosis.

Although it can happen in any bone, osteonecrosis most commonly affects the ends (epiphysis) of the femur, the bone extending from the knee joint to the hip joint. Other common sites include the upper arm bone, knees, shoulders, and ankles. The disease may affect just one bone, more than one bone at the same time, or more than one bone at different times. Osteonecrosis of the jaw (ONJ) is a rare condition that has been linked to the use of bisphosphonate medications. ONJ has different causes and treatments than osteonecrosis found in other parts of the skeleton.

The amount of disability that results from osteonecrosis depends on what part of the bone is affected, how large an area is involved, and how effectively the bone rebuilds itself. Normally, bone continuously breaks down and rebuilds—old bone is replaced with new bone. This process, which takes place after an injury as well as during normal growth, keeps the skeleton strong and helps it to maintain a balance of minerals. In the course of osteonecrosis, however, the healing process is usually ineffective and the bone tissues break down faster than the body can repair them. If left untreated, the disease progresses, the bone collapses, and the joint surface breaks down, leading to pain and arthritis.

What are the symptoms of osteonecrosis?

In the early stages of osteonecrosis, people may not have any symptoms. As the disease progresses, however, most experience joint pain. At first, the pain occurs only when putting weight on the affected joint. Later, it occurs even when resting. Pain usually develops gradually, and may be mild or severe. If osteonecrosis progresses and the bone and surrounding joint surface collapse, pain may develop or increase dramatically. Pain may be severe enough to limit range of motion in the affected joint. In some cases, particularly those involving the hip, disabling osteoarthritis may develop. The period between the first symptoms and loss of joint function is different for each person, but it typically ranges from several months to more than a year.

What treatments are available?

Appropriate treatment for osteonecrosis is necessary to keep joints from breaking down. Without treatment, most people with the disease will experience severe pain and limitation in movement. To determine the most appropriate treatment, the doctor considers the age of the patient, the stage of the disease (early or late), the location and whether bone is affected over a small or large area, and the underlying cause of osteonecrosis. With an ongoing cause such as corticosteroid or alcohol use, treatment may not work unless use of the substance is stopped.

The goal in treating osteonecrosis is to improve the patient's use of the affected joint, stop further damage to the bone, and ensure bone and joint survival. To reach these goals, the doctor may use one or more of the following surgical or nonsurgical treatments.

Nonsurgical treatments: Usually, doctors will begin with nonsurgical treatments, alone or in combination. Unfortunately, although these treatments may relieve pain or help in the short term, for most people they don't bring lasting improvement.

Nonsteroidal anti-inflammatory drugs (NSAIDs) are often prescribed to reduce pain. NSAIDs can cause stomach irritation or, less often, they can affect kidney function. The longer a person uses NSAIDs, the more likely he or she is to have side effects, ranging from mild to serious. Many other drugs cannot be taken when a patient is being treated with NSAIDs because NSAIDs alter the way the body uses or eliminates these other drugs. Check with your health care provider or pharmacist before you take NSAIDs. Also, NSAIDs sometimes are associated with serious gastrointestinal problems, including ulcers, bleeding, and perforation of the stomach or intestine. People age 65 and older, as well as those with any history of ulcers or gastrointestinal bleeding, should use NSAIDs with caution.

People with clotting disorders may be given blood thinners to reduce clots that block the blood supply to the bone. Cholesterol-lowering medications may be used to reduce fatty substances (lipids) that increase with corticosteroid treatment (a major risk factor for osteonecrosis).

If osteonecrosis is diagnosed early, the doctor may begin treatment by having the patient remove weight from the affected joint. The doctor may recommend limiting activities or using crutches. In some cases, reduced weight bearing can slow the damage caused by osteonecrosis and permit natural healing. When combined with pain medication, reduced weight bearing can be an effective way to avoid or delay surgery for some patients.

An exercise program involving the affected joints may help keep them mobile and increase their range of motion.

Electrical stimulation treatment has been used in several centers to induce bone growth, and in some studies has been helpful when used before femoral head collapse.

Surgical treatments: A number of different surgical procedures are used to treat osteonecrosis. Most people with osteonecrosis will eventually need surgery.

Core decompression removes the inner cylinder of bone, which reduces pressure within the bone, increases blood flow to the bone, and allows more blood vessels to form. Core decompression works best in people who are in the earliest stages of osteonecrosis, often before the collapse of the joint. This procedure sometimes reduces pain and slows the progression of bone and joint destruction.

Osteotomy involves reshaping the bone to reduce stress on the affected area. Recovery can be a lengthy process, requiring several months of very limited activities. This procedure is most effective for patients with early-stage osteonecrosis and those with a small area of affected bone.

Bone grafting is the transplantation of healthy bone from another part of the body. It is often used to support a joint after core decompression. In many cases, the surgeon will use what is called a vascular graft, which includes an artery and vein, to increase the blood supply to the affected area. Recovery from a bone graft can take several months.

Arthroplasty, or total joint replacement, is the treatment of choice in late-stage osteonecrosis and when the joint is destroyed. In this surgery, the diseased joint is replaced with artificial parts. Total joint replacement, or sometimes femoral head resurfacing, is often recommended for people for whom other efforts to preserve the joint have failed. Various types of replacements are available, and people should discuss specific needs with their doctor.

Chapter 13

Fibromyalgia

What is fibromyalgia?

Fibromyalgia is a disorder that causes aches and pain all over the body. People with fibromyalgia also have "tender points" throughout their bodies. Tender points are specific places on the neck, shoulders, back, hips, arms, and legs that hurt when pressure is put on them.

What are the symptoms of fibromyalgia?

In addition to pain, people with fibromyalgia could also have these symptoms:

- Cognitive and memory problems (sometimes called "fibro fog")
- Trouble sleeping
- Morning stiffness
- Headaches
- Irritable bowel syndrome
- Painful menstrual periods
- Numbness or tingling of hands and feet
- Restless legs syndrome

Excerpted from "Fibromyalgia Fact Sheet," Office on Women's Health (http://womenshealth.gov), U.S. Department of Health and Human Services, June 2010.

- Temperature sensitivity
- Sensitivity to loud noises or bright lights

How common is fibromyalgia? Who is mainly affected?

Fibromyalgia affects as many as five million Americans ages 18 and older. Most people with fibromyalgia are women (about 80–90 percent). However, men and children also can have the disorder. Most people are diagnosed during middle age.

Fibromyalgia can occur by itself, but people with certain other diseases, such as rheumatoid arthritis, lupus, and other types of arthritis, may be more likely to have it. Individuals who have a close relative with fibromyalgia are more likely to develop it themselves.

What causes fibromyalgia?

The causes of fibromyalgia are not known. Researchers think a number of factors might be involved. Fibromyalgia can occur on its own, but has also been linked to having a family history of fibromyalgia or being exposed to stressful or traumatic events, such as car accidents, injuries to the body caused by performing the same action over and over again (called *repetitive injuries*), infections or illnesses, or being sent to war.

How is fibromyalgia diagnosed?

People with fibromyalgia often see many doctors before being diagnosed. One reason for this may be that pain and fatigue, the main symptoms of fibromyalgia, also are symptoms of many other conditions. Therefore, doctors often must rule out other possible causes of these symptoms before diagnosing fibromyalgia. Fibromyalgia cannot be found by a lab test.

A doctor who knows about fibromyalgia, however, can make a diagnosis based upon two criteria:

- A history of widespread pain lasting more than three months. Pain must be present in both the right and left sides of the body as well as above and below the waist.

- Presence of tender points. The body has 18 sites that are possible tender points. For fibromyalgia diagnosis a person must have 11 or more tender points. For a point to be *tender*, the patient must feel pain when pressure is put on the site. People who have fibromyalgia may feel pain at other sites, too, but those 18 sites on the body are used for diagnosis.

Your doctor may try to rule out other causes of your pain and fatigue. Testing for some of these things may make sense to you. For instance, you may find it reasonable that your doctor wants to rule out rheumatoid arthritis, since that disease also causes pain. Testing for other conditions—such as lupus, multiple sclerosis, or sleep apnea—may make less sense to you. But fibromyalgia can mimic or even overlap many other conditions. Talk with your doctor. He or she can help you understand what each test is for and how each test is part of making a final diagnosis.

How is fibromyalgia treated?

Fibromyalgia can be hard to treat. It's important to find a doctor who has treated others with fibromyalgia. Many family doctors, general internists, or rheumatologists can treat fibromyalgia. Rheumatologists are doctors who treat arthritis and other conditions that affect the joints and soft tissues.

Treatment often requires a team approach. The team may include your doctor, a physical therapist, and possibly other health care providers. A pain or rheumatology clinic can be a good place to get treatment. Treatment for fibromyalgia may include the following components:

Pain management: Three medicines have been approved by the U.S. Food and Drug Administration (FDA) to treat fibromyalgia. These are pregabalin (Lyrica), duloxetine (Cymbalta), and milnacipran (Savella). Other medications are being developed and may also receive FDA approval in the future. Your doctor may also suggest nonnarcotic pain relievers, low-dose antidepressants, or other classes of medications that might help improve certain symptoms.

Sleep management: Getting the right amount of sleep at night may help improve your symptoms. Here are tips for good sleep:

- Keep regular sleep habits. Try to get to bed at the same time and get up at the same time every day—even on weekends and vacations.

- Avoid caffeine and alcohol in the late afternoon and evening.

- Time your exercise. Regular daytime exercise can improve nighttime sleep. But avoid exercising within three hours of bedtime, which can be stimulating, keeping you awake.

- Avoid daytime naps. Sleeping in the afternoon can interfere with nighttime sleep. If you feel you cannot get by without a nap, set an alarm for one hour. When it goes off, get up and start moving.

- Reserve your bed for sleeping. Watching the late news, reading a suspense novel, or working on your laptop in bed can stimulate you, making it hard to sleep.
- Keep your bedroom dark, quiet, and cool.
- Avoid liquids and spicy meals before bed. Heartburn and late-night trips to the bathroom do not lead to good sleep.
- Wind down before bed. Avoid working right up to bedtime. Do relaxing activities, such as listening to soft music or taking a warm bath, that get you ready to sleep. (A warm bath also may soothe aching muscles.)

Psychological support: Living with a chronic condition can be hard on you. If you have fibromyalgia, find a support group. Counseling sessions with a trained counselor may improve your understanding of your illness.

Other treatments: Complementary therapies may help you. Talk to your physician before trying any alternative treatments. Here are some examples of complementary therapies:

- Physical therapy
- Massage
- Myofascial release therapy
- Water therapy
- Light aerobics
- Acupressure
- Applying heat or cold
- Acupuncture
- Yoga
- Relaxation exercises
- Breathing techniques
- Aromatherapy
- Cognitive therapy
- Biofeedback
- Herbs
- Nutritional supplements
- Osteopathic or chiropractic manipulation

What can I do to try to feel better?

Besides taking medicine prescribed by your doctor, there are many things you can do to lessen the impact of fibromyalgia on your life:

Getting enough sleep: Getting enough sleep and the right kind of sleep can help ease the pain and fatigue of fibromyalgia. Most adults need seven to eight hours of restorative sleep per night. Restorative sleep leaves you feeling well-rested and ready for your day to start when you wake up. It is hard for people with fibromyalgia to get a good night's sleep. It is important to discuss any sleep problems with your doctor, who can recommend treatment for them.

Exercising: Although pain and fatigue may make exercise and daily activities difficult, it is crucial to be as physically active as possible. Research has repeatedly shown that regular exercise is one of the most effective treatments for fibromyalgia. People who have too much pain or fatigue to do hard exercise should just begin to move more and become more active in routine daily activities. Then they can begin with walking (or other gentle exercise) and build their endurance and intensity slowly.

Making changes at work: Most people with fibromyalgia continue to work, but they may have to make big changes to do so. For example, some people cut down the number of hours they work, switch to a less demanding job, or adapt a current job. If you face obstacles at work, such as an uncomfortable desk chair that leaves your back aching or difficulty lifting heavy boxes or files, your employer may make changes that will enable you to keep your job. An occupational therapist can help you design a more comfortable workstation or find more efficient and less painful ways to lift. A number of federal laws protect the rights of people with disabilities.

Eating well: Although some people with fibromyalgia report feeling better when they eat or avoid certain foods, no specific diet has been proven to influence fibromyalgia. Of course, it is important to have a healthy, balanced diet. Not only will proper nutrition give you more energy and make you generally feel better, it will also help you avoid other health problems.

Will fibromyalgia get better with time?

Fibromyalgia is a chronic condition, meaning it lasts a long time—possibly a lifetime. However, it may be comforting to know that fibromyalgia is not a progressive disease. It is never fatal, and it will not cause damage to the joints, muscles, or internal organs. In many people, the condition does improve over time.

What is the difference between fibromyalgia and chronic fatigue syndrome?

Chronic fatigue syndrome (CFS) and fibromyalgia are alike in many ways. In fact, it is not uncommon for a person to have both fibromyalgia and CFS. Some experts believe that fibromyalgia and CFS are in fact the same disorder, but expressed in slightly different ways. Both CFS and fibromyalgia have pain and fatigue as symptoms.

The main symptom of CFS is extreme tiredness. CFS often begins after having flu-like symptoms. But people with CFS do not have the tender points that people with fibromyalgia have.

What if I can't work because of fibromyalgia?

Many experts in fibromyalgia do not suggest patients go on disability. These experts have found that if patients stop working, they stop moving as much during the day, lose contact with co-workers, and lose a "sense of purpose" in life.

All of these things can make a patient feel more alone and depressed. These three things tend to make fibromyalgia symptoms worse. Deciding to go on disability is a hard choice that you should talk about with your doctor or nurse.

However, if you cannot work because of your fibromyalgia, contact the Social Security Administration for help with disability benefits. You may qualify for disability benefits through your employer or the federal government. Social Security Disability Insurance (SSDI) and Supplemental Security Insurance (SSI) are the largest federal programs providing financial assistance to people with disabilities. Although the medical requirements for eligibility are the same under the two programs, the way they are funded is different. SSDI is paid by Social Security taxes, and those who qualify for assistance receive benefits based on how much they have paid into the system. SSI is funded by general tax revenues, and those who qualify receive payments based on financial need. For information about the SSDI and SSI programs, contact the Social Security Administration at 800-772-1213 (or visit online at http://www.ssa.gov).

Chapter 14

Foot Pain

Foot pain is very common. About 75% of people in the United States have foot pain at some time in their lives. Most foot pain is caused by shoes that do not fit properly or that force the feet into unnatural shapes (such as pointed-toe, high-heeled shoes).

The foot is a complex structure of 26 bones and 33 joints, layered with an intertwining web of more than 120 muscles, ligaments, and nerves. It serves the following functions:

- Supports weight

- Acts as a shock absorber

- Serves as a lever to propel the leg forward

- Helps maintain balance by adjusting the body to uneven surfaces

Because the feet are very small compared with the rest of the body, the impact of each step exerts tremendous force upon them. This force is about 50% greater than the person's body weight. During a typical day, people spend about four hours on their feet and take 8,000–10,000 steps. This means that the feet support a combined force equivalent to several hundred tons every day.

Foot Problems and Their Locations

Foot pain generally starts in one of three places: the toes, the fore-foot, or the hindfoot.

Excerpted from "Foot Pain," © 2013 A.D.A.M., Inc.; reprinted with permission.

Toes: Toe problems most often occur because of the pressure imposed by ill-fitting shoes.

Forefoot: The forefoot is the front of the foot. Pain originating here usually involves one of the following bone groups:

- The metatarsal bones (five long bones that extend from the front of the arch to the bones in the toe)

- The sesamoid bones (two small bones embedded at the top of the first metatarsal bone, which connects to the big toe)

Hindfoot: The hindfoot is the back of the foot. Pain originating here can extend from the heel, across the sole (known as the plantar surface), to the ball of the foot (the metatarsophalangeal joint).

Corns and Calluses

A corn is a protective layer of dead skin cells that forms due to repeated friction. It is cone-shaped and has a knobby core that points inward. This core can put pressure on a nerve and cause sharp pain. Corns can develop on the top of, or between, toes. If a corn develops between the toes, it may be kept pliable by the moisture from perspiration and is therefore called a soft corn.

Corns develop as a result of friction from the toes rubbing together or against the shoe. They often occur from the following:

- Shoes, socks, or stockings that fit too tightly around the toes

- Pressure on the toes from high-heeled shoes

- Shoes that are too loose, due to the friction of the foot sliding within the shoe

- Deformed and crooked toes

Calluses are composed of the same material as corns. Calluses, however, develop on the ball or heel of the foot. The skin on the sole of the foot is ordinarily about 40 times thicker than the skin anywhere else on the body, but a callus can even be twice as thick. A protective callus layer naturally develops to guard against excessive pressure and chafing as people get older and the padding of fat on the bottom of the foot thins out. If calluses get too big or too hard, they may pull and tear the underlying skin.

Risk factors for calluses include the following:

- Poorly fitting shoes

- Walking regularly on hard surfaces

- Flat feet

Of note, in people with diabetes, the presence of calluses is a strong predictor of ulceration, particularly in those who have a history of foot ulcers.

Preventing Corns and Calluses and Relieving Discomfort

- Do not wear shoes that are too tight or too loose. Wear well-padded shoes with open toes or a deep toe box (the part of the shoe that surrounds the toes). If necessary, have a cobbler stretch the shoes in the area where the corn or callus is located.

- Wear thick socks to absorb pressure, but do not wear tight socks or stockings.

- Apply petroleum jelly or lanolin hand cream to corns or calluses to soften them.

- Use doughnut-shaped pads that fit over a corn and decrease pressure and friction. They are available at most drug stores.

- Place cotton, lamb's wool, or mole skin between the toes to cushion any corns in these areas.

Removing Corns and Calluses

To remove a corn or callus, soak it in very warm water for five minutes or more to soften the hardened tissue, then gently sand it with a pumice stone. Several treatments may be necessary. Do not trim corns or calluses with a razor blade or other sharp tool. Unsterile cutting tools can cause infection, and it is easy to slip and cut too deep, causing excessive bleeding or injury to the toe or foot.

Medicated Solutions and Pads

There are numerous over-the-counter pads, plasters, and medications for removing corns and calluses. These treatments commonly contain salicylic acid, which may cause irritation, burns, or infections that are more serious than the corn or callus. Use caution with these medications. The following people should not use them:

- Patients with diabetes

- Patients with reduced feeling in the feet due to circulation problems or neurological damage

- Patients who do not have the flexibility or eyesight to use them properly

Bunions

A bunion is a deformity that usually occurs at the end of one of the five long bones (the metatarsal bones) that extend from the arch of the foot and connect to the toes. Most often bunions develop in the first metatarsal bone (the one that attaches to the big toe). A bunion may also develop in the bone that joins the little toe to the foot (the fifth metatarsal bone), in which case it is known as either a bunionette or a tailor's bunion.

A bunion typically develops in the following way:

- The big toe or the fifth ("pinky") toe is forced in toward the other toes, causing the head of the metatarsal bone to jut out and rub against the side of the shoe.

- The underlying tissue becomes inflamed, and a painful bump forms.

- As this bony growth develops, a bunion is formed as the big toe is forced to grow at an increasing angle toward the rest of the toes. One important bunion deformity, hallux valgus, causes the bone and joint of the big toe to shift and grow inward, so that the second toe crosses over it.

People born with abnormal bones in their feet are more likely to form a bunion. In addition, wearing narrow-toed, high-heeled shoes, which put enormous pressure on the front of the foot, may also lead to a bunion formation. The condition may become painful as extra bone and a fluid-filled sac grow at the base of the big toe.

Flat feet, gout, arthritis, and occupations (such as ballet) that place undue stress on the feet can also increase the risk for bunions.

Shoes and Protective Pads

Pressure and pain from bunions and bunionettes can be relieved by wearing appropriate shoes, such as the following:

- Soft, wide, low-heeled leather shoes that lace up

- Athletic shoes with soft toe boxes

- Open shoes or sandals with straps that don't touch the irritated area

A thick doughnut-shaped, moleskin pad can protect the protrusion. In some cases, an orthotic can help redistribute weight and take pressure off the bunion. Nonsteroidal anti-inflammatory drugs (NSAIDs) or corticosteroid injections may offer some pain relief.

Surgery

If discomfort persists, surgery may be necessary, particularly for more serious conditions, such as hallux valgus. There are more than 100 surgical variations, ranging from removing the bump to realigning the toes.

The most common surgery, an office procedure known as bunionectomy, involves shaving down the bone of the big toe joint. In one procedure the surgeon uses a very small incision, through which the bone-shaving drill is inserted. The physician shaves off the bone, guided by feel or x-ray. This technique is not a cure, but patient satisfaction is high and results are long-lasting.

More extensive surgeries may be required to realign the toe joint. Although there are variations of each, they generally involve one or more of the following:

- **Osteotomy** (cutting and realigning the joint): Long-term studies on osteotomies report that 90% of patients are satisfied with the procedure.

- **Exostosectomy** (removal of the large bony growth): This technique is only useful when there is no shift in the toe bone itself.

- **Arthrodesis** (removal of damaged portion of the joint, followed by implantation of screws, wires, or plates to hold the bones together until they heal): This is the gold standard procedure for very severe cases or when previous procedures have failed. Most patients report good results.

- **Arthroplasty** (removal of damaged portion of the joint with the goal of achieving a flexible scar): This technique offers symptom relief and faster rehabilitation than arthrodesis, but it can cause deformity and some foot weakness. Arthroplasty tends to be used in older patients. Biological or synthetic implants for supporting the toes are showing promise as part of this procedure.

- **Tendon and ligament repair:** If tendons and ligaments have become too loose, the surgeon may tighten them.

In severe cases, surgeons are testing bone grafts to restore bone length in patients who have had previous bunion surgeries or damage from osteoarthritis.

Complications, though uncommon in even the most complex procedures, can include:

- Continued pain

- Infection

- Possible numbness

- Irritation from implants used to support the bone

- An excessively shortened metatarsal bone

Recovery from more invasive procedures, such as arthrodesis or osteotomy, may take six to eight weeks, and it can be that long before a patient can put full weight on the foot. In such cases, the patient will need to wear a cast or use crutches. Elderly patients may need wheelchairs.

Hammertoes

A hammertoe is a permanent deformity of the toe joint, in which the toe bends up slightly and then curls downward, resting on its tip. When forced into this position long enough, the tendons of the toe shrink, and the toe stiffens into a hammer- or claw-like shape.

Hammertoe is most common in the second toe, but it can develop in any or all of the three middle toes if they are pushed forward and do not have enough room to lie flat in the shoe. The risk is increased when the toes are already crowded by the pressure of a bunion. Conditions that increase the risk of hammertoe include:

- Diabetes

- Diseases that affect the nerves and muscles

Treatment for Hammertoe

At first, a hammertoe is flexible, and any pain it causes can usually be relieved by putting a toe pad, sold in drug stores, into the shoe. To help prevent and ease existing discomfort from hammertoes, shoes should have a deep, wide toe area. As the tendon becomes tighter and the toe stiffens, other treatments, including exercises, splints, and custom-made shoe inserts (orthotics) may help redistribute weight and ease the position of the toe.

Patients with severe cases of hammertoe may need surgery. If the toe is still flexible, only a simple procedure that releases the tendon may be involved. Such procedures sometimes require only a single stitch and a Band-Aid. If the toe has become rigid, surgery on the bone is necessary, but it can still be performed in the doctor's office. A procedure called PIP [proximal interphalangeal] arthroplasty involves releasing the ligaments at the joint and removing a small piece of toe bone, which restores the toe to its normal position. The toe is held in this position with a pin for about three weeks, and then the pin is removed. The procedure seems to have a high, lasting success rate.

Ingrown Toenails

Ingrown toenails can occur on any toe but are most common on the big toes. They usually develop when tight-fitting or narrow shoes put too much pressure on the toenail and force the nail to grow into the flesh of the toe. Incorrect toenail trimming can also contribute to the risk of developing an ingrown toenail. Other causes are:

- Injuries

- Abnormalities in the structure of the foot

- Repeated impact on the toenail from high-impact aerobic exercise

Caring for Toenails

Trim toenails straight across and keep them long enough so that the nail corner is not visible. If the nail is cut too short, it may grow inward. If the nail does grow inward, do not cut the nail corner at an angle. This only trains the nail to continue growing inward. When filing the nails, file straight across the nail in a single movement, lifting the file before the next stroke. Do not saw back and forth. A cuticle stick can be used to clean under the nail.

Treatments

To relieve pain from ingrown toenails, try wearing sandals or open-toed shoes. Soaking the toe for five minutes twice a day in a warm water solution of salt, Domeboro or Betadine can help. People who are at increased risk for infections, such as those with diabetes, should have professional treatment.

Antibiotic ointments may help treat ingrown toenails that are infected. Apply the ointment by working a wisp of cotton under the nail, especially the corners, to lift the nail up and drain the infection. The cotton will also help force the toenail to grow out correctly. Change the cotton daily, and use the antibiotic consistently.

In severe cases, more intensive treatments are needed. Surgery involves simply cutting away the sharp portion of ingrown nail, removing the nail bed, or removing a wedge of the affected tissue. Orthonyxia, a newer surgical technique that implants a small metal brace into the top of the nail, may be as effective as traditional surgical techniques for preventing ingrown toenails from recurring.

Nonsurgical methods can also treat ingrown toenails. One technique uses chemicals to remove the skin. Both sodium hydroxide and phenol may be used, but research shows that sodium hydroxide produces a better outcome and faster recovery than phenol. Other nonsurgical methods include using cauterization (heating), or lasers, to remove the skin.

Forefoot Pain

Forefoot pain refers to pain and discomfort felt toward the top of the foot. The rate of forefoot pain and deformity increases with age. When a cause cannot be determined, any pain on the ball of the foot is generally referred to as metatarsalgia.

Morton's Neuroma

A neuroma usually means a benign tumor of a nerve. However, Morton's neuroma, also called interdigital neuroma, is not actually a tumor. It is a thickening of the tissue surrounding the nerves leading to the toes. Morton's neuroma usually develops when the bones in the third and fourth toes pinch together, compressing a nerve. It can also occur in other locations. The nerve becomes enlarged and inflamed. The inflammation causes a burning or tingling sensation and cramping in the front of the foot. Other causes of this condition include:

- Tight, poorly-fitting shoes
- Injury
- Arthritis
- Abnormal bone structure

Treatment for neuromas: Pain from Morton's neuroma can be reduced by massaging the affected area. Roomier shoes (box-toed shoes), pads of various sorts, and cortisone injections in the painful area are also helpful. A combination of cortisone injections and shoe modifications provides better immediate relief than changes in footwear alone. Ultrasound-guided injection of alcohol might also provide relief from Morton's neuroma, research finds.

If these treatments are not effective, the enlarged area may need to be surgically removed. Success rates for this procedure seem to be high and provide long-term relief. Some numbness is common afterward, but it rarely bothers patients. Occasionally, the nerve tissue may re-grow and form another neuroma.

Sesamoiditis

Sesamoiditis is an inflammation of the tendons around the small, round bones that are embedded in the head of the first metatarsal bone, which leads to the big toe. Sesamoid bones bear much stress under ordinary circumstances; excessive stress can strain the surrounding tendons. Often there is no clear-cut cause, but sesamoid injuries are common among people who participate in jarring, high-impact activities, such as ballet, jogging, and aerobic exercise.

Treatment for sesamoiditis: Rest and reducing stress on the ball of the foot are the first lines of treatment for sesamoiditis. A low-heeled shoe with a stiff sole and soft padding inside is all that is usually required. In severe cases, surgery may be necessary.

Stress Fracture

A stress fracture in the foot, also called fatigue or march fracture, usually results from a break or rupture in any of the five metatarsal bones (mostly the second or third). These fractures are caused by overuse during strenuous exercise, particularly jogging and high-impact aerobics. Women are at higher risk for stress fracture than men.

A fracture in the first metatarsal bone, which leads to the big toe, is uncommon because of the thickness of this bone. If it occurs, however, it is more serious than a fracture in any of the other metatarsal bones because it dramatically changes the pattern of normal walking and weight bearing.

Treatment for stress fractures: Patients should seek treatment if pain persists for three weeks. Treatment after that time may reduce the chances of returning to previous level of functioning. Surgery may be needed if conservative measures fail. In most cases, however, stress fractures heal by themselves if you avoid rigorous activities. Some health care providers recommend moderate exercise, particularly swimming and walking. It is best to wear low-heeled shoes with stiff soles. Occasionally, a health care provider may recommend wearing a walking "boot" (brace) to reduce pain and facilitate healing.

Heel Pain

The heel is the largest bone in the foot. Heel pain is the most common foot problem and affects two million Americans every year. It can occur in the front, back, or bottom of the heel. Types of heel pain include:

- Achilles tendinitis

- Bursitis of the heel

- Excess pronation

- Haglund's deformity

- Heel spur syndrome

- Plantar fasciitis

Each type of heal pain is described in more detail below. General treatment guidelines are as follows:

- The American Orthopaedic Foot and Ankle Society (AOFAS) suggests shoe inserts, medications, and stretching as a first line of therapy for heel pain. One study found that 95% of women who used an insert and did simple stretching exercises for the Achilles tendon and plantar fascia experienced improvement after eight weeks.

- If these treatments fail, the patient may need prescription heel orthotics and extended physical therapy. Surgery may be an option if other methods have failed.

Achilles Tendinitis

Achilles tendinitis is an inflammation of the tendon that connects the calf muscles to the heel bone. It is caused by small tears in the tendon from overuse or injury. This condition is most common in people who engage in high-impact exercise, particularly jogging, racquetball, and tennis.

Of the people who engage in these activities, those at highest risk for this disorder are the ones with a shortened Achilles tendon. Such people tend to roll their feet too far inward when walking, and may bounce when they walk. A shortened tendon can be due to an inborn structural abnormality, or it can develop from regularly wearing high heels.

An inflamed or torn Achilles tendon causes intense pain and affects mobility.

Evidence is inconclusive about the best way to treat either acute or chronic Achilles tendinitis. Some approaches include:

Treatments to relieve pain and reduce inflammation: Nonsteroidal anti-inflammatory drugs (NSAIDs), such as aspirin or ibuprofen (Advil), may help ease pain and reduce inflammation. It is also helpful to apply ice for 20–30 minutes, four or five times a day. (Note: Corticosteroid injections are sometimes used, although evidence suggests they don't help very much, and they can pose a risk for rupture of the tendon.)

Gentle stretching: Gentle calf muscle stretches may also help reduce pain and spasms. If the calf is swollen, elevate the leg. Exercise is safe when the heel is no longer swollen or tender, even if pain is still present. If pain increases with exercise, stop immediately.

Surgery vs. nonsurgical treatment: Chronic inflammation may lead to rupture of the Achilles tendon. If pain continues, the ruptured tendon will require a cast and perhaps surgery, called tendon transfer. Although some experts believe a cast without surgery is a sufficient treatment for such rupture, there is a chance the tendon may rupture again in the future, even after it heals. Some experts suggest surgery for active people and nonsurgical treatment for older people.

Surgery requires a long incision with a postoperative period of immobilization that can average six weeks. Complications can include a significant surgical scar, infection, and muscle atrophy, although surgery reduces pain and preserves foot function in the long term.

Bursitis of the Heel

Bursitis of the heel is an inflammation of the bursa, a small sack of fluid beneath the heel bone. Nonsteroidal anti-inflammatory drugs (NSAIDs), such as aspirin or ibuprofen (Advil), and steroid injections will help relieve pain from bursitis. Applying ice and massaging the heel are also beneficial. A heel cup or soft padding in the heel of the shoe reduces direct impact when walking.

Excessive Pronation

Pronation is the normal motion that allows the foot to adapt to uneven walking surfaces and to absorb shock. Excessive pronation occurs when the foot has a tendency to turn inward and stretch and pull the fascia. It can cause not only heel pain, but also hip, knee, and lower back problems.

Haglund's Deformity

Haglund's deformity, known medically as posterior calcaneal exostosis, is a bony growth surrounded by tender tissue on the back of the heel bone. It develops when the back of the shoe repeatedly rubs against the back of the heel, aggravating the tissue and the underlying bone. It is commonly called pump bump because it's often linked to wearing high heels. (It can also develop in runners, however.)

Treatment for Haglund's deformity: Applying ice followed by moist heat will help ease discomfort from a pump bump. Nonsteroidal anti-inflammatory drugs (NSAIDs), such as aspirin or ibuprofen (Advil), will also reduce pain. Your doctor may recommend an orthotic device to control heel motion. Corticosteroid injections are not recommended because they can weaken the Achilles tendon.

In severe cases, surgery may be necessary to remove or reduce the bony growth. Studies show, however, that recovery from surgery is very long, and success rates vary. Experts advise patients to try all conservative measures before choosing surgery.

Plantar Fasciitis and Heel Spur Syndrome

Plantar fasciitis is a common foot problem that accounts for one million office visits per year. Plantar fasciitis occurs from small tears and inflammation in the wide band of tendons and ligaments that stretches from the heel to the ball of the foot. This band, much like the tensed string in a bow, forms the arch of the foot and helps serve as a shock absorber for the body.

The term plantar means the sole of the foot, and fascia refers to any fibrous connective tissue in the body. Most people with plantar fasciitis experience pain in the heel with their first steps in the morning. The pain also often spreads to the arch of the foot. The condition can be temporary, or it may become chronic if ignored. Resting can provide relief, but only temporarily.

Heel spurs are calcium deposits that can develop under the heel bone as a result of the inflammation that occurs with plantar fasciitis. Heel spurs and plantar fasciitis are sometimes blamed interchangeably for pain, but plantar fasciitis can occur without heel spurs, and spurs commonly develop without causing any symptoms at all.

Causes of plantar fasciitis: The cause of plantar fasciitis is often unknown. It is usually associated with overuse during high-impact exercise and sports. Plantar fasciitis accounts for up to 9% of all running injuries. Because the condition often occurs in only one foot, however, factors other than overuse are likely to be responsible in many cases. Other causes of this injury include poorly fitting shoes, lack of calf flexibility, or an uneven stride that causes an abnormal and stressful impact on the foot.

Treatment goals: The three major treatment goals for plantar fasciitis are:

* Reducing inflammation and pain
* Reducing pressure on the heel
* Restoring strength and flexibility

Embarking on an exercise program as soon as possible and using NSAIDs, splints, or heel pads, as needed, can help relieve the problem. Pain that does not subside with NSAIDs may require more intensive treatments, including leg supports and even surgery.

Exercises to restore strength and flexibility: Stretching the plantar fascia is the mainstay therapy for restoring strength and flexibility. One exercise involves the following:

* Put the hands on a wall and lean against them.
* Place the uninjured foot on the floor in front of the injured foot.
* Raise the heel of the injured foot.
* Gently stretch the injured leg and foot.

With stretching treatments, the plantar fascia nearly always heals by itself but it may take as long as a year, with pain occurring intermittently. A moderate amount of low-impact exercise (such as walking, swimming, or cycling) also seems to be beneficial.

Treatment: Inflammation and pain is most commonly treated with ice and over-the-counter nonsteroidal anti-inflammatory drugs (NSAIDs), such as aspirin or ibuprofen. NSAIDs reduce pain and disability in people with plantar fasciitis when used with other techniques, such as night splints and stretching.

Corticosteroids are powerful anti-inflammatory agents. An injection of a steroid plus a local anesthetic (such as Xylocaine) may provide relief in severe cases of plantar fasciitis. (Steroid injections are not used for pain that is only due to heel spurs). For athletes or performers who need immediate relief, an effective method is to administer the steroid dexamethasone using a procedure called iontophoresis, which introduces the drug into the foot's tissue using an electrical current.

Several non-drug approaches can relieve pressure on the heel, including:

- **Sturdy shoes and insoles:** It is important to wear comfortable but sturdy shoes that have thick soles, rubber heels, and a sole insole to relieve pressure. (An insole with an arch support might also be helpful.) Cutting a round hole about the size of a quarter in the sole cushion under the painful area may help support the rest of the heel while relieving pressure on the painful spot. Heel cups are not very useful. When combined with exercises that stretch the arch and heel cord, over-the-counter insoles may offer the same relief as prescribed orthotics.

- **Night splints:** Some evidence suggests that splints worn at night may be helpful for some people. One device, for example, uses an Ace bandage and an L-shaped fiberglass splint to keep the foot stretched while the patient is sleeping. This allows the muscle to heal. Although patient compliance may be better with custom-made prescribed orthotics than with tension night splints, it is believed that they are equally effective in improving pain. In addition, evidence suggests that nearly any splint, regardless of cost, is equally effective in about three-quarters of patients.

- **Elevated heels:** Some people report relief from mild symptoms with the use of shoes or cowboy boots that have elevated heels. This approach, however, may not work in some people and is not recommended for anyone with a moderate-to-severe condition. (Heel cups have not been proven to be very useful.)

- **Orthotics:** For severe conditions, such as fallen arches or structural problems that cause imbalance, special insoles, called orthotics, may help. Custom orthotics are made to fit the patient's foot and individual clinical needs.

- **Extracorporeal shock wave therapy (ESWT):** ESWT may be used as an alternative to surgery for patients who have not responded to other treatments. The therapy uses low-dose sound waves to injure the surrounding tissues in the heel, which is believed to trigger healing of the tissues that are causing the pain. Studies show that the treatment provides a very small reduction in heel pain without side effects. It can be considered as an option for patients who haven't responded well to extensive conservative treatment.

- **Surgery:** Surgery may be needed for some patients, typically those who have disabling heel pain that does not respond to other treatments for at least a year. A typical surgery is called instep plantar fasciotomy. It relieves pressure on the nerves that are causing pain by removing and therefore releasing part of the plantar fascia. A less invasive method uses a procedure called endoscopy, which requires smaller incisions. Wearing a below-the-knee walking cast after surgery for two weeks may reduce the need for pain relief and speed recovery time compared to the use of crutches.

- **Botox:** Studies show that injections of botulinum toxin (Botox), a protein used to temporarily paralyze certain muscles, reduce pain and improve patients' future ability to walk. More research is needed on this treatment.

Tarsal Tunnel Syndrome

Tarsal tunnel syndrome results from compression of a nerve that runs through a narrow passage behind the inner ankle bone down to the heel. It can cause pain anywhere along the bottom of the foot. It can occur with:

- Diabetes

- Back pain

- Arthritis

- Injury to the ankle

- Abnormal blood vessels

- Scar tissue that press against the nerve

Magnetic resonance imaging (MRI) and the dorsiflexion-eversion test can diagnose this syndrome.

Treatment for tarsal tunnel syndrome: Specially designed shoe inserts called orthotics can relieve pain from tarsal tunnel syndrome because they help redistribute weight and take pressure off the nerve. Corticosteroid injections may also help. Surgery is sometimes performed, particularly if symptoms persist for more than a year, although its benefits are a matter of debate. Tarsal tunnel syndrome caused by known conditions, such as tumors or cysts, may respond better to surgery than tarsal tunnel syndrome of unknown cause. It can take months after this surgery for a person to recover and resume normal activities. Only experienced surgeons should perform tarsal tunnel syndrome surgery.

Foot Injury

If you suspect that you have broken or fractured bones in a toe or foot, call a doctor, who will probably order x-rays. Even if you can walk, you still might have a fracture. People are often able to walk even if a foot bone has been fractured, particularly if it is a chipped bone or a toe fracture.

Over-the-counter pain relievers: Over-the-counter NSAIDs are commonly used to treat mild pain caused by muscle inflammation. Aspirin is the most common NSAID. Others include ibuprofen (Motrin, Advil, Nuprin, Rufen), ketoprofen (Actron, Orudis KT), naproxen (Aleve, Naprelan), and tolmetin (Tolectin). A gel containing ibuprofen can be applied to sore joints. Acetaminophen (Tylenol) is not an NSAID, and although it is a mild pain reliever, it will not reduce inflammation. It is important to note that high doses or long-term use of any NSAID can cause gastrointestinal disturbances with sometimes serious consequences, including dangerous bleeding. NSAIDs can also increase the risk of heart disease and stroke. This risk increases the longer you use them. No one should take NSAIDs for prolonged periods of time without consulting a doctor.

RICE: The acronym RICE stands for rest, ice, compression, and elevation—the four basic elements of immediate treatment for an injured foot.

- Rest: Patients should get off injured foot as soon as possible.

- Ice: This is particularly important to reduce swelling and promote recovery during the first 48 hours. Wrap a bag or towel containing ice around the injured area on a repetitive cycle of 20 minutes on, 40 minutes off.

- Compression: Lightly wrap an Ace bandage around the area.

- Elevation: Elevate the foot on several pillows.

Chapter 15

Growing Pains

Your eight-year-old son wakes up crying in the night complaining that his legs are throbbing. You rub them and soothe him as much as you can, but you're uncertain about whether to give him any medication or take him to the doctor.

Sound familiar? Your son probably is experiencing growing pains, a normal occurrence in about 25% to 40% of children. They generally strike during two periods: in early childhood among three- to five-year-olds and, later, in eight- to twelve-year-olds.

What Causes Them?

No firm evidence shows that the growth of bones causes pain. The most likely causes are the aches and discomforts resulting from the jumping, climbing, and running that active kids do during the day. The pains can occur after a child has had a particularly athletic day.

Signs and Symptoms

Growing pains always concentrate in the muscles, rather than the joints. Most kids report pains in the front of their thighs, in the calves,

About This Chapter: "Growing Pains," July 2012, reprinted with permission from www.kidshealth.org. This information was provided by KidsHealth®, one of the largest resources online for medically reviewed health information written for parents, kids, and teens. For more articles like this, visit www.KidsHealth.org, or www.TeensHealth.org. Copyright © 1995-2012 The Nemours Foundation. All rights reserved.

or behind the knees. Whereas joints affected by more serious diseases are swollen, red, tender, or warm, the joints of kids experiencing growing pains appear normal.

Although growing pains often strike in late afternoon or early evening before bed, pain can sometimes wake a sleeping child. The intensity of the pain varies from child to child, and most kids don't experience the pains every day.

Diagnosing Growing Pains

One symptom that doctors find most helpful in making a diagnosis of growing pains is how the child responds to touch while in pain. Kids who have pain from a serious medical disease don't like to be handled because movement tends to increase the pain. But those with growing pains respond differently—they feel better when they're held, massaged, and cuddled.

Growing pains are what doctors call a diagnosis of exclusion. This means that other conditions should be ruled out before a diagnosis of growing pains is made. A thorough medical history and physical exam by your doctor can usually accomplish this. In rare instances, blood and x-ray studies may be required before a final diagnosis of growing pains is made.

Helping Your Child

Some things that may help alleviate the pain include:

- massaging the area

- stretching

- placing a heating pad on the area

- giving ibuprofen or acetaminophen (Never give aspirin to a child under 12 due to its association with Reye syndrome, a rare but potentially fatal disease.)

When to Call the Doctor

Alert your doctor if any of the following symptoms occur with your child's pain:

- persistent pain, pain in the morning, or swelling or redness in one particular area or joint

- pain associated with a particular injury

- fever
- limping
- unusual rashes
- loss of appetite
- weakness
- tiredness
- uncharacteristic behavior

These signs are not due to growing pains and should be evaluated by the doctor.

Although growing pains often point to no serious illness, they can be upsetting to a child—or a parent. Because a child seems completely cured of the aches in the morning, parents sometimes suspect that the child faked the pains. However, this usually is not the case. Support and reassurance that growing pains will pass as kids grow up can help them relax.

Chapter 16

Knee Pain

What do the knees do? How do they work?

The knee is the joint where the bones of the upper leg meet the bones of the lower leg, allowing hinge-like movement while providing stability and strength to support the weight of the body. Flexibility, strength, and stability are needed for standing and for motions like walking, running, crouching, jumping, and turning.

Several kinds of supporting and moving parts, including bones, cartilage, muscles, ligaments, and tendons, help the knees do their job. Each of these structures is subject to disease and injury. When a knee problem affects your ability to do things, it can have a big impact on your life. Knee problems can interfere with many things, from participation in sports to simply getting up from a chair and walking.

What are the parts of the knee?

Like any joint, the knee is composed of bones and cartilage, ligaments, tendons, and muscles. Take a closer look at the different parts of the knee in the diagram below.

Excerpted from "Questions and Answers about Knee Problems," National Institute of Arthritis and Musculoskeletal and Skin Diseases (www.niams.nih.gov), NIH Publication No. 10-4912, updated May 2010.

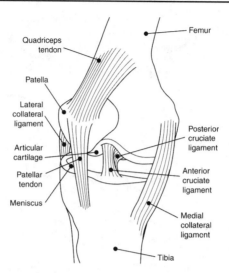

Figure 16.1. *Lateral View of the Knee (Source: National Institute of Arthritis and Musculoskeletal and Skin Diseases)*

Bones and cartilage: The knee joint is the junction of three bones: the femur (thigh bone or upper leg bone), the tibia (shin bone or larger bone of the lower leg), and the patella (kneecap). The patella is two to three inches wide and three to four inches long. It sits over the other bones at the front of the knee joint and slides when the knee moves. It protects the knee and gives leverage to muscles.

The ends of the three bones in the knee joint are covered with articular cartilage, a tough, elastic material that helps absorb shock and allows the knee joint to move smoothly. Separating the bones of the knee are pads of connective tissue called menisci. The menisci are two crescent-shaped discs, each called a meniscus, positioned between the tibia and femur on the outer and inner sides of each knee. The two menisci in each knee act as shock absorbers, cushioning the lower part of the leg from the weight of the rest of the body as well as enhancing stability.

Muscles: There are two groups of muscles at the knee. The four quadriceps muscles on the front of the thigh work to straighten the knee from a bent position. The hamstring muscles, which run along the back of the thigh from the hip to just below the knee, help to bend the knee.

Tendons and ligaments: The quadriceps tendon connects the quadriceps muscle to the patella and provides the power to straighten the knee. The following four ligaments connect the femur and tibia and give the joint strength and stability:

166

- The medial collateral ligament, which runs along the inside of the knee joint, provides stability to the inner (medial) part of the knee.

- The lateral collateral ligament, which runs along the outside of the knee joint, provides stability to the outer (lateral) part of the knee.

- The anterior cruciate ligament, in the center of the knee, limits rotation and the forward movement of the tibia.

- The posterior cruciate ligament, also in the center of the knee, limits backward movement of the tibia.

The knee capsule is a protective, fiber-like structure that wraps around the knee joint. Inside the capsule, the joint is lined with a thin, soft tissue called synovium.

What are some common knee injuries and problems?

There are many diseases and types of injuries that can affect the knee. These are some of the most common, along with their diagnoses and treatment.

Arthritis: There are some 100 different forms of arthritis, rheumatic diseases, and related conditions. Virtually all of them have the potential to affect the knees in some way. [For more information about how arthritis and rheumatic diseases are identified and treated, see Chapter 10.]

Chondromalacia: Chondromalacia, also called chondromalacia patellae, refers to softening of the articular cartilage of the kneecap. This disorder occurs most often in young adults and can be caused by injury, overuse, misalignment of the patella, or muscle weakness. Instead of gliding smoothly across the lower end of the thigh bone, the kneecap rubs against it, thereby roughening the cartilage underneath the kneecap. The damage may range from a slightly abnormal surface of the cartilage to a surface that has been worn away to the bone. Chondromalacia related to injury occurs when a blow to the kneecap tears off either a small piece of cartilage or a large fragment containing a piece of bone (osteochondral fracture).

The most frequent symptom of chondromalacia is a dull pain around or under the kneecap that worsens when walking down stairs or hills. A person may also feel pain when climbing stairs or when the knee bears weight as it straightens. The disorder is common in runners and is also seen in skiers, cyclists, and soccer players.

Your description of symptoms and an x-ray usually help the doctor make a diagnosis. Although arthroscopy can confirm the diagnosis, it's not performed unless conservative treatment has failed.

Many doctors recommend that people with chondromalacia perform low-impact exercises that strengthen muscles, particularly muscles of the inner part of the quadriceps, without injuring joints. Swimming, riding a stationary bicycle, and using a cross-country ski machine are examples of good exercises for this condition. Electrical stimulation may also be used to strengthen the muscles.

Increasingly, doctors are using osteochondral grafting, in which a plug of bone and healthy cartilage is harvested from one area and transplanted to the injury site. Another relatively new technique is known as autologous chondrocyte implantation (ACI). It involves harvesting healthy cartilage cells, cultivating them in a lab, and implanting them over the lesion.

If these treatments don't improve the condition, the doctor may perform arthroscopic surgery to smooth the surface of the cartilage and "wash out" the cartilage fragments that cause the joint to catch during bending and straightening. In more severe cases, surgery may be necessary to correct the angle of the kneecap and relieve friction between it and the cartilage, or to reposition parts that are out of alignment.

Meniscal injuries: The menisci can be easily injured by the force of rotating the knee while bearing weight. A partial or total tear may occur when a person quickly twists or rotates the upper leg while the foot stays still (for example, when dribbling a basketball around an opponent or turning to hit a tennis ball). If the tear is tiny, the meniscus stays connected to the front and back of the knee; if the tear is large, the meniscus may be left hanging by a thread of cartilage. The seriousness of a tear depends on its location and extent.

Generally, when people injure a meniscus, they feel some pain, particularly when the knee is straightened. If the pain is mild, the person may continue moving. Severe pain may occur if a fragment of the meniscus catches between the femur and the tibia. Swelling may occur soon after injury if there is damage to blood vessels. Swelling may also occur several hours later if there is inflammation of the joint lining (synovium). Sometimes, an injury that occurred in the past but was not treated becomes painful months or years later, particularly if the knee is injured a second time. After any injury, the knee may click, lock, feel weak, or give way. Although symptoms of meniscal injury may disappear on their own, they frequently persist or return and require treatment.

In addition to listening to your description of the onset of pain and swelling, the doctor may perform a physical examination and take x-rays of the knee. An magnetic resonance imaging (MRI) test may be recommended to confirm the diagnosis. Occasionally, the doctor may use arthroscopy to help diagnose a meniscal tear.

If the tear is minor and the pain and other symptoms go away, the doctor may recommend a muscle-strengthening program. The following exercises are designed to build up the quadriceps and hamstring muscles and increase flexibility and strength after injury to the meniscus:

- Warming up the joint by riding a stationary bicycle, then straightening and raising the leg (but not straightening it too much).

- Extending the leg while sitting (a weight may be worn on the ankle for this exercise).

- Raising the leg while lying on the stomach.

- Exercising in a pool (walking as fast as possible in chest-deep water, performing small flutter kicks while holding onto the side of the pool, and raising each leg to 90 degrees in chest-deep water while pressing the back against the side of the pool).

Before beginning any type of exercise program, consult your doctor or physical therapist to learn which exercises are appropriate for you and how to do them correctly, because doing the wrong exercise or exercising improperly can cause problems. A health care professional can also advise you on how to warm up safely and when to avoid exercising a joint affected by arthritis.

If your lifestyle is limited by the symptoms or the problem, the doctor may perform arthroscopic or open surgery to see the extent of injury and to remove or repair the tear. Most young athletes are able to return to active sports after meniscus repair.

Recovery after surgical repair takes several weeks. The best results of treatment for meniscal injury are achieved in people who do not show articular cartilage changes and who have an intact anterior cruciate ligament.

Cruciate ligament injuries: Cruciate ligament injuries are sometimes referred to as sprains. They don't necessarily cause pain, but they are disabling. The anterior cruciate ligament is most often stretched or torn (or both) by a sudden twisting motion (for example, when the feet are planted one way and the knees are turned another). The posterior cruciate ligament is most often injured by a direct impact, such as in an automobile accident or football tackle.

You may hear a popping sound, and the leg may buckle when you try to stand on it.

The doctor may perform several tests to see whether the parts of the knee stay in proper position when pressure is applied in different directions. A thorough examination is essential. An MRI is accurate in detecting a complete tear, but arthroscopy may be the only reliable means of detecting a partial one.

For an incomplete tear, the doctor may recommend an exercise program to strengthen surrounding muscles. He or she may also prescribe a brace to protect the knee during activity. For a completely torn anterior cruciate ligament in an active athlete and motivated person, the doctor is likely to recommend surgery. The surgeon may reconstruct the torn ligament by using a piece (graft) of healthy tissue from you (autograft) or from a cadaver (allograft). Although synthetic ligaments have been tried in experiments, the results have not been as good as with human tissue. One of the most important elements in a successful recovery after cruciate ligament surgery is a four-to-six-month exercise and rehabilitation program that may involve using special exercise equipment at a rehabilitation or sports center. Successful surgery and rehabilitation will allow the person to return to a normal lifestyle.

Medial and lateral collateral ligament injuries: The medial collateral ligament is more easily injured than the lateral collateral ligament. The cause of collateral ligament injuries is most often a blow to the outer side of the knee that stretches and tears the ligament on the inner side of the knee. Such blows frequently occur in contact sports such as football or hockey.

When injury to the medial collateral ligament occurs, you may feel a pop and the knee may buckle sideways. Pain and swelling are common.

A thorough examination is needed to determine the type and extent of the injury. In diagnosing a collateral ligament injury, the doctor exerts pressure on the side of the knee to determine the degree of pain and the looseness of the joint. An MRI is helpful in diagnosing injuries to these ligaments.

Most sprains of the collateral ligaments will heal if you follow a prescribed exercise program. In addition to exercise, the doctor may recommend ice packs to reduce pain and swelling, and a small sleeve-type brace to protect and stabilize the knee. A sprain may take two to four weeks to heal. A severely sprained or torn collateral ligament may be accompanied by a torn anterior cruciate ligament, which usually requires surgical repair.

Tendon injuries: Knee tendon injuries range from tendinitis (inflammation of a tendon) to a ruptured (torn) tendon. If a person overuses a tendon during certain activities such as dancing, cycling, or running, the tendon stretches and becomes inflamed. Tendinitis of the patellar tendon is sometimes called *jumper's knee* because in sports that require jumping, such as basketball, the muscle contraction and force of hitting the ground after a jump strain the tendon. After repeated stress, the tendon may become inflamed or tear.

People with tendinitis often have tenderness at the point where the patellar tendon meets the bone. In addition, they may feel pain during running, hurried walking, or jumping. A complete rupture of the quadriceps or patellar tendon is not only painful, but also makes it difficult for a person to bend, extend, or lift the leg against gravity.

If there is not much swelling, the doctor will be able to feel a defect in the tendon near the tear during a physical examination. An x-ray will show that the patella is lower than normal in a quadriceps tendon tear and higher than normal in a patellar tendon tear. The doctor may use an MRI to confirm a partial or total tear.

Initially, the treatment for tendinitis involves rest, elevating the knee, applying ice, and taking NSAID medications such as aspirin or ibuprofen to relieve pain and decrease inflammation and swelling. A series of rehabilitation exercises is also useful. If the quadriceps or patellar tendon is completely ruptured, a surgeon will reattach the ends. After surgery, a cast is worn for three to six weeks and crutches are used. For a partial tear, the doctor might apply a cast without performing surgery.

Rehabilitating a partial or complete tear of a tendon requires an exercise program that is similar to but less vigorous than that prescribed for ligament injuries. The goals of exercise are to restore the ability to bend and straighten the knee and to strengthen the leg to prevent repeat injury. A rehabilitation program may last six months, although people can resume many activities before then.

Osgood-Schlatter disease: Osgood-Schlatter disease is a condition caused by repetitive stress or tension on part of the growth area of the upper tibia (the apophysis). It is characterized by inflammation of the patellar tendon and surrounding soft tissues at the point where the tendon attaches to the tibia. The disease may also be associated with an injury in which the tendon is stretched so much that it tears away from the tibia and takes a fragment of bone with it. The disease most commonly affects active young people, particularly boys between the ages of 10 and 15, who play games or sports that include frequent running and jumping.

People with this disease experience pain just below the knee joint that usually worsens with activity and is relieved by rest. A bony bump that is particularly painful when pressed may appear on the upper edge of the tibia (below the kneecap). Usually, the motion of the knee is not affected. Pain may last a few months and may recur until the child's growth is completed.

Osgood-Schlatter disease is most often diagnosed by the symptoms. An x-ray may be normal, or show an injury, or, more typically, show that the growth area is in fragments.

Osgood-Schlatter disease is temporary and the pain usually goes away without treatment. Applying ice to the knee when pain begins helps relieve inflammation and is sometimes used along with stretching and strengthening exercises. The doctor may advise you to limit participation in vigorous sports. Children who wish to continue moderate or less stressful sports activities may need to wear knee pads for protection and apply ice to the knee after activity. If there is a great deal of pain, sports activities may be limited until the discomfort becomes tolerable.

Iliotibial band syndrome: Iliotibial band syndrome is an inflammatory condition caused when a band of tissue rubs over the outer bone (lateral condyle) of the knee. Although iliotibial band syndrome may be caused by direct injury to the knee, it is most often caused by the stress of long-term overuse, such as sometimes occurs in sports training and, particularly, in running.

A person with this syndrome feels an ache or burning sensation at the side of the knee during activity. Pain may be localized at the side of the knee or radiate up the side of the thigh. A person may also feel a snap when the knee is bent and then straightened. Swelling is usually absent, and knee motion is normal.

The diagnosis of this disorder is typically based on the symptoms, such as pain at the outer bone, and exclusion of other conditions with similar symptoms.

Usually, iliotibial band syndrome disappears if the person reduces activity and performs stretching exercises followed by muscle-strengthening exercises. In rare cases when the syndrome doesn't disappear, surgery may be necessary to split the tendon so it isn't stretched too tightly over the bone.

Osteochondritis dissecans: Osteochondritis dissecans results from a loss of the blood supply to an area of bone underneath a joint surface. It usually involves the knee. The affected bone and its covering of cartilage gradually loosen and cause pain. This problem usually arises spontaneously in an active adolescent or young adult. It may be caused by a slight blockage of a small artery or to an unrecognized injury or tiny fracture that damages the overlying cartilage. A person with this condition may eventually develop osteoarthritis.

Lack of a blood supply can cause bone to break down (osteonecrosis). The involvement of several joints or the appearance of osteochondritis dissecans in several family members may indicate that the disorder is inherited.

If normal healing doesn't occur, cartilage separates from the diseased bone and a fragment breaks loose into the knee joint, causing weakness, sharp pain, and locking of the joint.

An x-ray, MRI, or arthroscopy can determine the condition of the cartilage and can be used to diagnose osteochondritis dissecans.

If cartilage fragments have not broken loose, a surgeon may fix them in place with pins or screws that are sunk into the cartilage to stimulate a new blood supply. If fragments are loose, the surgeon may scrape down the cavity to reach fresh bone, add a bone graft, and fix the fragments in position. Fragments that cannot be mended are removed, and the cavity is drilled or scraped to stimulate new cartilage growth. Research is being done to assess the use of cartilage cell and other tissue transplants to treat this disorder.

Plica syndrome: Plica syndrome occurs when plicae (bands of synovial tissue) are irritated by overuse or injury. Synovial plicae are the remains of tissue pouches found in the early stages of fetal development. As the fetus develops, these pouches normally combine to form one large synovial cavity. If this process is incomplete, plicae remain as four folds or bands of synovial tissue within the knee. Injury, chronic overuse, or inflammatory conditions are associated with this syndrome.

Symptoms of plica syndrome include pain and swelling, a clicking sensation, and locking and weakness of the knee.

Because the symptoms are similar to those of some other knee problems, plica syndrome is often misdiagnosed. Diagnosis usually depends on excluding other conditions that cause similar symptoms.

The goal of treatment for plica syndrome is to reduce inflammation of the synovium and thickening of the plicae. The doctor usually prescribes medicine such as ibuprofen to reduce inflammation. People are also advised to reduce activity, apply ice and an elastic bandage to the knee, and do strengthening exercises. A cortisone injection into the plica folds helps about half of those treated. If treatment fails to relieve symptoms within three months, the doctor may recommend arthroscopic or open surgery to remove the plicae.

What about total knee replacement?

Joint replacement is becoming more common, and hips and knees are the most commonly replaced joints. In 2006, 542,000 total knee replacements and 231,000 total hip replacements were performed.

The new joint, called a prosthesis, can be made of plastic, metal, or both. It may be cemented into place or uncemented. An uncemented prosthesis is designed so that bones will grow into it.

First made available in the late 1950s, early total knee replacements did a poor job of mimicking the natural motion of the knee. For that reason, these procedures resulted in high failure and complication rates. Advances in total knee replacement technology in the past 10 to 15 years have enhanced the design and fit of knee implants.

Total knee replacement is often the answer for people when x-rays and other tests show joint damage; when moderate-to-severe, persistent pain does not improve adequately with nonsurgical treatment; and when the limited range of motion in their knee joint diminishes their quality of life.

In the past, patients between 60 and 75 years of age were considered to be the best candidates for total knee replacement. Over the past two decades, however, that age range has broadened to include more patients older than 75, who are likely to have other health issues, and patients younger than 60, who are generally more physically active and whose implants will probably be exposed to greater mechanical stress.

About 90 percent of patients appear to experience rapid and substantial reduction in pain, feel better in general, and enjoy improved joint function. Although most total knee replacement surgeries are successful, failure does occur and revision is sometimes necessary. Risk factors include being younger than 55 years old, being male, being obese, and having osteoarthritis, infection, or other illnesses.

What kinds of doctors evaluate and treat knee problems?

After an examination by your primary care doctor, he or she may refer you to a rheumatologist, an orthopaedic surgeon, or both. A rheumatologist specializes in nonsurgical treatment of arthritis and other rheumatic diseases. An orthopaedic surgeon, or orthopaedist, specializes in nonsurgical and surgical treatment of bones, joints, and soft tissues such as ligaments, tendons, and muscles.

You may also be referred to a physiatrist. Specializing in physical medicine and rehabilitation, physiatrists seek to restore optimal function to people with injuries to the muscles, bones, tissues, and nervous system.

Minor injuries or arthritis may be treated by an internist (a doctor trained to diagnose and treat nonsurgical diseases) or your primary care doctor.

Chapter 17

Muscle Pain

Chapter Contents

Section 17.1—Chronic Myofascial Pain 176

Section 17.2—Delayed Onset Muscle Soreness 179

Section 17.3—Muscle Cramps 184

Section 17.1

Chronic Myofascial Pain

"Chronic Myofascial Pain (CMP)," © 2013 The Cleveland Clinic Foundation, 9500 Euclid Avenue, Cleveland, OH 44195. All rights reserved. Reprinted with permission. Additional information is available from the Cleveland Clinic Health Information Center, 216-444-3771, toll-free 800-223-2273 extension 43771, or at http://my.clevelandclinic.org/health.

Chronic myofascial pain (CMP), also called myofascial pain syndrome, is a painful condition that affects the muscles and the sheath of the tissue—called the fascia—that surround the muscles. CMP can involve a single muscle or a group of muscles.

What are the symptoms of CMP?

The most notable feature of CMP is the presence of trigger points. Trigger points are highly sensitive areas within the muscle that are painful to touch and cause pain that can be felt in another area of the body, called referred pain.

Trigger points might be "active" or "latent." An active trigger point is always sore and can prevent the full use of the muscle, leading to weakness and decreased range of motion. A latent trigger point does not cause pain during normal activities, but is tender when touched and can be activated when the muscle is strained, fatigued, or injured.

Other symptoms associated with CMP include a sensation of muscle weakness, tingling, and stiffness. The pain associated with CMP might also lead to problems sleeping.

Is chronic myofascial pain the same thing as fibromyalgia syndrome?

CMP may resemble fibromyalgia syndrome (FMS) and has sometimes been referred to as "regional fibromyalgia." Both disorders are defined as having "tender points in muscles." However, CMP is believed to be a disorder of the muscle itself while FMS is believed to be a disorder in the way the brain processes pain signals. FMS is usually associated with more widespread pain and other symptoms that do not affect muscles including sleep disruption, irritable bowel syndrome, fatigue throughout the body, and headache.

What causes CMP?

No one is sure what causes CMP. Possible causes include mechanical factors — such as having one leg longer than the other—poor posture, stress, and overuse of muscles. Exercising or performing work activities using poor techniques can also put excessive strain on muscles, leading to CMP. In addition, anxiety and depression can cause increased muscle tension, leading to significant myofascial pain. Trigger points might be activated by overwork, fatigue, direct trauma, and cold.

How common is CMP?

Pain originating in the muscles and fascia is very common. Nearly everyone at some point suffers from this type of pain, known as myalgia fascitis or myofascitis. CMP, however, involves pain that is chronic, or long lasting, and is associated with specific trigger points.

CMP most often occurs in people between the ages of 30 and 60 years. It affects men and women equally.

How is CMP diagnosed?

Your health care provider usually begins with a thorough physical examination and medical history, including a review of symptoms. The provider will likely perform a detailed exam of the affected muscles, including strength and range of motion testing. He or she will rub the suspected trigger points to see if the muscles respond, or twitch, and cause pain in a predictable pattern or specific region.

Sometimes blood tests will be performed to look for medical causes of muscle pain, such as vitamin D deficiency or hypothyroidism.

How is CMP treated?

Treatment options might include:

- **Physical therapy:** A therapy program includes stretching, postural and strengthening exercises.

- **Medicine:** Non-steroidal anti-inflammatory drugs (NSAIDs), such as ibuprofen and naproxen, might be used to help reduce pain.

- **Massage therapy:** Therapeutic massage can loosen tight muscles and relieve cramping or spasms.

- **Injections:** This involves injecting a pain medicine (local anesthetic) directly into the trigger points.

It is also important to address any factors—such as poor posture, workplace ergonomics, or mechanical problems—that might be contributing to CMP pain.

What complications are associated with CMP?

In some cases, the pain of CMP can affect additional muscles. For example, a muscle can be stressed when another muscle is affected by CMP and is not functioning properly.

What is the outlook for people with CMP?

In general, the outlook is good. When properly diagnosed and treated, the pain associated with CMP often can be controlled.

Can CMP be prevented?

It might not be possible to prevent all episodes of CMP, but the following tips might help reduce their occurrence and speed recovery:

- Improve your posture
- Reduce your body weight
- Exercise regularly
- Eat a healthy, well-balanced diet
- Learn stress-management techniques
- Use proper techniques at work, and during exercise and sports

Resources

Borg-Stein J. Treatment of fibromyalgia, myofascial pain, and related disorders. *Phys Med Rehabil Clin N Am*. 2006 May; 17(2):491–510, viii.

Bernstein CD, Weiner DK. Chapter 123. Fibromyalgia and Myofascial Pain Syndromes. In: Halter JB, Ouslander JG, Tinetti ME, Studenski S, High KP, Asthana S, eds. *Hazzard's Geriatric Medicine and Gerontology. 6th ed*. New York: McGraw-Hill; 2009. http://www.accessmedicine.com/content.aspx?aID=5136432.

Langford CA. Chapter 336. Arthritis Associated with Systemic Disease, and Other Arthritides. In: Longo DL, Fauci AS, Kasper DL, Hauser SL, Jameson JL, Loscalzo J, eds. *Harrison's Principles of Internal Medicine. 18th ed.* New York: McGraw-Hill; 2012. http://www.accessmedicine.com/content.aspx?aID=9139559.

Yap E-C. Myofascial Pain: An Overview. *Ann Acad Med Singapore* 2007;36:43–8.

Childers MK, Feldman JB, Guo HM. Myofascial pain syndrome. In: Frontera, WR, Silver JK, Rizzo TD Jr, eds. *Essentials of Physical Medicine and Rehabilitation. 2nd ed.* Philadelphia, Pa: Saunders Elsevier; 2008:chap 96.

Annaswamy TM, DeLuigi AJ, O'Neill BJ, et al. Emerging Concepts in the Treatment of Myofascial Pain: A Review of Medications, Modalities, and Needle-based Interventions. *PM R* volume 3, issue 10 (October, 2011), p. 940–961.

Thompson JM. Exercise in muscle pain disorders. *PM R.* 2012 Nov;4(11):889–93.

Section 17.2

Delayed Onset Muscle Soreness

"Delayed Onset Muscle Soreness." Reprinted with permission from the American College of Sports Medicine. Copyright © 2011 American College of Sports Medicine. This brochure was created and updated by William Braun, Ph.D., and Gary Sforzo, Ph.D. It is a product of the ACSM's Consumer Information Committee. Visit ACSM online at www.acsm.org.

A Complete Physical Activity Program

A well-rounded physical activity program includes aerobic exercise and strength training exercise, but not necessarily in the same session. This blend helps maintain or improve cardiorespiratory and muscular fitness and overall health and function. Regular physical activity will provide more health benefits than sporadic, high intensity workouts, so choose exercises you are likely to enjoy and that you can incorporate into your schedule.

The American College of Sports Medicine (ACSM)'s physical activity recommendations for healthy adults, updated in 2011, recommend at least 30 minutes of moderate-intensity physical activity (working hard enough to break a sweat, but still able to carry on a conversation) five days per week, or 20 minutes of more vigorous activity three days per week. Combinations of moderate- and vigorous-intensity activity can be performed to meet this recommendation.

Examples of typical aerobic exercises are:

- Walking
- Stair climbing
- Rowing
- Swimming

- Running
- Cycling
- Cross country skiing

In addition, strength training should be performed a minimum of two days each week, with 8–12 repetitions of 8–10 different exercises that target all major muscle groups. This type of training can be accomplished using body weight, resistance bands, free weights, medicine balls or weight machines.

Delayed Onset Muscle Soreness (DOMS)

Any type of activity that places unaccustomed loads on muscle may lead to delayed onset muscle soreness (DOMS). This type of soreness is different from acute soreness, which is pain that develops during the actual activity. Delayed soreness typically begins to develop 12–24 hours after the exercise has been performed and may produce the greatest pain between 24–72 hours after the exercise has been performed.

While origins of the soreness and accompanying symptoms are complex, it is well-established that many types of physical activity can cause delayed soreness. Most believe soreness develops as a result of microscopic damage to muscle fibers involved the exercise. This type of damage likely results from novel stresses that were experienced during the exercise. One common misconception about DOMS is that it is due to lactic acid accumulation, but lactic acid is not a component of this process. DOMS appears to be a side effect of the repair process that develops in response to microscopic muscle damage.

Examples of activities that are known to cause DOMS include:

- Strength training exercise
- Jogging
- Jumping

- Walking down hills
- Step aerobics

Activities which cause DOMS all cause muscles to lengthen while force is applied. This is eccentric muscle action. Examples of eccentric muscle actions include the lowering phase of a bicep curl exercise or the lengthening of the thigh muscles while the limb brakes against your body's momentum as it walks or jogs down a hill. Jogging or running on a flat surface can also elicit DOMS symptoms for those who are unaccustomed to this type of activity.

The severity of soreness depends on the types of forces placed on the muscle. Running down a hill will place greater force on the muscle than walking down the same hill. The soreness that develops will likely be greater after running down a hill. A high number of repetitions will cause more damage and soreness than a low number of repetitions. As a result, work your way gradually into a new exercise program.

All people are susceptible to DOMS, even those who have been exercising for years. However, the severity of soreness normally becomes less as your body becomes adapted to work it regularly performs. Just one bout of soreness-producing exercise actually develops a partial protective effect that reduces the chance of developing soreness in that same activity for weeks or months into the future.

Does DMOS Only Cause Soreness?

There are numerous characteristics of DOMS beyond local muscle pain. Some of the most common symptoms include:

- Swelling of the affected limbs;
- Stiffness of the joint accompanied by temporary reduction in a joint's range of motion;
- Tenderness to the touch;
- Temporary reduction in strength of the affected muscles (lasting days);
- In rare and severe cases, muscle breakdown to the extent that the kidneys may be placed at risk; and
- Elevated creatine kinase (CK) enzyme in the blood, signaling muscle tissue damage.

Seeking Medical Treatment

DOMS symptoms do not typically necessitate the need for medical intervention. If the pain level becomes debilitating, if limbs experience heavy swelling or if urine becomes dark, then medical consultation is advisable.

DOMS Prevention

One of the best ways to reduce the severity of DOMS is to progress slowly in a new program. Allowing the muscle time to adapt to new stress should help to minimize the severity of symptoms, but it is unlikely that soreness can be avoided altogether. It is also important to allow the muscle time to recover from work that produces soreness, and participating in the same exercises on subsequent days should to be done judiciously.

Proper warmup is also important in preparing the muscle for the types of forces that may cause damage, but there is little evidence that warm-up will be effective in preventing DOMS symptoms. Stretching is sometimes done before exercise, but it is better to stretch after the body is warmed up and after exercise. Stretching has not been shown to reduce or prevent symptoms of DOMS, but DOMS should last only a few days (usually 3–5 days) and the involved muscles will be better prepared for future bouts of the same type of exercise.

Discontinuing Exercise

Often, symptoms diminish during activity, but they will return after recovery. Performing exercise while experiencing severe symptoms may make matters worse. On the other hand, light activity should not impair your recovery. However, there is also not much evidence that this will hasten your recovery. If you find that your symptoms make it difficult or too painful to perform the activity, then it is advisable to refrain from the activity for a few days and return to the activity as symptoms subside.

Easing DOMS Symptoms

There is little evidence that such treatment strategies will hasten recovery and return to normal function. If the primary goal is to reduce symptoms, then treatments such as ice pack application, massage, tender-point acupressure, and oral pain relief agents may be useful in easing pain. It is important to be aware that pain reduction does not represent recovery. Rather, these treatments may only be effective in reducing symptoms of pain, but underlying muscle damage and reduced function may persist.

No Pain, No Gain?

It is unlikely that you will avoid soreness altogether when beginning a new exercise program. However, pain does not need to be present to achieve gains in fitness status, and pain may indicate a need to reduce or refrain from an activity. While eccentric loading of muscle to achieve gains in muscle size appears to be important, gains in strength will occur without overemphasizing the eccentric component of a weight-lifting exercise. Pain that occurs during exercise (i.e., acute) signals a problem with the exercise (too intense, bad form, etc.) and should be halted before muscle or joint damage occurs.

Staying Active Pays Off!

Those who are physically active tend to live longer, healthier lives. Research shows that moderate physical activity—such as 30 minutes a day of brisk walking—significantly contributes to longevity. Even a person with risk factors like high blood pressure, diabetes, or even a smoking habit can gain real benefits from incorporating regular physical activity into their daily life.

As many dieters have found, exercise can help you stay on a diet and lose weight. What's more—regular exercise can help lower blood pressure, control blood sugar, improve cholesterol levels and build stronger, denser bones.

The First Step

Before you begin an exercise program, take a fitness test, or substantially increase your level of activity, make sure to answer the following questions. This physical activity readiness questionnaire (PAR-Q) will help determine if you're ready to begin an exercise routine or program.

- Has your doctor ever said that you have a heart condition or that you should participate in physical activity only as recommended by a doctor?

- Do you feel pain in your chest during physical activity?

- In the past month, have you had chest pain when you were not doing physical activity?

- Do you lose your balance from dizziness? Do you ever lose consciousness?

- Do you have a bone or joint problem that could be made worse by a change in your physical activity?

- Is your doctor currently prescribing drugs for your blood pressure or a heart condition?

- Do you know of any reason you should not participate in physical activity?

If you answered yes to one or more questions, if you are over 40 years of age and have recently been inactive, or if you are concerned about your health, consult a physician before taking a fitness test or substantially increasing your physical activity. If you answered no to each question, then it's likely that you can safely begin exercising.

Prior to Exercise

Prior to beginning any exercise program, including the activities depicted in this material, individuals should seek medical evaluation and clearance to engage in activity. Not all exercise programs are suitable for everyone, and some programs may result in injury. Activities should be carried out at a pace that is comfortable for the user. Users should discontinue participation in any exercise activity that causes pain or discomfort. In such event, medical consultation should be immediately obtained.

Section 17.3

Muscle Cramps

"Muscle Cramp," reproduced with permission from Your Orthopaedic Connection. © American Academy of Orthopaedic Surgeons, Rosemont, IL, reviewed May 2010.

Have you ever experienced a "charley horse"? If yes, you probably still remember the sudden, tight and intense pain caused by a muscle locked in spasm.

A cramp is an involuntary and forcibly contracted muscle that does not relax. Cramps can affect any muscle under your voluntary control (skeletal muscle). Muscles that span two joints are most prone to cramping. Cramps can involve part or all of a muscle, or several muscles in a group.

The most commonly affected muscle groups are:

- Back of lower leg/calf (gastrocnemius)

- Back of thigh (hamstrings)

- Front of thigh (quadriceps)

Cramps in the feet, hands, arms, abdomen, and along the rib cage are also very common.

Who Gets Cramps

Just about everyone will experience a muscle cramp sometime in life. It can happen while you play tennis or golf, bowl, swim, or do any exercise. It can also happen while you sit, walk, or even just sleep. Sometimes the slightest movement that shortens a muscle can trigger a cramp.

Some people are predisposed to muscle cramps and get them regularly with any physical exertion.

Those at greatest risk for cramps and other ailments related to excess heat include infants and young children, people over age 65, and those who are ill, overweight, overexert during work or exercise, or take drugs or certain medications.

Muscle cramps are very common among endurance athletes (i.e., marathon runners and triathletes) and older people who perform strenuous physical activities.

Athletes are more likely to get cramps in the preseason when the body is not conditioned and therefore more subject to fatigue. Cramps often develop near the end of intense or prolonged exercise, or 4–6 hours later.

Older people are more susceptible to muscle cramps due to normal muscle loss (atrophy) that begins in the mid-40s and accelerates with inactivity. As you age, your muscles cannot work as hard or as quickly as they used to. The body also loses some of its sense of thirst and its ability to sense and respond to changes in temperature.

Cause

Although the exact cause of muscle cramps is unknown (idiopathic), some researchers believe inadequate stretching and muscle fatigue leads to abnormalities in mechanisms that control muscle contraction. Other factors may also be involved, including poor conditioning, exercising or working in intense heat, dehydration, and depletion of salt and minerals (electrolytes).

Stretching and Muscle Fatigue

Muscles are bundles of fibers that contract and expand to produce movement. A regular program of stretching lengthens muscle fibers so they can contract and tighten more vigorously when you exercise.

When your body is poorly conditioned, you are more likely to experience muscle fatigue, which can alter spinal neural reflex activity. Overexertion depletes a muscle's oxygen supply, leading to build up of waste product and spasm. When a cramp begins, the spinal cord stimulates the muscle to keep contracting.

Heat, Dehydration, and Electrolyte Depletion

Muscle cramps are more likely when you exercise in hot weather because sweat drains your body's fluids, salt and minerals (i.e., potassium, magnesium and calcium). Loss of these nutrients may also cause a muscle to spasm.

Although most muscle cramps are benign, sometimes they can indicate a serious medical condition.

See your doctor if cramps are severe, happen frequently, respond poorly to simple treatments, or are not related to obvious causes like strenuous exercise. You could have problems with circulation, nerves, metabolism, hormones, medications, or nutrition.

Muscle cramps may be a part of many conditions that range from minor to severe, such as Lou Gehrig's disease (amyotrophic lateral sclerosis), spinal nerve irritation or compression (radiculopathy), hardening of the arteries, narrowing of the spinal canal (stenosis), thyroid disease, chronic infections, and cirrhosis of the liver.

Symptoms

Muscle cramps range in intensity from a slight tic to agonizing pain. A cramping muscle may feel hard to the touch and/or appear visibly distorted or twitch beneath the skin. A cramp can last a few seconds to 15 minutes or longer. It might recur multiple times before it goes away.

Doctor Examination

During your appointment, tell your doctor about your medical history including details about allergies, illnesses, injuries, surgeries, and medications.

Your doctor may ask you several questions. How long have you experienced cramps? Is there a family history of the problem? Do your cramps occur only after exercise, or do they happen while at rest? Does stretching relieve the cramps? Do you have muscle weakness or other symptoms? Your doctor may want to take a routine blood test to rule out diseases.

Treatment

Cramps usually go away on their own without seeing a doctor.

• Stop doing whatever activity triggered the cramp.

• Gently stretch and massage the cramping muscle, holding it in stretched position until the cramp stops.

• Apply heat to tense/tight muscles, or cold to sore/tender muscles.

Prevention

To avoid future cramps, work toward better overall fitness. Do regular flexibility exercises before and after you work out to stretch muscle groups most prone to cramping.

Warm Up

Always warm up before stretching. Good examples of warm-up activities are slowly running in place or walking briskly for a few minutes.

• **Calf muscle stretch:** You should feel this stretch in your calf and down toward your heel. Lean forward against a wall with one leg in front of the other. Straighten your back leg and press your heel into the floor. Your front knee is bent. Hold for 15 to 30 seconds. *Do:* Keep both heels flat on the floor. Point the toes of your back foot toward the heel of your front foot.

• **Hamstring muscle stretch:** You should feel this stretch at the back of your thighs and behind your knees. Sit up tall with both legs extended straight in front of you. Your feet are neutral—not pointed or flexed. Place your palms on the floor and slide your hands toward your ankles. Hold for 30 seconds. *Do:* Keep your chest open and back long. Reach from your hips. Stop sliding your palms forward when you feel the stretch. *Do not:* Round your back or try to bring your nose to your knees. Do not lock your knees.

• **Quadriceps muscle stretch:** You should feel this stretch in the front of your thigh. Hold on to a wall or the back of a chair for balance. Lift one foot and bring your heel up toward your buttocks. Grasp your ankle with your hand and pull your heel closer to your body. Hold the stretch for 30 seconds. *Do:* Keep your knees close together. Stop bringing your heel closer when you feel the stretch. *Do not:* Arch or twist your back.

Hold each stretch briefly, then release. Never stretch to the point of pain.

Chapter 18

Neck Pain

Chapter Contents

Section 18.1—What Causes a Pain in the Neck? 190

Section 18.2—Whiplash and Whiplash-Associated
Disorders... 193

Section 18.1

What Causes a Pain in the Neck?

From "Neck Pain," © 2013 A.D.A.M., Inc. Reprinted with permission.

Neck Pain

Neck pain is discomfort in any of the structures in the neck. These include muscles and nerves as well as spinal vertebrae and the cushioning disks in between.

When your neck is sore, you may have difficulty moving it, especially to one side. Many people describe this as having a stiff neck.

If neck pain involves nerves, you may feel numbness, tingling, or weakness in your arm, hand, or elsewhere.

Causes

A common cause of neck pain is muscle strain or tension. Usually, everyday activities are to blame. Such activities include bending over a desk for hours, having poor posture while watching TV or reading, placing your computer monitor too high or too low, sleeping in an uncomfortable position, or twisting and turning the neck in a jarring manner while exercising.

Extreme accidents or falls can cause severe neck injuries like vertebral fractures, whiplash, blood vessel injury, and even paralysis.

Other causes include:

- Other medical conditions, such as fibromyalgia

- Cervical arthritis or spondylosis

- Ruptured disk

- Small fractures to the spine from osteoporosis

- Spinal stenosis (narrowing of the spinal canal)

- Sprains

- Infection of the spine (osteomyelitis, diskitis, abscess)

- Cancer that involves the spine

Home Care

For minor, common causes of neck pain:

- Take over-the-counter pain relievers such as ibuprofen (Advil, Motrin IB) or acetaminophen (Tylenol).

- Apply heat or ice to the painful area. One good method is to use ice for the first 48–72 hours, then use heat after that. Heat may be applied with hot showers, hot compresses, or a heating pad. Do not fall asleep with a heating pad or ice bag.

- Stop normal physical activity for the first few days. This helps calm your symptoms and reduce inflammation.

- Perform slow range-of-motion exercises—up and down, side to side, and from ear to ear—to gently stretch the neck muscles.

- Have a partner gently massage the sore or painful areas.

- Try sleeping on a firm mattress without a pillow or with a special neck pillow.

- Use a soft neck collar for a short period of time to relieve discomfort. Using one too long can make your neck muscles weaker.

You may want to reduce your activity only for the first couple of days. Then slowly resume your usual activities. Do not perform activities that involve heavy lifting or twisting of your back or neck for the first six weeks after the pain begins. After two to three weeks, slowly resume exercise. A physical therapist can help you decide when to begin stretching and strengthening exercises and how to do them.

Avoid the following exercises during your initial recovery, unless your doctor or physical therapist says it is okay:

- Jogging
- Football
- Golf
- Ballet
- Weight lifting
- Leg lifts when lying on your stomach
- Sit-ups with straight legs (rather than bent knees)

When to Contact a Medical Professional

Seek immediate medical help if:

- You have a fever and headache, and your neck is so stiff that you cannot touch your chin to your chest. This may be meningitis. Call your local emergency number (such as 911) or get to a hospital.

- You have symptoms of a heart attack, such as shortness of breath, sweating, nausea, vomiting, or arm or jaw pain.

Call your health care provider if:

- Symptoms do not go away in one week with self care

- You have numbness, tingling, or weakness in your arm or hand

- Your neck pain was caused by a fall, blow, or injury—if you cannot move your arm or hand, have someone call 911

- You have swollen glands or a lump in your neck

- Your pain does not go away with regular doses of over-the-counter pain medication

- You have difficulty swallowing or breathing along with the neck pain

- The pain gets worse when you lie down or wakes you up at night

- Your pain is so severe that you cannot get comfortable

- You lose control over urination or bowel movements

Prevention

The following steps can prevent neck pain or help your neck pain improve:

- Use relaxation techniques and regular exercise to prevent unwanted stress and tension to the neck muscles.

- Learn stretching exercises for your neck and upper body. Stretch every day, especially before and after exercise. A physical therapist can help.

- Use good posture, especially if you sit at a desk all day. Keep your back supported. Adjust your computer monitor to eye level. This prevents you from continually looking up or down.

- If you work at a computer, stretch your neck every hour or so.

- Use a headset when on the telephone, especially if answering or using the phone is a main part of your job.

- When reading or typing from documents at your desk, place them in a holder at eye level.

- Evaluate your sleeping conditions. Make sure your pillow is properly and comfortably supporting your head and neck. You may need a special neck pillow. Make sure your mattress is firm enough.

- Use seat belts and bike helmets to prevent injuries.

Section 18.2

Whiplash and Whiplash-Associated Disorders

Printed with permission from: NASS Patient Education Committee. *Whiplash and Whiplash-Associated Disorders*. © 2003-2012 North American Spine Society. Available at: http://www.knowyourback.org.

What Is Whiplash?

The term *whiplash* might be confusing because it describes both a mechanism of injury and the symptoms caused by that injury. The most common symptom of whiplash is neck pain. The most common cause is a motor vehicle accident (MVA). In addition to neck pain, there may be pain in one or both arms, between the shoulder blades, the face and even the low back. Other symptoms—usually called *whiplash associated disorders* (WAD)—include heaviness or tingling in the arms, dizziness, ringing in the ears, vision changes, fatigue, poor concentration or memory and difficulty sleeping. If pain does not get better after several months, patients often get depressed.

What Causes Whiplash?

The most common cause of whiplash and WAD is a motor vehicle accident (MVA) in which one car (the struck vehicle) is hit from behind by another (the bullet vehicle). However, whiplash can also occur after side or front impact collisions. The energy of the impact passes through the bullet vehicle to the struck vehicle and then to the passengers. The amount of energy is determined by the weight of each vehicle and the speed at which they are traveling. If you are struck by a larger, faster vehicle, more energy will be transferred to you and your passengers and you are at greater risk for whiplash injury.

Outcome of Neck Pain Due to Whiplash

Most people who are in an MVA do not get neck pain or WAD. More important, most people who do get neck pain after an MVA will get better after a few weeks up to a few months. Only about one out of three patients does not totally recover—and even then, pain is usually mild, often comes and goes, and rarely interferes with daily activities or work. In general, after six months most people who are going to get better on their own will be better (although some patients do take longer to recover.) Just 10% of people who get neck pain after an MVA wind up with constant severe pain, but those are the patients who need the most medical care. Patients with pre-existing neck pain and those with abnormal x-rays at the time of the accident are at greater risk for chronic neck pain than others.

Anatomy of the Neck

The spine is a long chain of bones, discs, muscles and ligaments that extends from the base of the skull to the tip of the tailbone. The cervical spine (neck region) supports the head, protects the nerves and spinal cord, and allows for smooth function of the neck during activity. The major structural support is from the vertebrae (bone). Between two adjacent vertebrae is a disc. In the back of each vertebra are two facet joints, one on each side. The facet joints are designed to allow smooth motion for bending forward, backward, and rotating, but also limit excess motion. Muscles and ligaments surround and support the spinal column. All of these structures have nerve supplies, and injury to any one can cause pain.

What Causes Chronic Neck Pain?

It is usually not possible to know the exact cause of neck pain in the days or weeks after a car accident. We know the muscles and ligaments get strained and are probably inflamed, but they usually heal within six to ten weeks. Pain that lasts longer is usually due to deeper problems such as injury to the disc or facet joint, or both.

- **Facet joint pain** is the most common cause of chronic neck pain after a car accident. It may occur alone or along with disc pain. Facet joint pain is usually located to the right or left of the center back of the neck. The area might be tender to the touch, and facet pain may be mistaken for muscle pain. We cannot tell if a facet joint hurts by how it looks on an x-ray or MRI [magnetic resonance imaging] scan. The only way to tell if the joint is a cause of pain is to perform an injection called *medial branch block* (MBB), which is discussed below.

- **Disc injury** can also cause chronic neck pain. The disc allows motion of the neck, but at the same time keeps the neck from moving too much. The outer wall of the disc (called the anulus) can be torn by a whiplash injury. This usually heals, but in some people, the disc does not heal. In that case, it might get weaker and hurts when stressed during normal activities. The pain comes from the nerve endings in the anulus. The disc is the major cause of chronic neck pain in about 25% of patients, and there can be both disc pain and facet pain in some people. Less often, a disc can herniate and push on a nerve. This usually causes more arm pain than neck pain.

- **Muscle strain** of the neck and upper back can cause acute pain. However, there is no evidence that neck muscles are a primary cause of chronic neck pain, although muscles can hurt if they are working too hard to protect injured discs, joints, or the nerves of the neck or there is something else wrong that sustains the muscle pain, such as poor posture and work habits.

- Spinal nerves and the spinal cord can be compressed by a **herniated disc** or **bone spur.** This usually causes arm pain, but there can also be neck pain.

What Are the Symptoms?

What are the symptoms of whiplash and WAD?

- Headache due to neck problems is called cervicogenic or neck-related headache. It may be due to injury to an upper cervical disc, facet joint, or higher joints called the atlantooccipital or atlantoaxial joints. Cervicogenic headache can also make migraines worse.

- Arm pain and heaviness may be due to nerve compression from a herniated disc, which is easy for your health care professional to diagnose. More commonly, arm pain is "referred" from other parts of the neck. *Referred pain* is pain that is felt at a place away from the injured areas, but not due to pressure on a nerve.

- Pain between the shoulder blades is usually a type of referred pain.

- Low back pain is occasionally seen and is quite common after whiplash and may be due to injury to the discs, facet joints of the low back, or sacroiliac joints.

- Difficulties with concentration or memory can be due to pain itself, medications you are taking for the pain, depression, or mild brain injury. You might also experience irritability and depression.

- Sleep disturbance can be caused by pain or depression.

- Other symptoms might include blurry vision, ringing in the ears, tingling in the face, and fatigue.

How Is Whiplash Diagnosed?

Your health care professional will ask you about your symptoms and how the injury occurred and then perform a physical examination. This will allow the health care professional to know if you need any tests immediately or if they can wait, and also how to best treat your problem. In patients who do not get better after about 12 weeks, more detailed evaluation might be needed and some of the tests are described below. Not all patients need all tests.

- X-rays are used right after injury if the health care professional suspects there may be a fracture or that the spine is not stable. X-rays also show disc height and bone spurs. Otherwise they are often used in patients who do not get significantly better by about 12 weeks. If an MRI is performed, x-ray examination is usually also done to look at the bone anatomy.

- MRI scan is necessary if the health care professional suspects a disc herniation, disc injury or compression of a nerve or the spinal cord.

- Medial branch block (MBB) is an injection done to determine whether a facet joint is contributing to neck pain.

- Discography is an injection into the disc itself to determine if a disc may be contributing to the pain. Discography is only used for patients with severe pain that has not improved with good treatment, and for whom surgery is being considered.

- Computed tomography (CT scan), usually combined with myelogram (dye or contrast injected into the spinal canal) can also be used to help diagnose neck pain that does not respond to treatment.

- Electromyography and nerve conduction velocity (EMG/NCV) might be used if there is suspicion that a nerve is being trapped (such as in carpal tunnel syndrome) or there is nerve damage.

Treatment of Whiplash

The treatment of whiplash in the first few weeks and months usually involves strength training and body mechanics instruction. Patients who do not get better after about 12 weeks require specialized treatment, often from a spine specialist, based on the cause of the pain.

- Strength training is necessary to develop sufficient muscle strength to be able to hold the head and neck in positions of good posture at rest and during activity. Strengthening the muscles will also improve their range of motion.

- Body mechanics describes the interrelationship between the head, neck, upper body and low back during movement and at rest. Training in proper posture decreases the stress on muscles, discs and vertebrae, giving damaged tissue the chance to heal. Poor posture and body mechanics unbalances the spine and creates high stress on the neck, which may impede healing.

- Medications are helpful for symptom control. They never solve the problem and should be used as just one part of a total treatment program. There is no best medicine for neck pain. The choice of medication depends on the type, severity and duration of the pain as well as the general medical condition of the patient. Types of medications that are most often prescribed for acute neck pain include anti-inflammatory drugs and opioid (narcotic) pain relievers. Additionally, your health care professional may prescribe the use of muscle relaxants. For chronic and severe neck pain, the opioid analgesics and antidepressants are generally most helpful.

- Spinal injections can be helpful in carefully selected patients. Again, injections do not cure the problem and should be only one part of a comprehensive treatment program. Epidural injections into the spinal canal can provide short-term relief in cases of nerve compression with arm pain, but are rarely effective for pure disc pain without radiating symptoms. Facet (zygapophyseal) injections may help temporarily with neck pain and are usually tried before radiofrequency neurotomy. Radio-frequency neurotomy (RFN) is a procedure that heats the nerves to stop them from conducting pain signals but is only useful for facet joint pain. It can help for about nine to 18 months and then can be repeated if needed and should only be considered in chronic situations with significant pain.

- Spinal manipulative therapy (SMT) is usually provided by chiropractors, osteopaths or specially trained physical therapists. SMT can provide relief from symptoms for many patients, and is generally safe. SMT should be combined with strength training and body mechanics instruction.

- Surgery for chronic neck pain is hardly ever necessary. However, surgery can be helpful when there is severe pain arising from one or two discs and the patient is very disabled, psychologically healthy, and has not gotten better with nonoperative care. Surgery is done more often when there is pressure on a nerve or the spinal cord.

If You Have Whiplash ...

- A spine care specialist can help relieve the pain of whiplash and regain range of motion. Follow your health care professional's instructions carefully.

- Remain active and do the exercises that you are taught to improve your posture and reduce the strain on your neck.

- Remember that, with proper care and patience, you are likely to recover from whiplash.

Chapter 19

Repetitive Motion Disorders

Chapter Contents

Section 19.1—What Are Repetitive Motion Disorders? 200

Section 19.2—Bursitis and Tendinitis 201

Section 19.3—Carpal Tunnel Syndrome................................. 206

Section 19.1

What Are Repetitive Motion Disorders?

From "Repetitive Motion Disorders Information Page," National Institute of Neurological Disorders and Stroke (www.ninds.nih.gov), October 11, 2011.

Repetitive motion disorders (RMDs) are a family of muscular conditions that result from repeated motions performed in the course of normal work or daily activities. RMDs include carpal tunnel syndrome, bursitis, tendonitis, epicondylitis, ganglion cyst, tenosynovitis, and trigger finger. RMDs are caused by too many uninterrupted repetitions of an activity or motion, unnatural or awkward motions such as twisting the arm or wrist, overexertion, incorrect posture, or muscle fatigue. RMDs occur most commonly in the hands, wrists, elbows, and shoulders, but can also happen in the neck, back, hips, knees, feet, legs, and ankles. The disorders are characterized by pain, tingling, numbness, visible swelling or redness of the affected area, and the loss of flexibility and strength. For some individuals, there may be no visible sign of injury, although they may find it hard to perform easy tasks. Over time, RMDs can cause temporary or permanent damage to the soft tissues in the body—such as the muscles, nerves, tendons, and ligaments—and compression of nerves or tissue. Generally, RMDs affect individuals who perform repetitive tasks such as assembly line work, meatpacking, sewing, playing musical instruments, and computer work. The disorders may also affect individuals who engage in activities such as carpentry, gardening, and tennis.

Is there any treatment?

Treatment for RMDs usually includes reducing or stopping the motions that cause symptoms. Options include taking breaks to give the affected area time to rest, and adopting stretching and relaxation exercises. Applying ice to the affected area and using medications such as pain relievers, cortisone, and anti-inflammatory drugs can reduce pain and swelling. Splints may be able to relieve pressure on the muscles and nerves. Physical therapy may relieve the soreness and pain in the muscles and joints. In rare cases, surgery may be required to relieve symptoms and prevent permanent damage. Some employers have developed ergonomic programs to help workers adjust their pace of work and arrange office equipment to minimize problems.

What is the prognosis?

Most individuals with RMDs recover completely and can avoid re-injury by changing the way they perform repetitive movements, the frequency with which they perform them, and the amount of time they rest between movements. Without treatment, RMDs may result in permanent injury and complete loss of function in the affected area.

Section 19.2

Bursitis and Tendinitis

From "Questions and Answers about Bursitis and Tendinitis,"
National Institute of Arthritis and Musculoskeletal and Skin Diseases
(www.niams.nih.gov), NIH Publication No. 11-6240, March 2011.

What is bursitis and what is tendinitis?

Bursitis and tendinitis are both common conditions that involve inflammation of the soft tissue around muscles and bones, most often in the shoulder, elbow, wrist, hip, knee, or ankle.

A bursa is a small, fluid-filled sac that acts as a cushion between a bone and other moving parts: muscles, tendons, or skin. Bursae are found throughout the body. Bursitis occurs when a bursa becomes inflamed (redness and increased fluid in the bursa).

A tendon is a flexible band of fibrous tissue that connects muscles to bones. Tendinitis is inflammation of a tendon. Tendons transmit the pull of the muscle to the bone to cause movement. They are found throughout the body, including the hands, wrists, elbows, shoulders, hips, knees, ankles, and feet. Tendons can be small, like those found in the hand, or large, like the Achilles tendon in the heel.

What causes these conditions?

Bursitis is commonly caused by overuse or direct trauma to a joint. Bursitis may occur at the knee or elbow, from kneeling or leaning on the elbows longer than usual on a hard surface, for example. Tendinitis is most often the result of a repetitive injury or motion in the affected area. These conditions occur more often with age. Tendons become less flexible with age, and therefore, more prone to injury.

People such as carpenters, gardeners, musicians, and athletes who perform activities that require repetitive motions or place stress on joints are at higher risk for tendinitis and bursitis.

An infection, arthritis, gout, thyroid disease, and diabetes can also bring about inflammation of a bursa or tendon.

What parts of the body are affected?

Tendinitis causes pain and tenderness just outside a joint. Some common names for tendinitis identify with the sport or movement that typically increases risk for tendon inflammation. They include tennis elbow, golfer's elbow, pitcher's shoulder, swimmer's shoulder, and jumper's knee. Some common examples follow.

Tennis elbow and golfer's elbow: Tennis elbow refers to an injury to the outer elbow tendon. Golfer's elbow is an injury to the inner tendon of the elbow. These conditions can also occur with any activity that involves repetitive wrist turning or hand gripping, such as tool use, hand shaking, or twisting movements. Carpenters, gardeners, painters, musicians, manicurists, and dentists are at higher risk for these forms of tendinitis. Pain occurs near the elbow, sometimes radiating into the upper arm or down to the forearm. Another name for tennis elbow is lateral epicondylitis. Golfer's elbow is also called medial epicondylitis.

Shoulder tendinitis, bursitis, and impingement syndrome: Two types of tendinitis can affect the shoulder. Biceps tendinitis causes pain in the front or side of the shoulder and may travel down to the elbow and forearm. Pain may also occur when the arm is raised overhead. The biceps muscle, in the front of the upper arm, helps stabilize the upper arm bone (humerus) in the shoulder socket. It also helps accelerate and decelerate the arm during overhead movement in activities like tennis or pitching.

Rotator cuff tendinitis causes shoulder pain at the tip of the shoulder and the upper, outer arm. The pain can be aggravated by reaching, pushing, pulling, lifting, raising the arm above shoulder level, or lying on the affected side. The rotator cuff is primarily a group of four muscles that attach the arm to the shoulder joint and allow the arm to rotate and elevate. If the rotator cuff and bursa are irritated, inflamed, and swollen, they may become compressed between the head of the humerus and the acromion, the outer edge of the shoulder blade.

Repeated motion involving the arms, or the aging process involving shoulder motion over many years, may also irritate and wear down the tendons, muscles, and surrounding structures. Squeezing of the rotator cuff is called shoulder impingement syndrome.

Inflammation caused by rheumatoid arthritis may cause rotator cuff tendinitis and bursitis. Sports involving overuse of the shoulder and occupations requiring frequent overhead reaching are other potential causes of irritation to the rotator cuff or bursa, and may lead to inflammation and impingement.

Knee tendinitis or jumper's knee: If a person overuses a tendon during activities such as dancing, cycling, or running, it may elongate or undergo microscopic tears and become inflamed. Trying to break a fall may also cause the quadriceps muscles to contract and tear the quadriceps tendon above the knee cap (patella) or the patellar tendon below it. This type of injury is most likely to happen in older people whose tendons tend to be weaker and less flexible. Tendinitis of the patellar tendon is sometimes called jumper's knee because in sports that require jumping, such as basketball, the muscle contraction and force of hitting the ground after a jump strain the tendon. After repeated stress, the tendon may become inflamed or tear.

People with tendinitis of the knee may feel pain during running, hurried walking, or jumping. Knee tendinitis can increase risk for ruptures or large tears to the tendon. A complete rupture of the quadriceps or patellar tendon is not only painful, but also makes it difficult for a person to bend, extend, or lift the leg, or to bear weight on the involved leg.

Achilles tendinitis: Achilles tendon injuries involve an irritation, stretch, or tear to the tendon connecting the calf muscle to the back of the heel. Achilles tendinitis is a common overuse injury, but can also be caused by tight or weak calf muscles or any condition that causes the tendon to become less flexible and more rigid, such as reactive arthritis or normal aging.

Achilles tendon injuries can happen to anyone who regularly participates in an activity that causes the calf muscle to contract, like climbing stairs or using a stair-stepper, but are most common in middle-aged "weekend warriors" who may not exercise regularly or take time to warm up and stretch properly before an activity. Among professional athletes, most Achilles injuries seem to occur in quick-acceleration or jumping sports like football, tennis, and basketball, and almost always end the season's competition for the athlete.

Achilles tendinitis can be a chronic condition. It can also cause what appears to be a sudden injury. Tendinitis is the most common factor contributing to Achilles tendon tears. When a tendon is weakened by age or overuse, trauma can cause it to rupture. These injuries can be so sudden and agonizing that they have been known to bring down charging professional football players in shocking fashion.

How are these conditions diagnosed?

Diagnosis of tendinitis and bursitis begins with a medical history and physical examination. The patient will describe the pain and circumstances in which pain occurs. The location and onset of pain, whether it varies in severity throughout the day, and the factors that relieve or aggravate the pain are all important diagnostic clues. Therapists and physicians will use manual tests called selective tissue tension tests to determine which tendon is involved, and then will palpate (a form of touching the tendon) specific areas of the tendon to pinpoint the area of inflammation. X-rays do not show tendons or bursae, but may be helpful in ruling out problems in the bone or arthritis. In the case of a torn tendon, x-rays may help show which tendon is affected. In a knee injury, for example, an x-ray will show that the patella is lower than normal in a quadriceps tendon tear and higher than normal in a patellar tendon tear. The doctor may also use magnetic resonance imaging (MRI) to confirm a partial or total tear. MRIs detect both bone and soft tissues like muscles, tendons and their coverings (sheaths), and bursae.

An anesthetic-injection test is another way to confirm a diagnosis of tendinitis. A small amount of anesthetic (lidocaine hydrochloride) is injected into the affected area. If the pain is temporarily relieved, the diagnosis is confirmed.

To rule out infection, the doctor may remove and test fluid from the inflamed area.

How are bursitis and tendinitis treated?

A primary care physician or a physical therapist can treat the common causes of tendinitis and bursitis. Complicated cases or those resistant to conservative therapies may require referral to a specialist, such as an orthopaedist or rheumatologist.

Treatment focuses on healing the injured bursa or tendon. The first step in treating both of these conditions is to reduce pain and inflammation with rest, compression, elevation, and anti-inflammatory medicines such as aspirin, naproxen, or ibuprofen. Ice may also be used in acute injuries, but most cases of bursitis or tendinitis are considered chronic, and ice is not helpful. When ice is needed, an ice pack can be applied to the affected area for 15–20 minutes every four to six hours for three to five days. Longer use of ice and a stretching program may be recommended by a health care provider.

Activity involving the affected joint is also restricted to encourage healing and prevent further injury.

In some cases (for example, in tennis elbow), elbow bands may be used to compress the forearm muscle to provide some pain relief, limiting the pull of the tendon on the bone. Other protective devices, such as foot orthoses for the ankle and foot or splints for the knee or hand, may temporarily reduce stress to the affected tendon or bursa and facilitate quicker healing times, while allowing general activity levels to continue as usual.

The doctor or therapist may use ultrasound (gentle sound-wave vibrations) to warm deep tissues and improve blood flow. Iontophoresis may also be used. This involves using an electrical current to push a corticosteroid medication through the skin directly over the inflamed bursa or tendon. Gentle stretching and strengthening exercises are added gradually. Massage of the soft tissue may be helpful. These may be preceded or followed by use of an ice pack. The type of exercises recommended may vary depending on the location of the affected bursa or tendon.

If there is no improvement, the doctor may inject a corticosteroid medicine into the area surrounding the inflamed bursa or tendon. While corticosteroid injections are a common treatment, they must be used with caution because they may lead to weakening or rupture of the tendon (especially weight-bearing tendons such as the Achilles [ankle], posterior tibial [arch of the foot], and patellar [knee] tendons). If there is still no improvement after six to twelve months, the doctor may perform either arthroscopic or open surgery to repair damage and relieve pressure on the tendons and bursae.

If the bursitis is caused by an infection, the doctor will prescribe antibiotics.

If a tendon is completely torn, surgery may be needed to repair the damage. After surgery on a quadriceps or patellar tendon, for example, the patient will wear a cast for three to six weeks and use crutches. For a partial tear, the doctor might apply a cast without performing surgery.

Rehabilitating a partial or complete tear of a tendon requires an exercise program to restore the ability to bend and straighten the knee and to strengthen the leg to prevent repeat injury. A rehabilitation program may last six months, although the patient can return to many activities before then.

Can bursitis and tendinitis be prevented?

These tips can help prevent inflammation or reduce the severity of its recurrence:

- Warm up or stretch before physical activity.
- Strengthen muscles around the joint.
- Take breaks from repetitive tasks often.
- Cushion the affected joint. Use foam for kneeling or elbow pads. Increase the gripping surface of tools with gloves or padding. Apply grip tape or an oversized grip to golf clubs.
- Use two hands to hold heavy tools; use a two-handed backhand in tennis.
- Don't sit still for long periods.
- Practice good posture and position the body properly when going about daily activities.
- Begin new activities or exercise regimens slowly. Gradually increase physical demands following several well-tolerated exercise sessions.
- If a history of tendinitis is present, consider seeking guidance from your doctor or therapist before engaging in new exercises and activities.

Section 19.3

Carpal Tunnel Syndrome

From "Carpal Tunnel Syndrome Fact Sheet," National Institute of Neurological Disorders and Stroke (www.ninds.nih.gov), October 26, 2012.

You're working at your desk, trying to ignore the tingling or numbness you've had for months in your hand and wrist. Suddenly, a sharp, piercing pain shoots through the wrist and up your arm. Just a passing cramp? More likely you have carpal tunnel syndrome, a painful progressive condition caused by compression of a key nerve in the wrist.

What is carpal tunnel syndrome?

Carpal tunnel syndrome occurs when the median nerve, which runs from the forearm into the palm of the hand, becomes pressed or squeezed at the wrist. The median nerve controls sensations to the palm side of the thumb and fingers (although not the little finger), as well as impulses to some small muscles in the hand that allow the fingers and thumb to move. The carpal tunnel—a narrow, rigid passageway of ligament and bones at the base of the hand—houses the median nerve and tendons. Sometimes, thickening from irritated tendons or other swelling narrows the tunnel and causes the median nerve to be compressed. The result may be pain, weakness, or numbness in the hand and wrist, radiating up the arm. Although painful sensations may indicate other conditions, carpal tunnel syndrome is the most common and widely known of the entrapment neuropathies in which the body's peripheral nerves are compressed or traumatized.

What are the symptoms of carpal tunnel syndrome?

Symptoms usually start gradually, with frequent burning, tingling, or itching numbness in the palm of the hand and the fingers, especially the thumb and the index and middle fingers. Some carpal tunnel sufferers say their fingers feel useless and swollen, even though little or no swelling is apparent. The symptoms often first appear in one or both hands during the night, since many people sleep with flexed wrists. A person with carpal tunnel syndrome may wake up feeling the need to "shake out" the hand or wrist. As symptoms worsen, people might feel tingling during the day. Decreased grip strength may make it difficult to form a fist, grasp small objects, or perform other manual tasks. In chronic and/or untreated cases, the muscles at the base of the thumb may waste away. Some people are unable to tell between hot and cold by touch.

What are the causes of carpal tunnel syndrome?

Carpal tunnel syndrome is often the result of a combination of factors that increase pressure on the median nerve and tendons in the carpal tunnel, rather than a problem with the nerve itself. Most likely the disorder is due to a congenital predisposition— the carpal tunnel is simply smaller in some people than in others. Other contributing factors include trauma or injury to the wrist that cause swelling, such as sprain or fracture; overactivity of the pituitary gland; hypothyroidism; rheumatoid arthritis; mechanical problems in the wrist joint; work stress; repeated use of vibrating hand tools; fluid retention during pregnancy or menopause; or the development of a cyst or tumor in the canal. Carpal tunnel syndrome is also associated with pregnancy and diseases such as diabetes, thyroid disease, or rheumatoid arthritis. In some cases no cause can be identified.

There is little clinical data to prove whether repetitive and forceful movements of the hand and wrist during work or leisure activities can cause carpal tunnel syndrome. Repeated motions performed in the course of normal work or other daily activities can result in repetitive motion disorders such as bursitis and tendonitis. Writer's cramp—a condition in which a lack of fine motor skill coordination and ache and pressure in the fingers, wrist, or forearm is brought on by repetitive activity—is not a symptom of carpal tunnel syndrome.

Who is at risk of developing carpal tunnel syndrome?

Women are three times more likely than men to develop carpal tunnel syndrome, perhaps because the carpal tunnel itself may be smaller in women than in men. The dominant hand is usually affected first and produces the most severe pain. Persons with diabetes or other metabolic disorders that directly affect the body's nerves and make them more susceptible to compression are also at high risk. Carpal tunnel syndrome usually occurs only in adults.

The risk of developing carpal tunnel syndrome is not confined to people in a single industry or job, but is especially common in those performing assembly line work—manufacturing, sewing, finishing, cleaning, and meat, poultry, or fish packing. In fact, carpal tunnel syndrome is three times more common among assemblers than among data-entry personnel. A 2001 study by the Mayo Clinic found heavy computer use (up to seven hours a day) did not increase a person's risk of developing carpal tunnel syndrome.

During 1998, an estimated three of every 10,000 workers lost time from work because of carpal tunnel syndrome. Half of these workers missed more than 10 days of work. The average lifetime cost of carpal tunnel syndrome, including medical bills and lost time from work, is estimated to be about $30,000 for each injured worker.

How is carpal tunnel syndrome diagnosed?

Early diagnosis and treatment are important to avoid permanent damage to the median nerve. A physical examination of the hands, arms, shoulders, and neck can help determine if the patient's complaints are related to daily activities or to an underlying disorder, and can rule out other painful conditions that mimic carpal tunnel syndrome. The wrist is examined for tenderness, swelling, warmth, and discoloration. Each finger should be tested for sensation, and the muscles at the base of the hand should be examined for strength and signs of atrophy. Routine laboratory tests and x-rays can reveal diabetes, arthritis, and fractures.

Physicians can use specific tests to try to produce the symptoms of carpal tunnel syndrome. In the Tinel test, the doctor taps on or presses on the median nerve in the patient's wrist. The test is positive when tingling in the fingers or a resultant shock-like sensation occurs. The Phalen, or wrist-flexion, test involves having the patient hold his or her forearms upright by pointing the fingers down and pressing the backs of the hands together. The presence of carpal tunnel syndrome is suggested if one or more symptoms, such as tingling or increasing numbness, is felt in the fingers within one minute. Doctors may also ask patients to try to make a movement that brings on symptoms.

Often it is necessary to confirm the diagnosis by use of electrodiagnostic tests. In a nerve conduction study, electrodes are placed on the hand and wrist. Small electric shocks are applied and the speed with which nerves transmit impulses is measured. In electromyography, a fine needle is inserted into a muscle; electrical activity viewed on a screen can determine the severity of damage to the median nerve. Ultrasound imaging can show impaired movement of the median nerve. Magnetic resonance imaging (MRI) can show the anatomy of the wrist but to date has not been especially useful in diagnosing carpal tunnel syndrome.

How is carpal tunnel syndrome treated?

Treatments for carpal tunnel syndrome should begin as early as possible, under a doctor's direction. Underlying causes such as diabetes or arthritis should be treated first. Initial treatment generally involves resting the affected hand and wrist for at least two weeks, avoiding activities that may worsen symptoms, and immobilizing the wrist in a splint to avoid further damage from twisting or bending. If there is inflammation, applying cool packs can help reduce swelling.

Drugs: In special circumstances, various drugs can ease the pain and swelling associated with carpal tunnel syndrome. Nonsteroidal anti-inflammatory drugs, such as aspirin, ibuprofen, and other nonprescription pain relievers, may ease symptoms that have been present for a short time or have been caused by strenuous activity. Orally administered diuretics ("water pills") can decrease swelling. Corticosteroids (such as prednisone) or the drug lidocaine can be injected directly into the wrist or taken by mouth (in the case of prednisone) to relieve pressure on the median nerve and provide immediate, temporary relief to persons with mild or intermittent symptoms. (Caution: persons with diabetes and those who may be predisposed to diabetes should note that prolonged use of corticosteroids can make it difficult to regulate insulin levels. Corticosteroids should not be taken without a doctor's prescription.) Additionally, some studies show that vitamin B6 (pyridoxine) supplements may ease the symptoms of carpal tunnel syndrome.

Exercise: Stretching and strengthening exercises can be helpful in people whose symptoms have abated. These exercises may be supervised by a physical therapist, who is trained to use exercises to treat physical impairments, or an occupational therapist, who is trained in evaluating people with physical impairments and helping them build skills to improve their health and well-being.

Alternative therapies: Acupuncture and chiropractic care have benefited some patients but their effectiveness remains unproved. An exception is yoga, which has been shown to reduce pain and improve grip strength among patients with carpal tunnel syndrome.

Surgery: Carpal tunnel release is one of the most common surgical procedures in the United States. Generally recommended if symptoms last for six months, surgery involves severing the band of tissue around the wrist to reduce pressure on the median nerve. Surgery is done under local anesthesia and does not require an overnight hospital stay. Many patients require surgery on both hands.

Open release surgery, the traditional procedure used to correct carpal tunnel syndrome, consists of making an incision up to two inches in the wrist and then cutting the carpal ligament to enlarge the carpal tunnel. The procedure is generally done under local anesthesia on an outpatient basis, unless there are unusual medical considerations.

Endoscopic surgery may allow faster functional recovery and less postoperative discomfort than traditional open release surgery. The surgeon makes two incisions (about ½ inch each) in the wrist and palm, inserts a camera attached to a tube, observes the tissue on a screen, and cuts the carpal ligament (the tissue that holds joints together). This two-portal endoscopic surgery, generally performed under local anesthesia, is effective and minimizes scarring and scar tenderness, if any. Single portal endoscopic surgery for carpal tunnel syndrome is also available and can result in less postoperative pain and a minimal scar. It generally allows individuals to resume some normal activities in a short period of time.

Although symptoms may be relieved immediately after surgery, full recovery from carpal tunnel surgery can take months. Some patients may have infection, nerve damage, stiffness, and pain at the scar. Occasionally the wrist loses strength because the carpal ligament is cut. Patients should undergo physical therapy after surgery to restore wrist strength. Some patients may need to adjust job duties or even change jobs after recovery from surgery.

Recurrence of carpal tunnel syndrome following treatment is rare. The majority of patients recover completely.

How can carpal tunnel syndrome be prevented?

At the workplace, workers can do on-the-job conditioning, perform stretching exercises, take frequent rest breaks, wear splints to keep wrists straight, and use correct posture and wrist position. Wearing fingerless gloves can help keep hands warm and flexible. Workstations, tools and tool handles, and tasks can be redesigned to enable the worker's wrist to maintain a natural position during work. Jobs can be rotated among workers. Employers can develop programs in ergonomics, the process of adapting workplace conditions and job demands to the capabilities of workers. However, research has not conclusively shown that these workplace changes prevent the occurrence of carpal tunnel syndrome.

Chapter 20

Shoulder Pain

What are the most common shoulder problems?

The most movable joint in the body, the shoulder is also one of the most potentially unstable joints. As a result, it is the site of many common problems. They include sprains, strains, dislocations, separations, tendinitis, bursitis, torn rotator cuffs, frozen shoulder, fractures, and arthritis.

What are the structures of the shoulder and how does it function?

To better understand shoulder problems and how they occur, it helps to begin with an explanation of the shoulder's structure and how it functions.

The shoulder joint is composed of three bones: the clavicle (collarbone), the scapula (shoulder blade), and the humerus (upper arm bone). Two joints facilitate shoulder movement. The acromioclavicular (AC) joint is located between the acromion (part of the scapula that forms the highest point of the shoulder) and the clavicle. The glenohumeral joint, commonly called the shoulder joint, is a ball-and-socket-type joint that helps move the shoulder forward and backward and allows the arm to rotate in a circular fashion or hinge out and up away from the body. (The "ball," or humerus, is the top, rounded portion of the

Excerpted from "Questions and Answers about Shoulder Problems," National Institute of Arthritis and Musculoskeletal and Skin Diseases (www.niams.nih.gov), NIH Publication No. 10-4865, May 2010.

upper arm bone; the "socket," or glenoid, is a dish-shaped part of the outer edge of the scapula into which the ball fits.) The capsule is a soft tissue envelope that encircles the glenohumeral joint. It is lined by a thin, smooth synovial membrane.

In contrast to the hip joint, which more closely approximates a true ball-and-socket joint, the shoulder joint can be compared to a golf ball and tee, in which the ball can easily slip off the flat tee. Because the bones provide little inherent stability to the shoulder joint, it is highly dependent on surrounding soft tissues such as capsule ligaments and the muscles surrounding the rotator cuff to hold the ball in place. Whereas the hip joint is inherently quite stable because of the encircling bony anatomy, it also is relatively immobile. The shoulder, on the other hand, is relatively unstable but highly mobile, allowing an individual to place the hand in numerous positions. It is, in fact, one of the most mobile joints in the human body.

The bones of the shoulder are held in place by muscles, tendons, and ligaments. Tendons are tough cords of tissue that attach the shoulder muscles to bone and assist the muscles in moving the shoulder. Ligaments attach shoulder bones to each other, providing stability. For example, the front of the joint capsule is anchored by three glenohumeral ligaments. The rotator cuff is a structure composed of tendons that work along with associated muscles to hold the ball at the top of the humerus in the glenoid socket and provide mobility and strength to the shoulder joint. Two filmy sac-like structures called bursae permit smooth gliding between bones, muscles, and tendons. They cushion and protect the rotator cuff from the bony arch of the acromion.

What are the origins and causes of shoulder problems?

The shoulder is easily injured because the ball of the upper arm is larger than the shoulder socket that holds it. To remain stable, the shoulder must be anchored by its muscles, tendons, and ligaments.

Although the shoulder is easily injured during sporting activities and manual labor, the primary source of shoulder problems appears to be the natural age-related degeneration of the surrounding soft tissues such as those found in the rotator cuff. The incidence of rotator cuff problems rises dramatically as a function of age and is generally seen among individuals who are more than 60 years old. Often, the dominant and nondominant arm will be affected to a similar degree. Overuse of the shoulder can lead to more rapid age-related deterioration.

Shoulder pain may be localized or may be felt in areas around the shoulder or down the arm. Disease within the body (such as gallbladder, liver, or heart disease, or disease of the cervical spine of the neck) also may generate pain that travels along nerves to the shoulder.

How are shoulder problems diagnosed?

As with any medical issue, a shoulder problem is generally diagnosed using a three-part process: medical history, physical examination, and tests. Commonly used tests may include standard x-rays and some of the following:

- **Arthrogram:** A diagnostic record that can be seen on an x-ray after injection of a contrast fluid into the shoulder joint to outline structures such as the rotator cuff. In disease or injury, this contrast fluid may either leak into an area where it does not belong, indicating a tear or opening, or be blocked from entering an area where there normally is an opening.

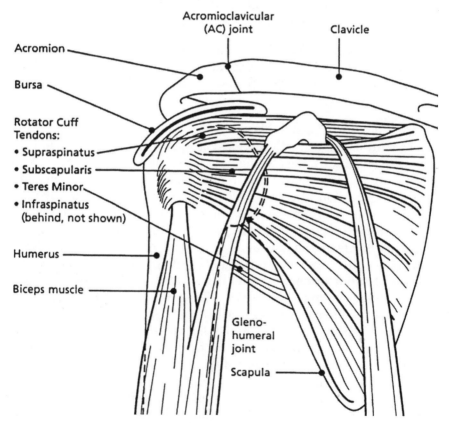

Figure 20.1. Structure of the Shoulder

- **Ultrasound:** A noninvasive, patient-friendly procedure in which a small, hand-held scanner is placed on the skin of the shoulder. Just as ultrasound waves can be used to visualize the fetus during pregnancy, they can also be reflected off the rotator cuff and other structures to form a high-quality image of them. The accuracy of ultrasound for the rotator cuff is particularly high.

- **MRI (magnetic resonance imaging):** A noninvasive procedure in which a machine with a strong magnet passes a force through the body to produce a series of cross-sectional images of the shoulder.

Other diagnostic tests, such as one that involves injecting an anesthetic into and around the shoulder joint, are discussed later in this chapter.

What should I know about specific shoulder problems, including their symptoms and treatment?

The symptoms of shoulder problems, as well as their diagnosis and treatment, vary widely, depending on the specific problem. The following is important information to know about some of the most common shoulder problems.

Dislocation: The shoulder joint is the most frequently dislocated major joint of the body. In a typical case of a dislocated shoulder, either a strong force pulls the shoulder outward (abduction) or extreme rotation of the joint pops the ball of the humerus out of the shoulder socket. Dislocation commonly occurs when there is a backward pull on the arm that either catches the muscles unprepared to resist or overwhelms the muscles. When a shoulder dislocates frequently, the condition is referred to as shoulder instability. A partial dislocation in which the upper arm bone is partially in and partially out of the socket is called a subluxation.

The shoulder can dislocate either forward, backward, or downward. When the shoulder dislocates, the arm appears out of position. Other symptoms include pain, which may be worsened by muscle spasms; swelling; numbness; weakness; and bruising. Problems seen with a dislocated shoulder are tearing of the ligaments or tendons reinforcing the joint capsule and, less commonly, bone and/or nerve damage.

Doctors usually diagnose a dislocation by a physical examination; x-rays may be taken to confirm the diagnosis and to rule out a related fracture.

216

Doctors treat a dislocation by putting the ball of the humerus back into the joint socket, a procedure called a closed reduction. The arm is then stabilized for several weeks in a sling or a device called a shoulder immobilizer. Usually the doctor recommends resting the shoulder and applying ice three or four times a day. After pain and swelling have been controlled, the patient enters a rehabilitation program that includes exercises. The goal is to restore the range of motion of the shoulder, strengthen the muscles, and prevent future dislocations. These exercises may progress from simple motion to the use of weights.

After treatment and recovery, a previously dislocated shoulder may remain more susceptible to reinjury, especially in young, active individuals. Ligaments may have been stretched or torn, and the shoulder may tend to dislocate again. A shoulder that dislocates severely or often, injuring surrounding tissues or nerves, usually requires surgical repair to tighten stretched ligaments or reattach torn ones.

Sometimes the doctor performs surgery through a tiny incision into which a small scope (arthroscope) is inserted to observe the inside of the joint. After this procedure, called arthroscopic surgery, the shoulder is generally stabilized for about six weeks. Full recovery takes several months. In other cases, the doctor may repair the dislocation using a traditional open surgery approach.

Separation: A shoulder separation occurs where the collarbone (clavicle) meets the shoulder blade (scapula). When ligaments that hold the joint together are partially or completely torn, the outer end of the clavicle may slip out of place, preventing it from properly meeting the scapula. Most often, the injury is caused by a blow to the shoulder or by falling on an outstretched hand.

Shoulder pain or tenderness and, occasionally, a bump in the middle of the top of the shoulder (over the AC joint) are signs that a separation may have occurred.

Doctors may diagnose a separation by performing a physical examination. They may confirm the diagnosis and determine the severity of the separation by taking an x-ray. While the x-ray is being taken, the patient makes the separation more pronounced by holding a light weight that pulls on the muscles.

A shoulder separation is usually treated conservatively by rest and wearing a sling. Soon after injury, an ice bag may be applied to relieve pain and swelling. After a period of rest, a therapist helps the patient perform exercises that put the shoulder through its range of motion. Most shoulder separations heal within two or three months without further intervention. However, if ligaments are severely torn, surgical repair may be required to hold the clavicle in place. A doctor may wait to see if conservative treatment works before deciding whether surgery is required.

Rotator cuff disease (tendinitis and bursitis): Tendinitis and bursitis are closely related and may occur alone or in combination. Tendinitis is inflammation (redness, soreness, and swelling) of a tendon. In tendinitis of the shoulder, the rotator cuff and/or biceps tendon become inflamed, usually as a result of being pinched by surrounding structures. The injury may vary from mild inflammation to involvement of most of the rotator cuff. When the rotator cuff tendon becomes inflamed and thickened, it may get trapped under the acromion. Squeezing of the rotator cuff is called impingement syndrome.

Bursitis, or inflammation of the bursa sacs that protect the shoulder, may accompany tendinitis and impingement syndrome. Inflammation caused by a disease such as rheumatoid arthritis may cause rotator cuff tendinitis and bursitis. Sports involving overuse of the shoulder and occupations requiring frequent overhead reaching are other potential causes of irritation to the rotator cuff or bursa and may lead to inflammation and impingement.

If the rotator cuff and bursa are irritated, inflamed, and swollen, they may become squeezed between the head of the humerus and the acromion. Repeated motion involving the arms, or the effects of the aging process on shoulder movement over many years, may also irritate and wear down the tendons, muscles, and surrounding structures.

Signs of these conditions include the slow onset of discomfort and pain in the upper shoulder or upper third of the arm and/or difficulty sleeping on the shoulder. Tendinitis and bursitis also cause pain when the arm is lifted away from the body or overhead. If tendinitis involves the biceps tendon (the tendon located in front of the shoulder that helps bend the elbow and turn the forearm), pain will occur in the front or side of the shoulder and may travel down to the elbow and forearm. Pain may also occur when the arm is forcefully pushed upward overhead.

Diagnosis of tendinitis and bursitis begins with a medical history and physical examination. X-rays do not show tendons or the bursae, but may be helpful in ruling out bony abnormalities or arthritis. The doctor may remove and test fluid from the inflamed area to rule out infection. Impingement syndrome may be confirmed when injection of a small amount of anesthetic (lidocaine hydrochloride) into the space under the acromion relieves pain.

The first step in treating these conditions is to reduce pain and inflammation with rest, ice, and anti-inflammatory medicines such

218

as aspirin and ibuprofen (for example, Advil or Motrin. (Brand names are provided as examples only, and their inclusion does not mean that these products are endorsed by the National Institutes of Health or any other government agency. Also, if a particular brand name is not mentioned, this does not mean or imply that the product is unsatisfactory.) In some cases, the doctor or therapist will use ultrasound (gentle soundwave vibrations) to warm deep tissues and improve blood flow. Gentle stretching and strengthening exercises are added gradually. These may be preceded or followed by use of an ice pack. If there is no improvement, the doctor may inject a corticosteroid medicine into the space under the acromion. Although steroid injections are a common treatment, they must be used with caution because they may lead to tendon rupture. If there is still no improvement after 6–12 months, the doctor may recommend either arthroscopic or open surgery to repair damage and relieve pressure on the tendons and bursae.

Torn rotator cuff: Rotator cuff tendons often become inflamed from overuse, aging, or a fall on an outstretched hand or another traumatic cause. Sports or occupations requiring repetitive overhead motion or heavy lifting can also place a significant strain on rotator cuff muscles and tendons. Over time, as a function of aging, tendons become weaker and degenerate. Eventually, this degeneration can lead to complete tears of both muscles and tendons. These tears are surprisingly common. In fact, a tear of the rotator cuff is not necessarily an abnormal situation in older individuals if there is no significant pain or disability. Fortunately, these tears do not lead to any pain or disability in most people. However, some individuals can develop very significant pain as a result of these tears and they may require treatment.

Typically, a person with a rotator cuff injury feels pain over the deltoid muscle at the top and outer side of the shoulder, especially when the arm is raised or extended out from the side of the body. Motions like those involved in getting dressed can be painful. The shoulder may feel weak, especially when trying to lift the arm into a horizontal position. A person may also feel or hear a click or pop when the shoulder is moved. Pain or weakness on outward or inward rotation of the arm may indicate a tear in a rotator cuff tendon. The patient also feels pain when lowering the arm to the side after the shoulder is moved backward and the arm is raised.

A doctor may detect weakness but may not be able to determine from a physical examination where the tear is located. X-rays, if taken, may appear normal. An MRI or ultrasound can help detect a full tendon tear or a partial tendon tear.

Doctors usually recommend that patients with a rotator cuff injury rest the shoulder, apply heat or cold to the sore area, and take medicine to relieve pain and inflammation. Other treatments might be added, such as electrical stimulation of muscles and nerves, ultrasound, or a cortisone injection near the inflamed area of the rotator cuff. If surgery is not an immediate consideration, exercises are added to the treatment program to build flexibility and strength and restore the shoulder's function. If there is no improvement with these conservative treatments and functional impairment persists, the doctor may perform arthroscopic or open surgical repair of the torn rotator cuff.

Treatment for a torn rotator cuff usually depends on the severity of the injury, the age and health status of the patient, and the length of time a given patient may have had the condition. Patients with rotator cuff tendinitis or bursitis that does not include a complete tear of the tendon can usually be treated without surgery. Nonsurgical treatments include the use of anti-inflammatory medication and occasional steroid injections into the area of the inflamed rotator cuff, followed by rehabilitative rotator cuff strengthening exercises. These treatments are best undertaken with the guidance of a health care professional such as a physical therapist, who works in conjunction with the treating physician.

Surgical repair of rotator cuff tears is best for younger patients, especially those with small tears. Surgery leads to a high degree of successful healing and reduces concerns about the tear getting worse over time. Surgery is also best for individuals whose rotator cuff tears are caused by an acute, severe injury. These people should seek immediate treatment that includes surgical repair of the tendon.

Generally speaking, individuals who are older and have had shoulder pain for a longer period of time can be treated with nonoperative measures even in the presence of a complete rotator cuff tear. These people are often treated similarly to those who have pain, but do not have a rotator cuff tear. Again, anti-inflammatory medication, use of steroid injections, and rehabilitative exercises can be very effective. When treated surgically, rotator cuff tears can be repaired by either arthroscopic or traditional open surgical techniques.

Frozen shoulder (adhesive capsulitis): As the name implies, movement of the shoulder is severely restricted in people with a frozen shoulder. This condition, which doctors call adhesive capsulitis, is frequently caused by injury that leads to lack of use due to pain. Rheumatic disease progression and recent shoulder surgery can also cause frozen shoulder. Intermittent periods of use may cause inflammation. Adhesions (abnormal bands of tissue) grow between the joint surfaces, restricting motion. There is also a lack of synovial fluid, which normally lubricates the gap between the arm bone and socket to help the shoulder joint move. It is this restricted space between the capsule and ball of the humerus that distinguishes adhesive capsulitis from a less complicated painful, stiff shoulder. People with diabetes, stroke, lung disease, rheumatoid arthritis, and heart disease, or those who have been in an accident, are at a higher risk for frozen shoulder. People between the ages of 40 and 70 are most likely to experience it.

With a frozen shoulder, the joint becomes so tight and stiff that it is nearly impossible to carry out simple movements, such as raising the arm. Stiffness and discomfort may worsen at night.

A doctor may suspect a frozen shoulder if a physical examination reveals limited shoulder movement. X-rays usually appear normal.

Treatment of this disorder focuses on restoring joint movement and reducing shoulder pain. Usually, treatment begins with nonsteroidal anti-inflammatory drugs and the application of heat, followed by gentle stretching exercises. These stretching exercises, which may be performed in the home with the help of a physical therapist, are the treatment of choice. In some cases, transcutaneous electrical nerve stimulation (TENS) with a small battery-operated unit may be used to reduce pain by blocking nerve impulses. If these measures are unsuccessful, an intra-articular injection of steroids into the glenoid humeral joint can result in marked improvement of the frozen shoulder in a large percentage of cases. In those rare people who do not improve from nonoperative measures, manipulation of the shoulder under general anesthesia and an arthroscopic procedure to cut the remaining adhesions can be highly effective in most cases.

Fracture: A fracture involves a partial or total crack through a bone. The break in a bone usually occurs as a result of an impact injury, such as a fall or blow to the shoulder. A fracture usually involves the clavicle or the neck (area below the ball) of the humerus.

A shoulder fracture that occurs after a major injury is usually accompanied by severe pain. Within a short time, there may be redness and bruising around the area. Sometimes a fracture is obvious because the bones appear out of position.

X-rays can confirm the diagnosis of a shoulder fracture and the degree of its severity.

When a fracture occurs, the doctor tries to bring the bones into a position that will promote healing and restore arm movement. If someone's clavicle is fractured, he or she must initially wear a strap and sling around the chest to keep the clavicle in place. After removing the strap and sling, the doctor will prescribe exercises to strengthen the shoulder and restore movement. Surgery is occasionally needed for certain clavicle fractures.

Fracture of the neck of the humerus is usually treated with a sling or shoulder stabilizer. If the bones are out of position, surgery may be necessary to reset them. Exercises are also part of restoring shoulder strength and motion.

Arthritis of the shoulder: Arthritis is a degenerative disease caused by either wear and tear of the cartilage (osteoarthritis) or an inflammation (rheumatoid arthritis) of one or more joints. Arthritis not only affects joints, but may also affect supporting structures such as muscles, tendons, and ligaments.

The usual signs of arthritis of the shoulder are pain, particularly over the acromioclavicular joint, and a decrease in shoulder motion.

A doctor may suspect the patient has arthritis when there is both pain and swelling in the joint. The diagnosis may be confirmed by a physical examination and x-rays. Blood tests may be helpful for diagnosing rheumatoid arthritis, but other tests may be needed as well. Analysis of synovial fluid from the shoulder joint may be helpful in diagnosing some kinds of arthritis. Although arthroscopy permits direct visualization of damage to cartilage, tendons, and ligaments, and may confirm a diagnosis, it is usually done only if a repair procedure is to be performed.

Treatment of shoulder arthritis depends in part on the type of arthritis. Osteoarthritis of the shoulder is usually treated with nonsteroidal anti-inflammatory drugs, such as aspirin and ibuprofen. Rheumatoid arthritis may require physical therapy and additional medications such as corticosteroids.

When nonoperative treatment of arthritis of the shoulder fails to relieve pain or improve function, or when there is severe wear and tear of the joint causing parts to loosen and move out of place, shoulder joint replacement (arthroplasty) may provide better results. In this operation, a surgeon replaces the shoulder joint with an artificial ball for the top of the humerus and a cap (glenoid) for the scapula. Passive shoulder exercises (where someone else moves the arm to rotate the shoulder joint) are started soon after surgery. Patients begin exercising on their own about three to six weeks after surgery. Eventually, stretching and strengthening exercises become a major part of the rehabilitation program. The success of the operation often depends on the condition of rotator cuff muscles prior to surgery and the degree to which the patient follows the exercise program.

Chapter 21

Sports Injuries

Introduction

In recent years, increasing numbers of people of all ages have been heeding their health professionals' advice to get active for all of the health benefits exercise has to offer. But for some people—particularly those who overdo or who don't properly train or warm up—these benefits can come at a price: sports injuries.

Fortunately, most sports injuries can be treated effectively, and most people who suffer injuries can return to a satisfying level of physical activity after an injury. Even better, many sports injuries can be prevented if people take the proper precautions.

What Are Sports Injuries?

The term sports injury, in the broadest sense, refers to the kinds of injuries that most commonly occur during sports or exercise. Some sports injuries result from accidents; others are due to poor training practices, improper equipment, lack of conditioning, or insufficient warmup and stretching.

Although virtually any part of your body can be injured during sports or exercise, the term is usually reserved for injuries that involve the musculoskeletal system, which includes the muscles, bones, and associated tissues like cartilage. Following are some of the most common sports injuries.

Excerpted from "Handout on Health: Sports Injuries," National Institute of Arthritis and Musculoskeletal and Skin Diseases (www.niams.nih.gov), April 2009.

Bruises

A bruise, or muscle contusion, can result from a fall or from contact with a hard surface, a piece of equipment, or another player while participating in sports. A bruise results when muscle fiber and connective tissue are crushed; torn blood vessels may cause a bluish appearance. Most bruises are minor, but some can cause more extensive damage and complications.

Sprains and Strains

A sprain is a stretch or tear of a ligament, the band of connective tissues that joins the end of one bone with another. Sprains are caused by trauma such as a fall or blow to the body that knocks a joint out of position and, in the worst case, ruptures the supporting ligaments. Sprains can range from first degree (minimally stretched ligament) to third degree (a complete tear). Areas of the body most vulnerable to sprains are ankles, knees, and wrists. Signs of a sprain include varying degrees of tenderness or pain; bruising; inflammation; swelling; inability to move a limb or joint; or joint looseness, laxity, or instability.

A strain is a twist, pull, or tear of a muscle or tendon, a cord of tissue connecting muscle to bone. It is an acute, noncontact injury that results from overstretching or overcontraction. Symptoms of a strain include pain, muscle spasm, and loss of strength. Although it's hard to tell the difference between mild and moderate strains, severe strains not treated professionally can cause damage and loss of function.

Knee Injuries

Knee injuries can range from mild to severe. Some of the less severe, yet still painful and functionally limiting, knee problems are runner's knee (pain or tenderness close to or under the knee cap at the front or side of the knee), iliotibial band syndrome (pain on the outer side of the knee), and tendinitis, also called tendinosis (marked by degeneration within a tendon, usually where it joins the bone). [See Chapter 16 for more information about knee injuries.]

Compartment Syndrome

In many parts of the body, muscles (along with the nerves and blood vessels that run alongside and through them) are enclosed in a "compartment" formed of a tough membrane called fascia. When muscles become swollen, they can fill the compartment to capacity, causing interference with nerves and blood vessels as well as damage to the muscles themselves. The resulting painful condition is referred to as compartment syndrome.

Compartment syndrome may be caused by a one-time traumatic injury (acute compartment syndrome), such as a fractured bone or a hard blow to the thigh, by repeated hard blows (depending upon the sport), or by ongoing overuse (chronic exertional compartment syndrome), which may occur, for example, in long-distance running.

Shin Splints

Although the term "shin splints" has been widely used to describe any sort of leg pain associated with exercise, the term actually refers to pain along the tibia or shin bone, the large bone in the front of the lower leg. This pain can occur at the front outside part of the lower leg, including the foot and ankle (anterior shin splints) or at the inner edge of the bone where it meets the calf muscles (medial shin splints).

Shin splints are primarily seen in runners, particularly those just starting a running program. Risk factors for shin splints include overuse or incorrect use of the lower leg; improper stretching, warmup, or exercise technique; overtraining; running or jumping on hard surfaces; and running in shoes that don't have enough support. These injuries are often associated with flat (over pronated) feet.

Achilles Tendon Injuries

An Achilles tendon injury results from a stretch, tear, or irritation to the tendon connecting the calf muscle to the back of the heel. These injuries can be so sudden and agonizing that they have been known to bring down charging professional football players in shocking fashion. [You can find additional information about Achilles tendon injuries in Chapter 14.]

Traumatic Brain and Spinal Cord Injuries

Traumatic brain and spinal cord injuries are relatively rare during sports or exercise. Traumatic brain injury (TBI) occurs when a sudden physical assault on the head causes damage to the brain. A closed injury occurs when the head suddenly and violently hits an object, but the object does not break through the skull. A penetrating injury occurs when an object pierces the skull and enters the brain tissue.

Several types of traumatic injuries can affect the head and brain. A skull fracture occurs when the bone of the skull cracks or breaks. A depressed skull fracture occurs when pieces of the broken skull press into the tissue of the brain. This can cause bruising of the brain tissue, called a contusion. A contusion can also occur in response to shaking of the brain within the confines of the skull. Damage to a major blood vessel within the head can cause a hematoma, or heavy bleeding into or around the brain. The severity of a TBI can range from a mild concussion to the extremes of coma or even death.

For anything more than the most superficial injury, call for emergency medical assistance immediately. Observe symptoms so that you can report when help arrives. Do not allow the person to continue the activity. In more serious cases, do not move the person unless there is danger.

Spinal cord injury (SCI) occurs when a traumatic event results in damage to cells in the spinal cord or severs the nerve tracts that relay signals up and down the spinal cord. The most common types of SCI include contusion (bruising of the spinal cord) and compression (caused by pressure on the spinal cord). Other types include lacerations (severing or tearing of nerve fibers) and central cord syndrome (specific damage to the cervical region of the spinal cord).

In some cases, drugs called corticosteroids can minimize cell damage from a spinal cord injury. To be effective, they must be given within eight hours of the injury. For this reason, it is important to call for emergency medical assistance immediately. Any person suspected of sustaining such a spinal cord injury should not be moved unless it is absolutely essential to keep the airway open so the person can breathe or to maintain circulation.

Common Types of Sports Injuries

Fractures

A fracture is a break in the bone that can occur from either a quick, one-time injury to the bone (acute fracture) or from repeated stress to the bone over time (stress fracture).

Acute fractures can be simple (a clean break with little damage to the surrounding tissue) or compound (a break in which the bone pierces the skin with little damage to the surrounding tissue). Most acute fractures are emergencies. One that breaks the skin is especially dangerous because there is a high risk of infection.

Stress fractures occur largely in the feet and legs and are common in sports that require repetitive impact, primarily running/jumping sports such as gymnastics or track and field. Running creates forces two to three times a person's body weight on the lower limbs.

The most common symptom of a stress fracture is pain at the site that worsens with weight-bearing activity. Tenderness and swelling often accompany the pain.

Dislocations

When the two bones that come together to form a joint become separated, the joint is described as being dislocated. Contact sports such as football and basketball, as well as high-impact sports and sports that can result in excessive stretching or falling, cause the majority of dislocations. A dislocated joint is an emergency situation that requires medical treatment.

The joints most likely to be dislocated are some of the hand joints. Aside from these joints, the joint most frequently dislocated is the shoulder. Dislocations of the knees, hips, and elbows are uncommon.

Acute vs. Chronic Injuries

Regardless of the specific structure affected, sports injuries can generally be classified in one of two ways: acute or chronic.

Acute injuries, such as a sprained ankle, strained back, or fractured hand, occur suddenly during activity. Signs of an acute injury include sudden, severe pain, swelling, inability to place weight on a lower limb, extreme tenderness in an upper limb, inability to move a joint through its full range of motion, extreme limb weakness, and a visible dislocation or break of a bone.

Chronic injuries usually result from overusing one area of the body while playing a sport or exercising over a long period. Signs of a chronic injury include pain when performing an activity, a dull ache when at rest, and swelling. [For more information on repetitive motion disorders, see Chapter 19.]

What Should I Do if I Suffer an Injury?

Whether an injury is acute or chronic, there is never a good reason to try to "work through" the pain of an injury. When you have pain from a particular movement or activity, STOP! Continuing the activity only causes further harm.

Some injuries require prompt medical attention, while others can be self-treated. Here's what you need to know about both types:

When to Seek Medical Treatment

You should call a health professional if the injury causes severe pain, swelling, or numbness; if you can't tolerate any weight on the area; or if the pain or dull ache of an old injury is accompanied by increased swelling or joint abnormality or instability.

If you don't have any of those symptoms, it's probably safe to treat the injury at home—at least at first. If pain or other symptoms worsen, it's best to check with your health care provider. Use the RICE method to relieve pain and inflammation and speed healing. Follow these four steps immediately after injury and continue for at least 48 hours.

- **Rest:** Reduce regular exercise or activities of daily living as needed. If you cannot put weight on an ankle or knee, crutches may help. If you use a cane or one crutch for an ankle injury, use it on the uninjured side to help you lean away and relieve weight on the injured ankle.

- **Ice:** Apply an ice pack to the injured area for 20 minutes at a time, four to eight times a day. A cold pack, ice bag, or plastic bag filled with crushed ice and wrapped in a towel can be used. To avoid cold injury and frostbite, do not apply the ice for more than 20 minutes. (Note: Do not use heat immediately after an injury. This tends to increase internal bleeding or swelling. Heat can be used later on to relieve muscle tension and promote relaxation.)

- **Compression:** Compression of the injured area may help reduce swelling. Compression can be achieved with elastic wraps, special boots, air casts, and splints. Ask your health care provider for advice on which one to use.

- **Elevation:** If possible, keep the injured ankle, knee, elbow, or wrist elevated on a pillow, above the level of the heart, to help decrease swelling.

Although severe injuries will need to be seen immediately in an emergency room, particularly if they occur on the weekend or after office hours, most sports injuries can be evaluated and, in many cases, treated by your primary health care provider.

Depending on your preference and the severity of your injury or the likelihood that your injury may cause ongoing, long-term problems, you may want to see, or have your primary health care professional refer you to, one of the following:

- **Orthopaedic surgeon:** A doctor specializing in the diagnosis and treatment of the musculoskeletal system, which includes bones, joints, ligaments, tendons, muscles, and nerves.

- **Physical therapist/physiotherapist:** A health care professional who can develop a rehabilitation program. Your primary care physician may refer you to a physical therapist after you begin to recover from your injury to help strengthen muscles and joints and prevent further injury.

Treating Sports Injuries

Although using the RICE technique described previously can be helpful for any sports injury, RICE is often just a starting point. Here are some other treatments your doctor or other health care provider may administer, recommend, or prescribe to help your injury heal.

Nonsteroidal anti-inflammatory drugs (NSAIDs): The moment you are injured, chemicals are released from damaged tissue cells. This triggers the first stage of healing: inflammation. Inflammation causes tissues to become swollen, tender, and painful. Although inflammation is needed for healing, it can actually slow the healing process if left unchecked.

To reduce inflammation and pain, doctors and other health care providers often recommend taking an over-the-counter (OTC) nonsteroidal anti-inflammatory drug (NSAID) such as aspirin, ibuprofen (Advil, Motrin IB, Nuprin), ketoprofen (Actron, Orudis KT), or naproxen sodium (Aleve). For more severe pain and inflammation, doctors may prescribe one of several dozen NSAIDs available in prescription strength.

Brand names included are provided as examples only, and their inclusion does not mean that these products are endorsed by the National Institutes of Health or any other government agency. Also, if a particular brand name is not mentioned, this does not mean or imply that the product is unsatisfactory.

Like all medications, NSAIDs can have side effects. The list of possible adverse effects is long, but major problems are few. The intestinal tract heads the list with nausea, abdominal pain, vomiting, and diarrhea. Changes in liver function frequently occur in children (but not in adults) who use aspirin. Changes in liver function are rare in children using the other NSAIDs. Questions about the appropriate use of NSAIDs should be directed toward your health care provider or pharmacist.

Though not an NSAID, another commonly used OTC medication, acetaminophen (Tylenol), may relieve pain. It has no effect on inflammation, however.

Immobilization: Immobilization is a common treatment for sports injuries that may be done immediately by a trainer or paramedic. Immobilization involves reducing movement in the area to prevent further damage. By enabling the blood supply to flow more directly to the injury (or the site of surgery to repair damage from an injury), immobilization reduces pain, swelling, and muscle spasm and helps the healing process begin. Following are some devices used for immobilization:

- Slings, to immobilize the upper body, including the arms and shoulders.

- Splints and casts, to support and protect injured bones and soft tissue. Casts can be made from plaster or fiberglass. Splints can be custom made or ready-made. Standard splints come in a variety of shapes and sizes and have Velcro straps that make them easy to put on and take off or adjust. Splints generally offer less support and protection than a cast, and therefore may not always be a treatment option.

- Leg immobilizers, to keep the knee from bending after injury or surgery. Made from foam rubber covered with fabric, leg immobilizers enclose the entire leg, fastening with Velcro straps.

Surgery: In some cases, surgery is needed to repair torn connective tissues or to realign bones with compound fractures. The vast majority of sports injuries, however, do not require surgery.

Rehabilitation (exercise): A key part of rehabilitation from sports injuries is a graduated exercise program designed to return the injured body part to a normal level of function.

With most injuries, early mobilization—getting the part moving as soon as possible—will speed healing. Generally, early mobilization starts with gentle range-of-motion exercises and then moves on to stretching and strengthening exercise when you can without increasing pain. For example, if you have a sprained ankle, you may be able to work on range of motion for the first day or two after the sprain by gently tracing letters with your big toe. Once your range of motion is fairly good, you can start doing gentle stretching and strengthening exercises. When you are ready, weights may be added to your exercise routine to further strengthen the injured area. The key is to avoid movement that causes pain.

As damaged tissue heals, scar tissue forms, which shrinks and brings torn or separated tissues back together. As a result, the injury site becomes tight or stiff, and damaged tissues are at risk of reinjury. That's why stretching and strengthening exercises are so important. You should continue to stretch the muscles daily and as the first part of your warmup before exercising.

When planning your rehabilitation program with a health care professional, remember that progression is the key principle. Start with just a few exercises, do them often, and then gradually increase how much you do. A complete rehabilitation program should include exercises for flexibility, endurance, and strength; instruction in balance and proper body mechanics related to the sport; and a planned return to full participation.

Throughout the rehabilitation process, avoid painful activities and concentrate on those exercises that will improve function in the injured part. Don't resume your sport until you are sure you can stretch the injured tissues without any pain, swelling, or restricted movement, and monitor any other symptoms. When you do return to your sport, start slowly and gradually build up to full participation.

Rest: Although it is important to get moving as soon as possible, you must also take time to rest following an injury. All injuries need time to heal; proper rest will help the process. Your health care professional can guide you regarding the proper balance between rest and rehabilitation.

Other Therapies

Other therapies commonly used in rehabilitating sports injuries include the following. Most of these therapies are administered or supervised by a licensed health care professional.

Electrostimulation: Mild electrical current provides pain relief by preventing nerve cells from sending pain impulses to the brain. Electrostimulation may also be used to decrease swelling, and to make muscles in immobilized limbs contract, thus preventing muscle atrophy and maintaining or increasing muscle strength.

Cold/cryotherapy: Ice packs reduce inflammation by constricting blood vessels and limiting blood flow to the injured tissues. Cryotherapy eases pain by numbing the injured area. It is generally used for only the first 48 hours after injury.

Heat/thermotherapy: Heat, in the form of hot compresses, heat lamps, or heating pads, causes the blood vessels to dilate and increase blood flow to the injury site. Increased blood flow aids the healing process by removing cell debris from damaged tissues and carrying healing nutrients to the injury site. Heat also helps to reduce pain. It should not be applied within the first 48 hours after an injury.

Ultrasound: High-frequency sound waves produce deep heat that is applied directly to an injured area. Ultrasound stimulates blood flow to promote healing.

Massage: Manual pressing, rubbing, and manipulation soothe tense muscles and increase blood flow to the injury site.

Recent Advances in Treating Sports Injuries

Today, the outlook for an injured athlete is far more optimistic than in the past. Sports medicine has developed some near-miraculous ways to help athletes heal and, in most cases, return to sports. Following are some procedures that have greatly advanced the treatment of sports injuries:

Arthroscopy

Most doctors agree that the single most important advance in sports medicine has been the development of arthroscopic surgery, or arthroscopy. Arthroscopy uses a small fiberoptic scope inserted through a small incision in the skin to see inside a joint. It is primarily a diagnostic tool, allowing surgeons to view joint problems without major surgery. Depending on the problem found, surgeons may use small tools inserted through additional incisions to repair the damage, such as a torn meniscus or a torn ligament that fails to heal naturally. Using arthroscopy, for example, a surgeon may reattach the torn ends of a ligament or reconstruct the ligament by using a piece (graft) of healthy ligament from the patient or from a cadaver.

Because arthroscopy uses tiny incisions, it results in less trauma, swelling, and scar tissue than conventional surgery, which in turn decreases hospitalization and rehabilitation times. Problems can be diagnosed earlier and treated without serious health risks or more invasive procedures. Furthermore, because injuries are often addressed at an earlier stage, operations are more likely to be successful.

Tissue Engineering

When joint cartilage is damaged by an injury, it doesn't heal on its own the way other tissues do. In recent years, however, the field of sports medicine and orthopaedic surgery has begun to develop techniques such as transplantation of one's own healthy cartilage or cells to improve healing. At present, this technique is used for small cartilage defects. Questions remain about its usefulness and cost.

Targeted Pain Relief

For people with painful sports injuries, new pain-killing medicated patches can be applied directly to the injury site. The patch is an effective method of delivering pain relief, especially for many people who prefer to put their pain medication exactly where it's needed rather than throughout their entire system.

Part Three

Other Pain-Related Injuries and Disorders

Chapter 22

Burns

Chapter Contents

Section 22.1—Facts about Burns 236

Section 22.2—Burn Pain... 238

Section 22.1

Facts about Burns

From "Burns Fact Sheet," National Institute of General Medical Sciences (www.nigms.nih.gov), August 2012.

What is a burn?

A burn is tissue damage caused by heat, chemicals, electricity, sunlight, or nuclear radiation. The most common burns are those caused by scalds, building fires, and flammable liquids and gases.

- First-degree burns affect only the outer layer (the epidermis) of the skin.

- Second-degree burns damage the epidermis and the layer beneath it (the dermis).

- Third-degree burns involve damage or complete destruction of the skin to its full depth and damage to underlying tissues.

How does the body react to a severe burn?

The swelling and blistering characteristic of burns is caused by the loss of fluid from damaged blood vessels. In severe cases, such fluid loss can cause shock. Burns often lead to infection, due to damage to the skin's protective barrier.

How are burns treated?

In many cases, topical antibiotics (skin creams or ointments) are used to prevent infection. For third-degree burns and some second-degree ones, immediate blood transfusion and/or extra fluids are needed to maintain blood pressure. Grafting with natural or artificial materials speeds the post-burn healing process.

What is skin grafting?

There are two types of skin grafts. An autologous skin graft transfers skin from one part of the body to another while an allograft transfers skin from another person, sometimes even a cadaver. Scientists typically take cells from the epidermal layer of skin and then grow them into large sheets of cells in the laboratory. They do not yet know how to grow the lower, dermal layer of skin in the lab. For this reason, surgeons, after removing burned skin, first cover the area with an artificial material and then add the cell sheets on top. This procedure helps encourage the growth of new skin.

What is the prognosis for severe burn victims?

A few decades ago, burns covering half the body were often fatal. Now, thanks to research, many people with burns covering 90 percent of their bodies can survive, although they often have permanent impairments and scars.

Where are people treated for burns?

Over half of burn patients in the United States are treated in specialized burn centers, and most hospitals have trauma teams that care exclusively for patients with traumatic injuries that may accompany burns.

How has basic research improved burn care?

Remarkable improvements in burn care have resulted from basic research funded by the National Institutes of Health. The results have led to the best approaches for fluid resuscitation, wound cleaning, skin replacement, infection control and nutritional support.

Section 22.2

Burn Pain

"Managing Pain after Burn Injury," Copyright © 2011 Model Systems Knowledge Translation Center (MSKTC). Reprinted with permission. This publication was produced by the Burn Injury Model Systems in collaboration with the University of Washington Model Systems Knowledge Translation Center.

Introduction

Pain and discomfort are an unfortunate part of burn injury and recovery. Many of our patients tell us that ongoing pain continues to be a problem long after discharge from the hospital.

Continued pain can interfere with every aspect of your life, including:

- **Sleep:** Pain can make it difficult for you to fall or stay asleep.

- **Ability to work:** Pain can limit your ability to function or concentrate on the job.

- **Mood:** Pain can cause depression and anxiety, especially when the pain is severe and lasts a long time.

- **Quality of life:** Pain can keep you from being able to enjoy time with loved ones or do activities that are meaningful.

- **Healing:** Pain can get in the way of healing if it keeps you from being able to sleep, eat or exercise enough.

If you are having pain, tell your physician.

Things to Remember

- Burn pain is complex and requires careful assessment by your health care provider in order to find the best treatment.

- Pain management often requires a multidisciplinary approach that may include both medication and non-medication treatments and involve a team of health providers, such as psychologists or physical therapists, working with your physician.

- Pain severity is not necessarily related to the size or seriousness of the injury. Small burns can be very painful, and some large burns not as painful.

Step 1: Understanding Your Pain

There are many different types of burn pain, and each person's pain is unique. Understanding the type, intensity, and duration of your pain is important for getting the best treatment.

Your health care provider will ask you about several types of pain:

- **Acute pain:** Short-term intense pain that typically happens during a procedure like dressing changes or physical therapy.

- **Breakthrough pain:** Pain that comes and goes throughout the day, often due to wound healing, contractures (tightened muscles) or repositioning.

- **Resting pain:** "Background" pain that is almost always present.

- **Chronic pain:** Ongoing pain that lasts for six months or longer after the wound has healed.

- **Neuropathic pain:** Pain that is caused by damage to and/or regeneration (re-growing) of nerve endings in your skin.

You might also be asked to describe the pain in the following ways:

- **Intensity:** How strong the pain is, often rated on a scale of 0–10, with 0 as "no pain" and 10 as "worst pain imaginable."

- **Duration:** How long it lasts (for example: hours, days, etc).

- **Timing:** When it gets worse (during the day, night, or during certain activities).

- **Quality:** How the pain feels (for example: stinging, throbbing, itching, aching, shooting).

- **Impact:** How the pain affects your emotions and your ability to do things.

- **Itching:** Whether pain is related to itching, which may be a sign that the skin is still healing.

Other important information that can help your health care providers plan the best treatments for your pain:

- Your experiences with either acute pain or chronic pain before your burn injury.

- Your experiences with insomnia, depression, or anxiety before or after your burn injury.

- Pain medications you have taken in the past.

- How much your pain limits your ability to do certain things.

- Any activities that make your pain worse or better.

Step 2: Treating Your Pain

Medications

- **Opiates** are the most common medications given in the hospital setting. Opiates may be less effective for chronic pain, however. Side effects, such as constipation and low mood, can also become a problem. For this reason, your physician will help you taper off opiates when appropriate to avoid withdrawal symptoms.

- **Over-the-counter pain medications** such as non-steroidal anti-inflammatory drugs (NSAIDs; ibuprofen is one example) can be used for long term pain relief. These medications are more effective than opiates for treating muscle pain. Use of NSAIDs for long term pain management may cause serious side-effects and should be used only under the supervision of your health care provider.

- **Anticonvulsant medications,** such as gabapentin and pre-gablin, have been useful for managing neuropathic pain in some situations, but their helpfulness varies considerably from person to person. These medications work by changing the way the body experiences pain.

- **Sleep medications:** If pain is interfering with sleep, talk to your physician about safe medications for sleep.

- **Antidepressants:** Some antidepressants provide pain relief for some people, even if they are not depressed. Anti-depressants can also help with sleep. You might talk to your health care provider about trying antidepressants as one way to manage your chronic pain.

Behavioral Approaches

Rarely do medications take away all of the pain. You may also need to use behavioral approaches to help make pain more manageable. A psychologist with expertise in pain management can work with you to find non-medication approaches that can help. These may include:

- **Relaxation:** A burn injury puts immense stress on the body that continues for many months during the recovery phase. This stress causes muscle tension that can increase pain. Relaxation techniques can be used to lessen the stress placed on your body.

  - Cognitive (thinking) relaxation techniques use the power of your thoughts to relieve stress. These techniques include meditation and a process called "cognitive restructuring," which helps you change the way you think about your pain and reassure yourself that the pain is temporary and manageable.

  - Somatic relaxation techniques use physical methods, such as deep breathing, yoga, and progressive muscle relaxation, to relieve tension in your muscles.

- **Hypnosis** has been shown to be a powerful tool in relieving both acute and chronic pain. A psychologist can teach you how to do self-hypnosis so you can include it in your daily routine.

- **Pacing of activities:** Daily activity and regular exercise are crucial in order to rebuild your strength and stamina and increase your range of motion. But pushing yourself too far can increase your pain. Pace yourself by gradually increasing your physical activity over time. If you are too sore to move comfortably the day after an activity, you have probably pushed yourself too hard. It is best to reduce your activity level until you are more comfortable. This is a difficult balance as burn recovery can be painful, and some pain may be necessary in order to progress to your previous level of function. Work closely with your physical and occupational therapists to set up an activity program that is appropriate for you.

Step 3: Coping with Pain

People have different ways of coping with difficult situations or physical discomfort. Your coping "style" can have a large impact on how much pain you feel or how much the pain bothers you.

In any difficult situation, a person can react by choosing to either change the situation, change themselves, or simply "give up." The first two options are considered "active" coping styles and are highly effective in managing stress. The third option often results in withdrawal or depression.

Research has shown that it is best to determine how much of the situation is under your control, and then pick the appropriate coping style. If the situation is out of your control, changing how you think about and respond to it can be the best coping style. A psychologist can work with you on developing this kind of coping skill.

It is also important to look for aspects of the situation that are under your control. For example, you cannot change the fact that you have suffered a burn injury that has resulted in ongoing pain. "Wishing" the injury had not occurred and dwelling on the "what-ifs" won't help your pain and may lead to feeling more helpless and depressed. However, focusing on the part of the situation that you can control—such as your own rehabilitation, time spent in physical therapy, doing your daily range-of-motion exercises, and following the pain management strategies suggested by your doctor—can be a highly effective coping strategy.

For More Information

- The Phoenix Society for Burn Survivors
  (http://www.phoenix-society.org)

References

Wiechman-Askay, S., Sharar, S., Mason, S.T, & Patterson, D. (2009) Pain, Pruritus, and Sleep Following Burn Injury. *International Journal of Psychiatry* 21(6):522–30.

Chapter 23

Cancer Pain

What You Should Know about Treating Cancer Pain

You don't have to accept pain.

People who have cancer don't always have pain. Everyone is different. But if you do have cancer pain, you should know that you don't have to accept it. Cancer pain can almost always be relieved. Palliative care and pain specialists can help.

Cancer pain can be reduced so that you can enjoy your normal routines and sleep better. It may help to talk with a palliative care or pain specialist. These may be oncologists, anesthesiologists, neurologists, surgeons, other doctors, nurses, or pharmacists. If you have a pain control team, it may also include psychologists and social workers.

Pain and palliative care specialists are experts in pain control. Palliative care specialists treat the symptoms, side effects, and emotional problems of both cancer and its treatment. They will work with you to find the best way to manage your pain. Ask your doctor or nurse to suggest someone or contact your cancer center, your local hospital or medical center, your primary care provider, or people who belong to pain support groups in your area for help finding a specialist. The Center to Advance Palliative Care (www.getpalliativecare.org) lists of providers in each state.

Excerpted from "Pain Control: Support for People with Cancer," National Cancer Institute (www.cancer.gov), updated July 16, 2012.

When cancer pain is not treated properly, you may be tired, depressed, angry, worried, lonely, or stressed. When cancer pain is managed properly, you can enjoy being active, sleep better, enjoy family and friends, improve your appetite, enjoy sexual intimacy, and prevent depression.

Types and Causes of Cancer Pain

Cancer pain can range from mild to very severe. Some days it can be worse than others. It can be caused by the cancer itself, the treatment, or both.

You may also have pain that has nothing to do with your cancer. Some people have other health issues or headaches and muscle strains. But always check with your doctor before taking any over-the-counter medicine to relieve everyday aches and pains. This will help ensure that there will be no interactions with other drugs or safety concerns to know about.

Here are the common terms used to describe different types of pain:

- **Acute pain** ranges from mild to severe. It comes on quickly and lasts a short time.

- **Chronic pain** ranges from mild to severe. It either won't go away or comes back often.

- **Breakthrough pain** is an intense rise in pain that occurs suddenly or is felt for a short time. It can occur by itself or in relation to a certain activity. It may happen several times a day, even when you're taking the right dose of medicine. For example, it may happen as the current dose of your medicine is wearing off.

Major causes of cancer pain include the following:

- **Pain from medical tests:** Some methods used to diagnose cancer or see how well treatment is working are painful. Examples may be a biopsy, spinal tap, or bone marrow test. If you are told you need the procedure, don't let concerns about pain stop you from having it done. Talk with your doctor ahead of time about what will be done to lessen any pain you may have.

- **Pain from a tumor:** If the cancer grows bigger or spreads, it can cause pain by pressing on the tissues around it. For example, a tumor can cause pain if it presses on bones, nerves, the spinal cord, or body organs.

- **Spinal cord compression:** When a tumor spreads to the spine, it can press on the spinal cord and cause spinal cord compression.

The first sign of this is often back or neck pain, or both. Coughing, sneezing, or other motions may make it worse.

- **Pain from treatment:** Chemotherapy, radiation therapy, surgery, and other treatments may cause pain for some people. Some examples of pain from treatment are neuropathic and phantom pain:

  - **Neuropathic pain:** This is pain that may occur if treatment damages the nerves. The pain is often burning, sharp, or shooting. The cancer itself can also cause this kind of pain.

  - **Phantom pain:** You may still feel pain or other discomfort coming from a body part that has been removed by surgery. Doctors aren't sure why this happens, but it's real.

How much pain you feel depends on different things. These include where the cancer is in your body, what kind of damage it is causing, and how you experience the pain in your body. Everyone is different.

Talking about Your Pain

Controlling pain is a key part of your overall cancer treatment. The most important member of the team is you. You're the only one who knows what your pain feels like. Talking about pain is important. It gives your health care team the feedback they need to help you feel better.

Some people with cancer don't want to talk about their pain. They think that they'll distract their doctors from working on ways to help treat their cancer. Or they worry that they won't be seen as "good" patients. They also worry that they won't be able to afford pain medicine. As a result, people sometimes get so used to living with their pain that they forget what it's like to live without it.

But your health care team needs to know details about your pain and whether it's getting worse. This helps them understand how the cancer and its treatment are affecting your body. And it helps them figure out how to best control the pain.

Try to talk with your health care team and your loved ones about what you are feeling. This means telling them where you have pain, what it feels like (sharp, dull, throbbing, constant, burning, or shooting), how strong your pain is, how long it lasts, what lessens your pain or makes it worse, when it happens (what time of day, what you're doing, and what's going on), and if it gets in the way of daily activities. You will be asked to describe and rate your pain. This provides a way to assess your pain threshold and measure how well your pain control plan is working.

Your doctor may ask you to describe your pain in a number of ways. A pain scale is the most common way. The scale uses the numbers 0 to 10, where 0 is no pain, and 10 is the worst. You can also use words to describe pain, like pinching, stinging, or aching. Some doctors show their patients a series of faces and ask them to point to the face that best describes how they feel. [See Chapter 41—Diagnosing and Evaluating Pain for more information about pain scales.]

Your Pain Control Plan

Some people don't want to take medicine, even when it's prescribed by the doctor. Taking it may be against religious or cultural beliefs. Or there may be other personal reasons why someone won't take medicine. If you feel any of these ways about pain medicine, it's important to share your views with your health care team. If you prefer, ask a friend or family member to share them for you. Talking openly about your beliefs will help your health care team find a plan that works best for you.

Your pain control plan will be designed for you and your body. Everyone has a different pain control plan. Even if you have the same type of cancer as someone else, your plan may be different.

Take your pain medicine dose on schedule to keep the pain from starting or getting worse. This is one of the best ways to stay on top of your pain. Don't skip doses. Once you feel pain, it's harder to control and may take longer to get better.

The best way to control pain is to stop it before it starts or prevent it from getting worse. Don't wait until the pain gets bad or unbearable before taking your medicine. Pain is easier to control when it's mild. And you need to take pain medicine often enough to stay ahead of your pain. Follow the dose schedule your doctor gives you. Don't try to "hold off" between doses. If you wait your pain could get worse, it may take longer for the pain to get better or go away, and you may need larger doses to bring the pain under control.

If you are still having pain that is hard to control, you may want to talk with your health care team about seeing a pain or palliative care specialist. Whatever you do, don't give up. If one medicine doesn't work, there is almost always another one to try. Also, new medicines are created all the time. And unlike other medicines, there is no "right" dose for many pain medicines. Your dose may be more or less than someone else's. The right dose is the one that relieves your pain and makes you feel better.

Medicines to Treat Cancer Pain

Your doctor prescribes medicine based on the kind of pain you have and how severe it is. In studies, these medicines have been shown to help control cancer pain. Doctors use three main groups of drugs for pain: nonopioids, opioids, and other types. You may also hear the term analgesics used for these pain relievers. Some are stronger than others. It helps to know the different kinds of medicines, why and how they're used, how you take them, and what side effects you might expect.

Nonopioids

Nonopioids are drugs used to treat mild to moderate pain, fever, and swelling. On a scale of 0 to 10, a nonopioid may be used if you rate your pain from 1 to 4. These medicines are stronger than most people realize. In many cases, they are all you'll need to relieve your pain. You just need to be sure to take them regularly.

You can buy most nonopioids without a prescription. But you still need to talk with your doctor before taking them. Some of them may have things added to them that you need to know about. And they do have side effects. Common ones, such as nausea, itching, or drowsiness, usually go away after a few days. Do not take more than the label says unless your doctor tells you to do so.

Nonopioids include acetaminophen, which you may know as Tylenol. Acetaminophen reduces pain. It is not helpful with inflammation. Most of the time, people don't have side effects from a normal dose of acetaminophen. But taking large doses of this medicine every day for a long time can damage your liver. Drinking alcohol with the typical dose can also damage the liver.

Make sure you tell the doctor that you're taking acetaminophen. Sometimes it is used in other pain medicines, so you may not realize that you're taking more than you should. Also, your doctor may not want you to take acetaminophen too often if you're getting chemotherapy. The medicine can cover up a fever, hiding the fact that you might have an infection.

Nonsteroidal anti-inflammatory drugs (NSAIDs), such as ibuprofen (which you may know as Advil or Motrin) and aspirin, help control pain and inflammation. With NSAIDs, the most common side effect is stomach upset or indigestion, especially in older people. Eating food or drinking milk when you take these drugs may stop this from happening. NSAIDs may also keep blood from clotting the way it should. This means that it's harder to stop bleeding after you've hurt yourself. NSAIDs can also sometimes cause bleeding in the stomach. Tell your doctor if your stools become darker than normal, you notice bleeding from your rectum, you have an upset stomach, you have heartburn symptoms, or you cough up blood.

Some people have conditions that NSAIDs can make worse. In general, you should avoid these drugs if you are allergic to aspirin, are getting chemotherapy, are on steroid medicines, have stomach ulcers or a history of ulcers, gout, or bleeding disorders, are taking prescription medicines for arthritis, have kidney problems, have heart problems, are planning surgery within a week, or are taking blood-thinning medicine (such as heparin or Coumadin).

Opioids

If you're having moderate to severe pain, your doctor may recommend that you take stronger drugs called opioids. Opioids are sometimes called narcotics. You must have a doctor's prescription to take them. They are often taken with aspirin, ibuprofen, and acetaminophen. Common opioids include the following:

- Codeine
- Fentanyl
- Hydromorphone (for example, Dilaudid)
- Levorphanol
- Meperidine (for example, Demerol)
- Methadone
- Morphine
- Oxycodone (for example, OxyContin)
- Oxymorphone

Over time, people who take opioids for pain sometimes find that they need to take larger doses to get relief. This is caused by more pain, the cancer getting worse, or medicine tolerance. When a medicine doesn't give you enough pain relief, your doctor may increase the dose and how often you take it. He or she can also prescribe a stronger drug. Both methods are safe and effective under your doctor's care. Do not increase the dose of medicine on your own.

Some pain medicines may cause constipation (trouble passing stools), drowsiness (feeling sleepy), nausea (upset stomach), or vomiting (throwing up). Other less common side effects include dizziness, confusion, breathing problems, itching, and trouble urinating. Side effects vary with each person. It's important to talk to your doctor often about any side effects you're having. If needed, he or she can change your medicines or the doses you're taking. They can also add other medicines to your pain control plan to help your side effects.

Almost everyone taking opioids has some constipation. This happens because opioids cause the stool to move more slowly through your system, so your body takes more time to absorb water from the stool. The stool then becomes hard. Keep in mind that constipation will only go away if it's treated. But don't let any side effects stop you from getting your pain controlled. Your health care team can talk with you about other ways to relieve them. There are solutions to getting your pain under control.

You may be able to take less medicine when the pain gets better. You may even be able to stop taking opioids. But it's important to stop taking opioids slowly, with your doctor's advice. When pain medicines are taken for long periods of time, your body gets used to them. If the medicines are stopped or suddenly reduced, a condition called withdrawal may occur. This is why the doses should be lowered slowly. This has no relation to being addicted.

Stopping your pain medicines slowly prevents withdrawal symptoms. But if you stop taking opioids suddenly, you may start feeling like you have the flu. You may sweat and have diarrhea or other symptoms. If this happens, tell your doctor or nurse. He or she can treat these symptoms, which usually resolve quickly.

Other Types of Pain Medicine

Doctors also prescribe other types of medicine to relieve cancer pain. They can be used along with nonopioids and opioids. Here are some examples:

- **Antidepressants:** Some drugs can be used for more than one purpose. For example, antidepressants are used to treat depression, but they may also help relieve tingling and burning pain. Nerve damage from radiation, surgery, or chemotherapy can cause this type of pain.

- **Antiseizure medicines (anticonvulsants):** Like antidepressants, anticonvulsants or antiseizure drugs can also be used to help control tingling or burning from nerve injury.

- **Steroids:** Steroids are mainly used to treat pain caused by swelling.

Be sure to ask your health care team about the common side effects of these medicines.

Medicine Tolerance and Addiction

When treating cancer pain, addiction is rarely a problem.

Addiction is when people can't control their seeking or craving for something. They continue to take medicine, or perform a certain action, even when it causes them harm. Often people take medicines when they don't have pain. They take it for psychological reasons, not physical. But people with cancer need strong medicine to help control their pain. Yet some people are so afraid of becoming addicted to pain medicine that they won't take it. Family members may also worry that their loved ones will get addicted to pain medicine. Therefore, they sometimes encourage loved ones to "hold off" between doses. But even if they mean well, it's best to take your medicine as prescribed.

Tolerance to pain medicine sometimes happens. Some people think that they have to save stronger medicines for later. They're afraid that their bodies will get used to the medicine and that it won't work anymore. But medicine doesn't stop working—it just doesn't work as well as it once did. As you keep taking a medicine over time, you may need a change in your pain control plan to get the same amount of pain relief. This is called tolerance. Tolerance is a common issue in cancer pain treatment. Medicine tolerance is not the same as addiction.

Medicine tolerance happens when your body gets used to the medicine you're taking. The result is that the dose no longer works as well. Each person's body is different. Many people don't develop a tolerance to opioids. But if tolerance happens to you, under your doctor's care, you can increase your dose, add a new kind of medicine, or change the kind of medicine that you're taking for pain. The goal is to relieve your pain. Increasing the dose to overcome tolerance does not lead to addiction.

Other Ways to Relieve Pain

Medicine doesn't always relieve pain in some people. In these cases, doctors use other treatments to reduce pain:

- **Radiation therapy:** Different forms of radiation energy are used to shrink the tumor and reduce pain. Often one treatment is enough to help with the pain. But sometimes several treatments are needed.

- **Neurosurgery:** A surgeon cuts the nerves that carry pain messages to your brain.

- **Nerve blocks:** Anesthesiologists inject pain medicine into or around the nerve or into the spine to relieve pain.

- **Surgery:** A surgeon removes all or part of a tumor to relieve pain. This is especially helpful when a tumor presses on nerves or other parts of the body.

- **Chemotherapy:** Anticancer drugs are used to reduce the size of a tumor, which may help with the pain.

- **Transcutaneous electric nerve stimulation (TENS):** TENS uses a gentle electric current to relieve pain. The current comes from a small power pack that you can hold or attach to yourself.

Complementary Medicine

Your health care team may also suggest you try other methods to control your pain. However, unlike pain medicine, some of these methods have not been tested in cancer pain studies. But they may help improve your quality of life by helping you with your pain, as well as stress, anxiety, and coping with cancer. Some of these methods are called complementary or integrative. Before trying these therapies, talk with your health care team to make sure it's safe for your type of cancer.

These treatments include everything from cold packs, massage, acupuncture, hypnosis, and imagery to biofeedback, meditation, and therapeutic touch. Once you learn how, you can do some of them by yourself. For others, you may have to see a specialist to receive these treatments. If you do, ask if they are licensed experts.

- **Acupuncture:** Acupuncture is a form of Chinese medicine. It involves inserting very thin, metal needles into the skin at certain points of the body. (Applying pressure to these points with just the thumbs or fingertips is called acupressure.) The goal is to change the body's energy flow so it can heal itself. Make sure that you see a licensed expert when trying acupuncture.

- **Biofeedback:** Biofeedback uses machines to teach you how to control certain body functions, such as heart rate, breathing, and muscle tension.

- **Distraction:** Distraction is simply turning your focus to something other than the pain. It may be used alone to manage mild pain, or used with medicines to help with acute pain, such as pain related to procedures or tests. Or you may try it while waiting for your pain medicine to start working.

- **Heat and cold:** Heat may relieve sore muscles, while cold may numb the pain. However, ask your doctor if it is safe to use either during treatment. Do not use them for more than 10 minutes at a time. And do not use heat or cold over any area where circulation is poor.

- **Hypnosis:** Hypnosis is a trance-like state of relaxed and focused attention. Hypnosis can be used to block the awareness of pain or to help you change the sensation of pain to a more pleasant one. Make sure that you see a licensed expert when trying hypnosis.

- **Imagery:** Imagery is like a daydream. You close your eyes and create images in your mind to help you relax, feel less anxious, and sleep.

- **Massage:** Massage may help reduce pain and anxiety. It may also help with fatigue and stress. For pain, a steady, circular motion near the pain site may work best. Massage may also help relieve tension and increase blood flow. Deep or intense pressure should not be used with cancer patients unless their healthcare team says it's okay to do so. Make sure that you see a licensed expert when trying massage.

- **Meditation:** Meditation is a form of mind-body medicine used to help relax the body and quiet the mind. It may help with pain, as well as with worry, stress, or depression.

- **Relaxation:** Relaxation reduces pain or keeps it from getting worse by getting rid of tension in your muscles. It may help you sleep and give you more energy. Relaxation may also reduce anxiety and help you cope with stress.

Other Methods

Here are some other ways people have tried to find relief from cancer pain.

- **Physical therapy:** Exercises or methods used to help restore strength, increase movement to muscles, and relieve pain. Make sure that you see a licensed expert when trying physical therapy.

- **Reiki:** A form of energy medicine in which the provider places his or her hands on or near the patient. The intent is to transmit what is believed to be a life force energy called qi (or chi).

- **Tai chi:** A mind-body practice that is a series of slow, gentle movements with a focus on breathing and concentration. The thought is that it helps what is believed to be a life force energy (called qi) flow through the body.

- **Yoga:** Systems of stretches and poses with special focus given to breathing. It is meant to calm the nervous system and balance the body, mind, and spirit. There are different types of yoga, so ask about which ones would be best for you.

Chapter 24

Chest Pain

Chapter Contents

Section 24.1—Signs and Symptoms of a Heart Attack............ 254

Section 24.2—Angina.. 256

Section 24.3—Costochondritis.. 264

Section 24.1

Signs and Symptoms of a Heart Attack

"What Are the Signs and Symptoms of a Heart Attack?" National Heart
Lung and Blood Institute (www.nhlbi.nih.gov), March 1, 2011.

Not all heart attacks begin with the sudden, crushing chest pain
that often is shown on TV or in the movies. In one study, for example,
one-third of the patients who had heart attacks had no chest pain.
These patients were more likely to be older, female, or diabetic.

The warning signs and symptoms of a heart attack aren't the same
for everyone. Many heart attacks start slowly as mild pain or discomfort.
Some people don't have symptoms at all. Heart attacks that occur without any symptoms or very mild symptoms are called silent heart attacks.

Chest Pain or Discomfort

The most common heart attack symptom is chest pain or discomfort.
This includes new chest pain or discomfort or a change in the pattern
of existing chest pain or discomfort.

Most heart attacks involve discomfort in the center or left side of
the chest that often lasts for more than a few minutes or goes away
and comes back. The discomfort can feel like uncomfortable pressure,
squeezing, fullness, or pain. The feeling can be mild or severe.

Heart attack pain sometimes feels like indigestion or heartburn.

The symptoms of angina can be similar to the symptoms of a heart
attack. Angina is chest pain that occurs in people who have coronary
heart disease, usually when they're active. Angina pain usually lasts
for only a few minutes and goes away with rest.

Chest pain or discomfort that doesn't go away or changes from its
usual pattern (for example, occurs more often or while you're resting)
can be a sign of a heart attack.

All chest pain should be checked by a doctor.

Other Common Signs and Symptoms

Other common signs and symptoms of a heart attack include new
onset of indicators:

- Upper body discomfort in one or both arms, the back, neck, jaw, or upper part of the stomach

- Shortness of breath, which may occur with or before chest discomfort

- Nausea (feeling sick to your stomach), vomiting, light-headedness or sudden dizziness, or breaking out in a cold sweat

- Sleep problems, fatigue (tiredness), or lack of energy

Not everyone having a heart attack has typical symptoms. If you've already had a heart attack, your symptoms may not be the same for another one. However, some people may have a pattern of symptoms that recur.

The more signs and symptoms you have, the more likely it is that you're having a heart attack.

Act Fast

The signs and symptoms of a heart attack can develop suddenly. However, they also can develop slowly—sometimes within hours, days, or weeks of a heart attack.

Know the warning signs of a heart attack so you can act fast to get treatment for yourself or someone else. The sooner you get emergency help, the less damage your heart will sustain.

Call 9-1-1 for help right away if you think you or someone else may be having a heart attack. You also should call for help if your chest pain doesn't go away as it usually does when you take medicine prescribed for angina.

Do not drive to the hospital or let someone else drive you. Call an ambulance so that medical personnel can begin life-saving treatment on the way to the emergency room.

Section 24.2

Angina

Excerpted from "What Is Angina?" National Heart Lung
and Blood Institute (www.nhlbi.nih.gov), June 1, 2011.

What is angina?

Angina (which can be pronounced "an-JI-nuh" or "AN-juh-nuh") is
chest pain or discomfort that occurs if an area of your heart muscle
doesn't get enough oxygen-rich blood. Angina may feel like pressure
or squeezing in your chest. The pain also can occur in your shoulders,
arms, neck, jaw, or back. Angina pain may even feel like indigestion.

Angina isn't a disease; it's a symptom of an underlying heart problem. Angina usually is a symptom of coronary heart disease (CHD).
CHD is the most common type of heart disease in adults. It occurs if
a waxy substance called plaque builds up on the inner walls of your
coronary arteries. These arteries carry oxygen-rich blood to your heart.
Plaque narrows and stiffens the coronary arteries. This reduces the
flow of oxygen-rich blood to the heart muscle, causing chest pain.
Plaque buildup also makes it more likely that blood clots will form in
your arteries. Blood clots can partially or completely block blood flow,
which can cause a heart attack.

Angina also can be a symptom of coronary microvascular disease
(MVD). This is heart disease that affects the heart's smallest coronary
arteries. In coronary MVD, plaque doesn't create blockages in the arteries like it does in CHD. Studies have shown that coronary MVD is
more likely to affect women than men. Coronary MVD also is called
cardiac syndrome X and nonobstructive CHD.

The major types of angina are stable, unstable, variant (Prinzmet-
al's), and microvascular. Knowing how the types differ is important.
This is because they have different symptoms and require different
treatments.

- Stable angina is the most common type of angina. It occurs when
  the heart is working harder than usual. Stable angina has a regular pattern. ("Pattern" refers to how often the angina occurs, how

severe it is, and what factors trigger it.) If you have stable angina, you can learn its pattern and predict when the pain will occur. The pain usually goes away a few minutes after you rest or take your angina medicine. Stable angina isn't a heart attack, but it suggests that a heart attack is more likely to happen in the future.

- Unstable angina doesn't follow a pattern. It may occur more often and be more severe than stable angina. Unstable angina also can occur with or without physical exertion, and rest or medicine may not relieve the pain. Unstable angina is very dangerous and requires emergency treatment. This type of angina is a sign that a heart attack may happen soon.

- Variant angina is rare. A spasm in a coronary artery causes this type of angina. Variant angina usually occurs while you're at rest, and the pain can be severe. It usually happens between midnight and early morning. Medicine can relieve this type of angina.

- Microvascular angina can be more severe and last longer than other types of angina. Medicine may not relieve this type of angina.

What causes angina?

Angina usually is a symptom of coronary heart disease (CHD). This means that the underlying causes of angina generally are the same as the underlying causes of CHD. Research suggests that CHD starts when certain factors damage the inner layers of the coronary arteries. These factors include smoking, high amounts of certain fats and cholesterol in the blood, high blood pressure, and high amounts of sugar in the blood due to insulin resistance or diabetes.

Plaque may begin to build up where the arteries are damaged. When plaque builds up in the arteries, the condition is called atherosclerosis. Plaque narrows or blocks the arteries, reducing blood flow to the heart muscle. Some plaque is hard and stable and causes the arteries to become narrow and stiff. This can greatly reduce blood flow to the heart and cause angina. Other plaque is soft and more likely to rupture (break open) and cause blood clots. Blood clots can partially or totally block the coronary arteries and cause angina or a heart attack.

Many factors can trigger angina pain, depending on the type of angina you have.

Physical exertion is the most common trigger of stable angina. Severely narrowed arteries may allow enough blood to reach the heart when the demand for oxygen is low, such as when you're sitting. However, with physical exertion—like walking up a hill or climbing

257

stairs—the heart works harder and needs more oxygen. Other triggers of stable angina include emotional stress, exposure to very hot or cold temperatures, heavy meals, and smoking.

Blood clots that partially or totally block an artery cause unstable angina. If plaque in an artery ruptures, blood clots may form. This creates a blockage. A clot may grow large enough to completely block the artery and cause a heart attack. Blood clots may form, partially dissolve, and later form again. Angina can occur each time a clot blocks an artery.

A spasm in a coronary artery causes variant angina. The spasm causes the walls of the artery to tighten and narrow. Blood flow to the heart slows or stops. Variant angina can occur in people who have CHD and in those who don't. The coronary arteries can spasm as a result of exposure to cold, emotional stress, medicines that tighten or narrow blood vessels, smoking, and cocaine use.

Microvascular angina may be a symptom of coronary microvascular disease (MVD). Coronary MVD is heart disease that affects the heart's smallest coronary arteries. Reduced blood flow in the small coronary arteries may cause microvascular angina. Plaque in the arteries, artery spasms, or damaged or diseased artery walls can reduce blood flow through the small coronary arteries.

What are the signs and symptoms of angina?

Pain and discomfort are the main symptoms of angina. Angina often is described as pressure, squeezing, burning, or tightness in the chest. The pain or discomfort usually starts behind the breastbone. Pain from angina also can occur in the arms, shoulders, neck, jaw, throat, or back. The pain may feel like indigestion. Some people say that angina pain is hard to describe or that they can't tell exactly where the pain is coming from.

Signs and symptoms such as nausea (feeling sick to your stomach), fatigue (tiredness), shortness of breath, sweating, light-headedness, and weakness also may occur. Women are more likely to feel discomfort in the neck, jaw, throat, abdomen, or back. Shortness of breath is more common in older people and those who have diabetes. Weakness, dizziness, and confusion can mask the signs and symptoms of angina in elderly people.

Symptoms also vary based on the type of angina you have. Because angina has so many possible symptoms and causes, all chest pain should be checked by a doctor. Chest pain that lasts longer than a few minutes and isn't relieved by rest or angina medicine may be a sign of a heart attack. Call 9-1-1 right away.

With stable angina, the pain or discomfort occurs when the heart must work harder, usually during physical exertion. It doesn't come as a surprise, and episodes of pain tend to be alike. The pain usually lasts a short time (five minutes or less) and is relieved by rest or medicine. The pain may feel like gas or indigestion. It may feel like chest pain that spreads to the arms, back, or other areas.

The pain or discomfort associated with unstable angina often occurs at rest, while sleeping at night, or with little physical exertion. It comes as a surprise and is more severe and lasts longer than stable angina (as long as 30 minutes). The pain usually isn't relieved by rest or medicine and may get worse over time. It may mean that a heart attack will happen soon.

The pain or discomfort associated with variant angina usually occurs at rest and during the night or early morning hours. It tends to be severe and is relieved by medicine.

The pain or discomfort associated with microvascular angina may be more severe and last longer than other types of angina pain. It may occur with shortness of breath, sleep problems, fatigue, and lack of energy. It often is first noticed during routine daily activities and times of mental stress.

How is angina diagnosed?

The most important issues to address when you go to the doctor with chest pain are what's causing the chest pain and whether you're having or are about to have a heart attack.

If you have chest pain, your doctor will want to find out whether it's angina. He or she also will want to know whether the angina is stable or unstable. If it's unstable, you may need emergency medical treatment to try to prevent a heart attack.

To diagnose chest pain as stable or unstable angina, your doctor will do a physical exam, ask about your symptoms, and ask about your risk factors for and your family history of CHD or other heart diseases. Your doctor also may ask questions about your symptoms, such as these:

- What brings on the pain or discomfort and what relieves it?

- What does the pain or discomfort feel like (for example, heaviness or tightness)?

- How often does the pain occur?

- Where do you feel the pain or discomfort?

- How severe is the pain or discomfort?

- How long does the pain or discomfort last?

If your doctor thinks that you have unstable angina or that your angina is related to a serious heart condition, he or she may recommend one or more tests.

EKG: An EKG (electrocardiogram) is a simple, painless test that detects and records the heart's electrical activity. The test shows how fast the heart is beating and its rhythm (steady or irregular). An EKG also records the strength and timing of electrical signals as they pass through the heart. An EKG can show signs of heart damage due to CHD and signs of a previous or current heart attack. However, some people who have angina have normal EKGs.

Stress testing: During stress testing, you exercise to make your heart work hard and beat fast while heart tests are done. If you can't exercise, you may be given medicine to make your heart work hard and beat fast. When your heart is working hard and beating fast, it needs more blood and oxygen. Plaque-narrowed arteries can't supply enough oxygen-rich blood to meet your heart's needs. A stress test can show possible signs and symptoms of CHD, such as abnormal changes in your heart rate or blood pressure, shortness of breath or chest pain, or abnormal changes in your heart rhythm or your heart's electrical activity. As part of some stress tests, pictures are taken of your heart while you exercise and while you rest. These imaging stress tests can show how well blood is flowing in various parts of your heart. They also can show how well your heart pumps blood when it beats.

Chest x-ray: A chest x-ray takes pictures of the organs and structures inside your chest, such as your heart, lungs, and blood vessels. A chest x-ray can reveal signs of heart failure. It also can show signs of lung disorders and other causes of symptoms not related to CHD. However, a chest x-ray alone is not enough to diagnose angina or CHD.

Coronary angiography and cardiac catheterization: Your doctor may recommend coronary angiography if he or she suspects you have CHD. This test uses dye and special x-rays to show the inside of your coronary arteries. To get the dye into your coronary arteries, your doctor will use a procedure called cardiac catheterization. A thin, flexible tube called a catheter is put into a blood vessel in your arm, groin (upper thigh), or neck. The tube is threaded into your coronary arteries, and the dye is released into your bloodstream. Special x-rays are taken while the dye is flowing through your coronary arteries. The dye lets your doctor study the flow of blood through your heart and blood vessels. Cardiac catheterization usually is done in a hospital. You're awake during the procedure. It usually causes little or no pain, although you may feel some soreness in the blood vessel where your doctor inserts the catheter.

Computed tomography angiography: Computed tomography angiography (CTA) uses dye and special x-rays to show blood flow through the coronary arteries. This test is less invasive than coronary angiography with cardiac catheterization. For CTA, a needle connected to an intravenous (IV) line is put into a vein in your hand or arm. Dye is injected through the IV line during the scan. You may have a warm feeling when this happens. The dye highlights your blood vessels on the CT scan pictures. Sticky patches called electrodes are put on your chest. The patches are attached to an EKG machine to record your heart's electrical activity during the scan. The CT scanner is a large machine that has a hollow, circular tube in the middle. You lie on your back on a sliding table. The table slowly slides into the opening of the machine. Inside the scanner, an x-ray tube moves around your body to take pictures of different parts of your heart. A computer puts the pictures together to make a three-dimensional (3D) picture of the whole heart.

Blood tests: Blood tests check the levels of certain fats, cholesterol, sugar, and proteins in your blood. Abnormal levels may show that you have risk factors for CHD. Your doctor may recommend a blood test to check the level of a protein called C-reactive protein (CRP) in your blood. Some studies suggest that high levels of CRP in the blood may increase the risk for CHD and heart attack.

Your doctor also may recommend a blood test to check for low levels of hemoglobin in your blood. Hemoglobin is an iron-rich protein in red blood cells. It helps the blood cells carry oxygen from the lungs to all parts of your body. If your hemoglobin level is low, you may have a condition called anemia.

How is angina treated?

Treatments for angina include lifestyle changes, medicines, medical procedures, cardiac rehabilitation (rehab), and other therapies. The main goals of treatment are to reduce pain and discomfort and how often it occurs and prevent or lower your risk for heart attack and death by treating your underlying heart condition.

Lifestyle changes and medicines may be the only treatments needed if your symptoms are mild and aren't getting worse. If lifestyle changes and medicines don't control angina, you may need medical procedures or cardiac rehab. Unstable angina is an emergency condition that requires treatment in a hospital.

What lifestyle changes can help prevent episodes of angina?

- Slow down or take rest breaks if physical exertion triggers angina.

- Avoid large meals and rich foods that leave you feeling stuffed if heavy meals trigger angina.

- Try to avoid situations that make you upset or stressed if emotional stress triggers angina. Learn ways to handle stress that can't be avoided.

You also can make lifestyle changes that help lower your risk for coronary heart disease. One of the most important changes is to quit smoking. Smoking can damage and tighten blood vessels and raise your risk for CHD. Talk with your doctor about programs and products that can help you quit. Also, try to avoid secondhand smoke.

Following a healthy diet is another important lifestyle change. A healthy diet can prevent or reduce high blood pressure and high blood cholesterol and help you maintain a healthy weight. A healthy diet includes a variety of fruits and vegetables (including beans and peas). It also includes whole grains, lean meats, poultry without skin, seafood, and fat-free or low-fat milk and dairy products. A healthy diet also is low in sodium (salt), added sugars, solid fats, and refined grains.

Other important lifestyle changes include being physically active and maintaining a healthy weight. Check with your doctor to find out how much and what kinds of activity are safe for you. If you're overweight or obese, work with your doctor to create a reasonable weight-loss plan. Also, be sure to take all medicines as your doctor prescribes, especially if you have diabetes.

What medicines are used to treat angina?

Nitrates are the medicines most commonly used to treat angina. They relax and widen blood vessels. This allows more blood to flow to the heart, while reducing the heart's workload.

Nitroglycerin is the most commonly used nitrate for angina. Nitroglycerin that dissolves under your tongue or between your cheek and gum is used to relieve angina episodes. Nitroglycerin pills and skin patches are used to prevent angina episodes. However, pills and skin patches act too slowly to relieve pain during an angina attack.

Other medicines also are used to treat angina, such as beta blockers, calcium channel blockers, ACE inhibitors, oral antiplatelet medicines, or anticoagulants (blood thinners). These medicines can help lower blood pressure and cholesterol levels, slow the heart rate, relax blood vessels, reduce strain on the heart, and prevent blood clots from forming. People who have stable angina may be advised to get annual flu shots.

What medical procedures are used to treat angina?

If lifestyle changes and medicines don't control angina, you may need a medical procedure to treat the underlying heart disease. Both angioplasty and coronary artery bypass grafting (CABG) are commonly used to treat heart disease.

Angioplasty opens blocked or narrowed coronary arteries. During angioplasty, a thin tube with a balloon or other device on the end is threaded through a blood vessel to the narrowed or blocked coronary artery. Once in place, the balloon is inflated to push the plaque outward against the wall of the artery. This widens the artery and restores blood flow. Angioplasty can improve blood flow to your heart and relieve chest pain. A small mesh tube called a stent usually is placed in the artery to help keep it open after the procedure.

During CABG, healthy arteries or veins taken from other areas in your body are used to bypass (that is, go around) your narrowed coronary arteries. Bypass surgery can improve blood flow to your heart, relieve chest pain, and possibly prevent a heart attack. You will work with your doctor to decide which treatment is better for you.

What is cardiac rehabilitation?

Your doctor may recommend cardiac rehabilitation (rehab) for angina or after angioplasty, CABG, or a heart attack. Cardiac rehab is a medically supervised program that can help improve the health and well-being of people who have heart problems. The cardiac rehab team may include doctors, nurses, exercise specialists, physical and occupational therapists, dietitians or nutritionists, and psychologists or other mental health specialists. Rehab has two parts:

- **Exercise training:** This part helps you learn how to exercise safely, strengthen your muscles, and improve your stamina. Your exercise plan will be based on your personal abilities, needs, and interests.

- **Education, counseling, and training:** This part of rehab helps you understand your heart condition and find ways to reduce your risk for future heart problems. The rehab team will help you learn how to adjust to a new lifestyle and deal with your fears about the future.

What is enhanced external counterpulsation therapy?

Enhanced external counterpulsation (EECP) therapy is helpful for some people who have angina. Large cuffs, similar to blood pressure cuffs, are put on your legs. The cuffs are inflated and deflated in sync with your heartbeat. EECP therapy improves the flow of oxygen-rich blood to your heart muscle and helps relieve angina. You typically get 35 one-hour treatments over seven weeks.

Section 24.3

Costochondritis

"Costochondritis," October 2011, reprinted with permission from www.kidshealth.org. This information was provided by KidsHealth®, one of the largest resources online for medically reviewed health information written for parents, kids, and teens. For more articles like this, visit www.KidsHealth.org, or www.TeensHealth.org. Copyright © 1995-2012 The Nemours Foundation. All rights reserved.

A few months into the school year, Sophie noticed a sharp pain in her chest. She freaked out, worried she was having a heart attack. Sophie and her mom called the doctor to find out what was going on.

The doctor asked Sophie to come into the office. He asked about her symptoms, what she'd been doing before she felt the pain, and what kinds of exercising she'd been doing. The doctor told Sophie she had a condition called costochondritis.

What is costochondritis?

Costochondritis is an inflammation of the cartilage that attaches a rib to your breastbone (sternum). Costochondritis is a fairly common cause of chest pain. It usually affects girls more than guys.

The sternum is the hard bone that goes down the center of your chest, from the bottom of your neck to the top of your abdomen. Your ribs are connected to the sternum by rubbery cartilage at points called costosternal joints. These joints are where someone with costochondritis feels pain. Costochondritis can affect one or more of these joints.

Costochondritis can hurt, but it's really harmless. It usually goes away on its own after a week or so. Sometimes it can last for a few months, though.

You may hear medical staff call costochondritis by other names—like chest wall pain or costosternal syndrome—but it's all the same thing.

Top Things to Know about Costochondritis

- It's a non-serious condition caused by an inflammation of cartilage in the chest.

- Costochondritis can be scary because it can cause sharp pain in the chest that may make people think they are having a heart attack.

- If you have sharp chest pain that doesn't go away, call a doctor or get to an emergency room just in case it's a sign of something serious.

What causes costochondritis?

It's not always obvious what causes costochondritis. Doctors think it's usually caused by hard exercise or a minor injury from something like lifting a heavy object or coughing.

What are the signs?

The main signs of costochondritis are pain and tenderness on one side of the chest. The pain is usually sharp. It's often on the left side of the sternum (although it is possible to have pain on both sides).

If you have costochondritis, the pain may get worse when you take deep breaths, cough, move your upper body, or press on the sore area. The pain may lessen when you stop moving or take shallower breaths, but it usually doesn't go away entirely.

Costochondritis pain can be scary. Lots of teens worry that they're having a heart attack. So it can help to remember that heart attacks are extremely rare in teens. You'll still want to get checked out by a doctor to find out what's going on, though.

How is it diagnosed?

If you have sharp chest pain that doesn't go away, call a doctor or go to a hospital emergency room. In rare cases, chest pain can be an emergency situation that requires immediate medical attention.

To diagnose costochondritis, a doctor or nurse practitioner will ask questions about the pain, then feel along your sternum for areas that are tender.

It's usually not possible to see costochondritis on chest x-rays or other imaging tests. Still, your doctor might order these tests to rule out other possible causes of chest pain, such as pneumonia.

How is it treated?

Costochondritis usually goes away on its own within a few days or weeks, but in some cases it can go on longer. To help ease the pain until costochondritis goes away, doctors may recommend over-the-counter pain medications such as ibuprofen.

What can you do at home?

Here are some things doctors recommend for dealing with costochondritis:

- Try to get plenty of rest.

- Avoid activities that make the pain worse.

- When you're feeling better, you can do some of your usual activities. But be careful not to overdo things. Too much exercise can sometimes make costochondritis pain worse.

- Using a heating pad on the low setting or putting warm compresses on the painful area can provide some relief.

Can you prevent costochondritis?

It's not really possible to prevent costochondritis, since it's not always clear what causes it. You can take steps to avoid some of the known causes, though:

- If you know that some activities may cause you to have costochondritis-like pain, do your best to avoid them. You might want to work with a doctor or trainer to come up with an exercise program that doesn't cause symptoms to flare up.

- Minimize the amount of heavy lifting you do.

- If you have to carry lots of books, use a backpack or a bookbag that spreads the weight out evenly. Students who frequently carry heavy school bags may have an increased risk of costochondritis, especially if they carry a bag over one shoulder.

The good news about costochondritis is that it's not serious. But it definitely can be scary. That's why it helps to talk to a doctor. That way, if the doctor says you have costochondritis, you can relax and take the steps you need to feel better.

Chapter 25

Dental and Facial Pain

Chapter Contents

Section 25.1—Tooth Pain.. 268

Section 25.2—Temporomandibular Joint Disorders 270

Section 25.3—Trigeminal Neuralgia... 274

Section 25.1

Tooth Pain

"Tooth Pain," © 2013 American Association of Endodontists (www.aae.org). All rights reserved. Reprinted with permission.

Symptom: Momentary sensitivity to hot or cold foods.

Possible problem: If this discomfort lasts only moments, sensitivity to hot and cold foods generally does not signal a serious problem. The sensitivity may be caused by a small decay, a loose filling, or by minimal gum recession that exposes small areas of the root surface.

What to do: Try using toothpastes made for sensitive teeth. Brush up and down with a soft brush; brushing sideways wears away exposed root surfaces. If this is unsuccessful, see your general dentist. If the sensitivity is coming from a decay, you should see your general dentist.

Symptom: Sensitivity to hot or cold foods after dental treatment.

Possible problem: Dental work may inflame the pulp inside the tooth causing temporary sensitivity.

What to do: Wait two to four weeks. If the pain persists or worsens, see your general dentist.

Symptom: Sharp pain when biting down on food.

Possible problem: There are several possible causes of this type of pain: decay, a loose filling, or crack in the tooth. There may also be damage to the pulp tissue inside the tooth.

What to do: See a dentist for evaluation. If the problem is pulp tissue damage, your dentist may send you to an endodontist. Endodontists are dentists who specialize in pulp-related procedures. Your endodontist will perform a procedure that cleans out the damaged pulp and fills and seals the remaining space. This procedure is commonly called a "root canal."

Symptom: **Lingering pain after eating hot or cold foods.**

Possible problem: This probably means the pulp has been damaged by deep decay or physical trauma.

What to do: See your dentist or endodontist to save the tooth with root canal treatment.

Symptom: **Constant and severe pain and pressure, swelling of gum and sensitivity to touch.**

Possible problem: A tooth may have become abscessed, causing an infection in the surrounding gingival tissue and bone.

What to do: See your endodontist for evaluation and treatment to relieve the pain and save the tooth.

Symptom: **Dull ache and pressure in upper teeth and jaw.**

Possible problem: The pain of a sinus headache is often felt in the face and teeth. Grinding of teeth, a condition known as bruxism, can also cause this type of ache.

What to do: For sinus headache, see your physician. For bruxism, consult your dentist. If pain is severe and chronic, see your endodontist for evaluation.

Section 25.2

Temporomandibular Joint Disorders

Excerpted from "TMJ Disorders," National Institute of Dental and Cranio-facial Research (www.nidcr.nih.gov), NIH Pub. No. 13-3487, January 2013.

Temporomandibular joint and muscle disorders, commonly called "TMJ," are a group of conditions that cause pain and dysfunction in the jaw joint and the muscles that control jaw movement. We don't know for certain how many people have TMJ disorders, but some estimates suggest that over 10 million Americans are affected. The condition appears to be more common in women than men.

For most people, pain in the area of the jaw joint or muscles does not signal a serious problem. Generally, discomfort from these conditions is occasional and temporary, often occurring in cycles. The pain eventually goes away with little or no treatment. Some people, however, develop significant, long-term symptoms.

If you have questions about TMJ disorders, you are not alone. Researchers, too, are looking for answers to what causes these conditions and what the best treatments are. Until we have scientific evidence for safe and effective treatments, it's important to avoid, when possible, procedures that can cause permanent changes in your bite or jaw.

What is the temporomandibular joint?

The temporomandibular joint connects the lower jaw, called the mandible, to the bone at the side of the head—the temporal bone. If you place your fingers just in front of your ears and open your mouth, you can feel the joints. Because these joints are flexible, the jaw can move smoothly up and down and side to side, enabling us to talk, chew and yawn. Muscles attached to and surrounding the jaw joint control its position and movement.

When we open our mouths, the rounded ends of the lower jaw, called condyles, glide along the joint socket of the temporal bone. The condyles slide back to their original position when we close our mouths. To keep this motion smooth, a soft disc lies between the condyle and the temporal bone. This disc absorbs shocks to the jaw joint from chewing and other movements.

The temporomandibular joint is different from the body's other joints. The combination of hinge and sliding motions makes this joint among the most complicated in the body. Also, the tissues that make up the temporomandibular joint differ from other load-bearing joints, like the knee or hip. Because of its complex movement and unique makeup, the jaw joint and its controlling muscles can pose a tremendous challenge to both patients and health care providers when problems arise.

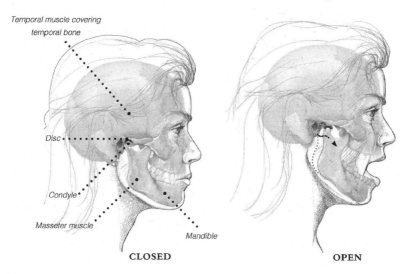

Figure 25.1. The Temporomandibular Joint

What are TMJ disorders?

Disorders of the jaw joint and chewing muscles—and how people respond to them—vary widely. Researchers generally agree that the conditions fall into three main categories:

- Myofascial pain involves discomfort or pain in the muscles that control jaw function.

- Internal derangement of the joint involves a displaced disc, dislocated jaw, or injury to the condyle.

- Arthritis refers to a group of degenerative/inflammatory joint disorders that can affect the temporomandibular joint.

A person may have one or more of these conditions at the same time. Some people have other health problems that co-exist with TMJ disorders, such as chronic fatigue syndrome, sleep disturbances, or fibromyalgia, a painful condition that affects muscles and other soft tissues throughout the body. These disorders share some common symptoms, which suggests that they may share similar underlying mechanisms of disease. However, it is not known whether they have a common cause.

Rheumatic disease, such as arthritis, may also affect the temporomandibular joint as a secondary condition. Rheumatic diseases refer to a large group of disorders that cause pain, inflammation, and stiffness in the joints, muscles, and bone. Arthritis and some TMJ disorders involve inflammation of the tissues that line the joints. The exact relationship between these conditions is not known.

How jaw joint and muscle disorders progress is not clear. Symptoms worsen and ease over time, but what causes these changes is not known. Most people have relatively mild forms of the disorder. Their symptoms improve significantly, or disappear spontaneously, within weeks or months. For others, the condition causes long-term, persistent and debilitating pain.

What are the signs and symptoms?

A variety of symptoms may be linked to TMJ disorders. Pain, particularly in the chewing muscles and/or jaw joint, is the most common symptom. Other likely symptoms include radiating pain in the face, jaw, or neck; jaw muscle stiffness; limited movement or locking of the jaw; painful clicking, popping or grating in the jaw joint when opening or closing the mouth; and a change in the way the upper and lower teeth fit together.

How are TMJ disorders treated?

Because more studies are needed on the safety and effectiveness of most treatments for jaw joint and muscle disorders, experts strongly recommend using the most conservative, reversible treatments possible. Conservative treatments do not invade the tissues of the face, jaw, or joint, or involve surgery. Reversible treatments do not cause permanent changes in the structure or position of the jaw or teeth. Even when TMJ disorders have become persistent, most patients still do not need aggressive types of treatment.

Because the most common jaw joint and muscle problems are temporary and do not get worse, simple treatment may be all that is necessary to relieve discomfort. There are steps you can take that may be helpful in easing symptoms, such as eating soft foods, applying ice packs, avoiding extreme jaw movements (such as wide yawning, loud singing, and gum chewing), learning techniques for relaxing and reducing stress, and practicing gentle jaw stretching and relaxing exercises that may help increase jaw movement. Your health care provider or a physical therapist can recommend exercises if appropriate for your particular condition.

For many people with TMJ disorders, short-term use of over-the-counter pain medicines or nonsteroidal anti-inflammatory drugs (NSAIDs), such as ibuprofen, may provide temporary relief from jaw discomfort. When necessary, your dentist or physician can prescribe stronger pain or anti-inflammatory medications, muscle relaxants, or anti-depressants to help ease symptoms.

Your physician or dentist may recommend an oral appliance, also called a stabilization splint or bite guard, which is a plastic guard that fits over the upper or lower teeth. Stabilization splints are the most widely used treatments for TMJ disorders. Studies of their effectiveness in providing pain relief, however, have been inconclusive. If a stabilization splint is recommended, it should be used only for a short time and should not cause permanent changes in the bite. If a splint causes or increases pain, or affects your bite, stop using it and see your health care provider.

The conservative, reversible treatments described are useful for temporary relief of pain—they are not cures for TMJ disorders. If symptoms continue over time, come back often, or worsen, tell your doctor.

About Botox: Botox (botulinum toxin type A) is a drug made from the same bacterium that causes food poisoning. Used in small doses, Botox injections can actually help alleviate some health problems and have been approved by the U.S. Food and Drug Administration (FDA) for certain disorders. However, Botox is currently not approved by the FDA for use in TMJ disorders. Results from recent clinical studies are inconclusive regarding the effectiveness of Botox for treatment of chronic TMJ disorders. Additional research is under way to learn how Botox specifically affects jaw muscles and their nerves. The findings will help determine if this drug may be useful in treating TMJ disorders.

What are irreversible treatments?

Irreversible treatments that have not been proven to be effective—and may make the problem worse—include orthodontics to change the bite; crown and bridge work to balance the bite; grinding down teeth to bring the bite into balance, called "occlusal adjustment"; and repositioning splints, also called orthotics, which permanently alter the bite.

Surgery: Other types of treatments, such as surgical procedures, invade the tissues. Surgical treatments are controversial, often irreversible, and should be avoided where possible. There have been no long-term clinical trials to study the safety and effectiveness of surgical treatments for TMJ disorders. Nor are there standards to identify people who would most likely benefit from surgery. Failure to respond to conservative treatments,

273

for example, does not automatically mean that surgery is necessary. If surgery is recommended, be sure to have the doctor explain to you, in words you can understand, the reason for the treatment, the risks involved, and other types of treatment that may be available.

Implants: Surgical replacement of jaw joints with artificial implants may cause severe pain and permanent jaw damage. Some of these devices may fail to function properly or may break apart in the jaw over time. If you have already had temporomandibular joint surgery, be very cautious about considering additional operations. Persons undergoing multiple surgeries on the jaw joint generally have a poor outlook for normal, pain-free joint function. Before undergoing any surgery on the jaw joint, it is extremely important to get other independent opinions and to fully understand the risks.

Report problems: The U.S. Food and Drug Administration (FDA) monitors the safety and effectiveness of medical devices implanted in the body, including artificial jaw joint implants. Patients and their health care providers can report serious problems with TMJ implants to the FDA through MedWatch at www.fda.gov/medwatch or telephone toll-free at 800-332-1088.

Section 25.3

Trigeminal Neuralgia

Excerpted from "Trigeminal Neuralgia Fact Sheet," National Institute of Neurological Disorders and Stroke (www.ninds.nih.gov), NIH Pub. No. 06-5116, updated November 30, 2012.

What is trigeminal neuralgia?

Trigeminal neuralgia (TN), also called tic douloureux, is a chronic pain condition that affects the trigeminal (or 5th cranial) nerve, one of the largest nerves in the head. The disorder causes extreme, sporadic, sudden burning or shock-like face pain that lasts anywhere from a few seconds to as long as two minutes per episode. These attacks can occur in quick succession. The intensity of pain can be physically and mentally incapacitating.

The trigeminal nerve is one of 12 pairs of cranial nerves that originate at the base of the brain. The nerve has three branches that conduct sensations from the upper, middle, and lower portions of the face, as well as the oral cavity, to the brain. The ophthalmic, or upper, branch supplies sensation to most of the scalp, forehead, and front of the head. The maxillary, or middle, branch passes through the cheek, upper jaw, top lip, teeth and gums, and to the side of the nose. The nerve's mandibular, or lower, branch passes through the lower jaw, teeth, gums, and bottom lip. More than one nerve branch can be affected by the disorder.

What causes trigeminal neuralgia?

The presumed cause of TN is a blood vessel pressing on the trigeminal nerve as it exits the brainstem. This compression causes the wearing away of the protective coating around the nerve (the myelin sheath). TN may be part of the normal aging process—as blood vessels lengthen they can come to rest and pulsate against a nerve. TN symptoms can also occur in people with multiple sclerosis, a disease caused by the deterioration of myelin throughout the body, or may be caused by damage to the myelin sheath by compression from a tumor. This deterioration causes the nerve to send abnormal signals to the brain. In some cases the cause is unknown.

What are its symptoms?

TN is characterized by a sudden, severe, electric shock-like, stabbing pain that is typically felt on one side of the jaw or cheek. Pain may occur on both sides of the face, although not at the same time. The attacks of pain, which generally last several seconds and may repeat in quick succession, come and go throughout the day. These episodes can last for days, weeks, or months at a time and then disappear for months or years. In the days before an episode begins, some patients may experience a tingling or numbing sensation or a somewhat constant and aching pain.

The intense flashes of pain can be triggered by vibration or contact with the cheek (such as when shaving, washing the face, or applying makeup), brushing teeth, eating, drinking, talking, or being exposed to the wind. The pain may affect a small area of the face or may spread. The bouts of pain rarely occur at night, when the patient is sleeping.

Patients are considered to have type 1 TN if more than 50 percent of the pain they experience is sudden, intermittent, sharp and stabbing, or shock-like. These patients may also have some burning sensation. Type 2 TN involves pain that is constant, aching, or burning more than 50 percent of the time.

TN is typified by attacks that stop for a period of time and then come back. The attacks often worsen over time, with fewer and shorter pain-free periods before they recur. The disorder is not fatal, but can be debilitating. Due to the intensity of the pain, some patients may avoid daily activities because they fear an impending attack.

How is TN diagnosed?

There is no single test to diagnose TN. Diagnosis is generally based on the patient's medical history and description of symptoms, a physical exam, and a thorough neurological examination by a physician. Other disorders, such as post-herpetic neuralgia, can cause similar facial pain, as do syndromes such as cluster headaches. Injury to the trigeminal nerve (perhaps the result of sinus surgery, oral surgery, stroke, or facial trauma) may produce neuropathic pain, which is characterized by dull, burning, and boring pain. Because of overlapping symptoms, and the large number of conditions that can cause facial pain, obtaining a correct diagnosis is difficult, but finding the cause of the pain is important as the treatments for different types of pain may differ.

Most TN patients undergo a standard magnetic resonance imaging scan to rule out a tumor or multiple sclerosis as the cause of their pain. This scan may or may not clearly show a blood vessel on the nerve. Magnetic resonance angiography, which can trace a colored dye that is injected into the bloodstream prior to the scan, can more clearly show blood vessel problems and any compression of the trigeminal nerve close to the brainstem.

How is it treated?

Treatment options include medicines, surgery, and complementary approaches.

Anticonvulsant medicines—used to block nerve firing—are generally effective in treating TN. These drugs include carbamazepine, oxcarbazepine, topiramate, clonazepam, phenytoin, lamotrigine, and valproic acid. Gabapentin or baclofen can be used as a second drug to treat TN and may be given in combination with other anticonvulsants.

Tricyclic antidepressants such as amitriptyline or nortriptyline are used to treat pain described as constant, burning, or aching. Typical analgesics and opioids are not usually helpful in treating the sharp, recurring pain caused by TN. If medication fails to relieve pain or produces intolerable side effects such as excess fatigue, surgical treatment may be recommended.

Several neurosurgical procedures are available to treat TN. The choice among the various types depends on the patient's preference, physical well-being, previous surgeries, presence of multiple sclerosis, and area of trigeminal nerve involvement (particularly when the upper/ophthalmic branch is involved). Some procedures are done on an outpatient basis, while others may involve a more complex operation that is performed under general anesthesia. Some degree of facial numbness is expected after most of these procedures, and TN might return despite the procedure's initial success. Depending on the procedure, other surgical risks include hearing loss, balance problems, infection, and stroke.

A rhizotomy is a procedure in which select nerve fibers are destroyed to block pain. A rhizotomy for TN causes some degree of permanent sensory loss and facial numbness. Several forms of rhizotomy are available to treat TN:

• Balloon compression works by injuring the insulation on nerves that are involved with the sensation of light touch on the face. The procedure is performed in an operating room under general anesthesia. A tube called a cannula is inserted through the cheek and guided to where one branch of the trigeminal nerve passes through the base of the skull. A soft catheter with a balloon tip is threaded through the cannula and the balloon is inflated to squeeze part of the nerve against the hard edge of the brain covering (the dura) and the skull. After one minute the balloon is deflated and removed, along with the catheter and cannula. Balloon compression is generally an outpatient procedure, although sometimes the patient may be kept in the hospital overnight.

• Glycerol injection is generally an outpatient procedure in which the patient is sedated intravenously. A thin needle is passed through the cheek, next to the mouth, and guided through the opening in the base of the skull to where all three branches of the trigeminal nerve come together. The glycerol injection bathes the ganglion (the central part of the nerve from which the nerve impulses are transmitted) and damages the insulation of trigeminal nerve fibers.

• Radiofrequency thermal lesioning is usually performed on an outpatient basis. The patient is anesthetized and a hollow needle is passed through the cheek to where the trigeminal nerve exits through a hole at the base of the skull. The patient is awakened and a small electrical current is passed through the needle, causing tingling. When the needle is positioned so that the tingling occurs in the area of TN pain, the patient is then sedated and that part of the nerve is gradually heated with an electrode, injuring the nerve fibers. The electrode and needle are then removed and the patient is awakened.

- Stereotactic radiosurgery uses computer imaging to direct highly focused beams of radiation at the site where the trigeminal nerve exits the brainstem. This causes the slow formation of a lesion on the nerve that disrupts the transmission of pain signals to the brain. Pain relief from this procedure may take several months. Patients usually leave the hospital the same day or the next day following treatment.

Microvascular decompression is the most invasive of all surgeries for TN, but it also offers the lowest probability that pain will return. This inpatient procedure, which is performed under general anesthesia, requires that a small opening be made behind the ear. While viewing the trigeminal nerve through a microscope, the surgeon moves away the vessels that are compressing the nerve and places a soft cushion between the nerve and the vessels. Unlike rhizotomies, there is usually no numbness in the face after this surgery. Patients generally recuperate for several days in the hospital following the procedure.

A neurectomy, which involves cutting part of the nerve, may be performed during microvascular decompression if no vessel is found to be pressing on the trigeminal nerve. Neurectomies may also be performed by cutting branches of the trigeminal nerve in the face. When done during microvascular decompression, a neurectomy will cause permanent numbness in the area of the face that is supplied by the nerve or nerve branch that is cut. However, when the operation is performed in the face, the nerve may grow back and in time sensation may return.

Some patients choose to manage TN using complementary techniques, usually in combination with drug treatment. These therapies offer varying degrees of success. Options include acupuncture, biofeedback, vitamin therapy, nutritional therapy, and electrical stimulation of the nerves.

Chapter 26

Ear Pain

A Close Look at the Ear

Next to the common cold, ear infections are the most commonly diagnosed childhood illness in the United States. More than three out of four kids have had at least one ear infection by the time they reach three years of age.

To understand how ear infections develop, let's review how the ear works.

Think about how you can feel speakers vibrate as you listen to your favorite CD in the car or how you feel your throat vibrate when you speak. Sound, which is made up of invisible waves of energy, causes these vibrations. Every time you hear a sound, the various structures of the ear have to work together to make sure the information gets to the brain.

The ear is responsible for hearing and balance and is made up of three parts—the outer ear, middle ear, and inner ear. Hearing begins when sound waves that travel through the air reach the outer ear, or pinna, which is the part of the ear that's visible. The sound waves then travel from the pinna through the ear canal to the middle ear, which includes the eardrum (a thin layer of tissue) and three tiny bones called ossicles. When the eardrum vibrates, the ossicles amplify these vibrations and carry them to the inner ear.

"Middle Ear Infections," October 2011, reprinted with permission from www .kids health.org. This information was provided by KidsHealth®, one of the largest resources online for medically reviewed health information written for parents, kids, and teens. For more articles like this, visit www.KidsHealth.org, or www.Teens Health.org. Copyright © 1995-2012 The Nemours Foundation. All rights reserved.

The inner ear translates the vibrations into electric signals and sends them to the auditory nerve, which connects to the brain. When these nerve impulses reach the brain, they're interpreted as sound.

The Eustachian Tube

To function properly, the middle ear must be at the same pressure as the outside world. This is taken care of by the eustachian tube, a small passage that connects the middle ear to the back of the throat behind the nose.

By letting air reach the middle ear, the eustachian tube equalizes the air pressure in the middle ear to the outside air pressure. (When your ears "pop" while yawning or swallowing, the eustachian tubes are adjusting the air pressure in your middle ears.) The eustachian tube also allows for drainage of mucus from the middle ear into the throat.

Sometimes, the eustachian tube may malfunction. For example, when someone has a cold or an allergy affecting the nasal passages, the eustachian tube may become blocked by congestion in its lining or by mucus within the tube. This blockage will allow fluid to build up within the normally air-filled middle ear.

Bacteria or viruses that have entered the middle ear through the eustachian tube also can get trapped in this way. These germs can breed in the trapped fluid, eventually leading to an ear infection.

About Middle Ear Infections

Inflammation in the middle ear area is known as otitis media. When referring to an ear infection, doctors most likely mean "acute otitis media" rather than the common ear infection called swimmer's ear, or otitis externa.

Acute otitis media is the presence of fluid, typically pus, in the middle ear with symptoms of pain, redness of the eardrum, and possible fever.

Other forms of otitis media are either more chronic (fluid is in the middle ear for six or more weeks) or the fluid in the middle ear is temporary and not necessarily infected (called otitis media with effusion).

Doctors try to distinguish between the different forms of otitis because this affects treatment options. Not all forms of otitis need to be treated with antibiotics.

Causes

Kids develop ear infections more frequently in the first two to four years of life for several reasons:

- Their eustachian tubes are shorter and more horizontal than those of adults, which allows bacteria and viruses to find their way into the middle ear more easily. Their tubes are also narrower and less stiff, which makes them more prone to blockage.

- The adenoids, which are gland-like structures located in the back of the upper throat near the eustachian tubes, are large in children and can interfere with the opening of the eustachian tubes.

A number of other factors can contribute to kids getting ear infections, such as exposure to cigarette smoke, bottle-feeding, and day-care attendance.

Ear infections also occur more commonly in boys than girls, in kids whose families have a history of ear infections, and during the winter season when upper respiratory tract infections or colds are frequent.

Signs and Symptoms

The signs and symptoms of acute otitis media may range from very mild to severe:

- The fluid in the middle ear may push on the eardrum, causing ear pain. An older child may complain of an earache, but a younger child may tug at the ear or simply act irritable and cry more than usual.

- Lying down, chewing, and sucking can also cause painful pressure changes in the middle ear, so a child may eat less than normal or have trouble sleeping.

- If the pressure from the fluid buildup is high enough, it can cause the eardrum to rupture, resulting in drainage of fluid from the ear. This releases the pressure behind the eardrum, usually bringing relief from the pain.

Signs of Hearing Difficulties

Fluid buildup in the middle ear also blocks sound, which can lead to temporary hearing difficulties. A child may:

- not respond to soft sounds
- turn up the television or radio
- talk louder
- appear to be inattentive at school

Other symptoms of acute otitis media can include:

- fever
- vomiting
- nausea
- dizziness

However, otitis media with effusion often has no symptoms. In some kids, the fluid that's in the middle ear may create a sensation of ear fullness or "popping." As with acute otitis media, the fluid behind the eardrum can block sound, so mild temporary hearing loss can happen, but might not be obvious.

Ear infections are also frequently associated with upper respiratory tract infections and, therefore, with their common signs and symptoms, such as a runny or stuffy nose or a cough.

Contagiousness

Ear infections are not contagious, though the cold that may lead to one can be.

Duration

Middle ear infections often go away on their own within two or three days, even without any specific treatment. If your doctor decides to prescribe antibiotics, a 10-day course is usually recommended.

For kids six years of age and older with a mild to moderate infection, a shortened course of antibiotics (five to seven days) may be appropriate.

But even after antibiotic treatment for an episode of acute otitis media, fluid may remain in the middle ear for up to several months.

Diagnosis and Treatment

A child who might have an ear infection should visit a doctor, who should be able to make a diagnosis by taking a medical history and doing a physical exam.

To examine the ear, doctors use an otoscope, a small instrument similar to a flashlight, through which they can see the eardrum.

There's no single best approach for treating all middle ear infections. In deciding how to manage your child's ear infection, a doctor will consider many factors, including:

- the type and severity of the ear infection
- how often your child has ear infections
- how long this infection has lasted

- your child's age

- risk factors your child may have

- whether the infection affects your child's hearing

The fact that most ear infections can clear on their own has led a number of physician associations to recommend a "wait-and-see" approach, which involves giving the child pain relief without antibiotics for a few days.

Another important reason to consider this type of approach are the limitations of antibiotics, which:

- won't help an infection caused by a virus

- won't eliminate middle ear fluid

- may cause side effects

- typically do not relieve pain in the first 24 hours and have only a minimal effect after that

Also, frequent use of antibiotics can lead to the development of antibiotic-resistant bacteria, which can be much more difficult to treat.

When Antibiotics Are Required

However, kids who get a lot of ear infections may be prescribed daily antibiotics by their doctor to help prevent future infections. And younger children or those with more severe illness may require antibiotics right from the start.

The "wait-and-see" approach also might not apply to children with other concerns, such as cleft palate, genetic conditions such as Down syndrome, underlying illnesses such as immune system disorders, or a history of recurrent acute otitis media.

Kids with persistent otitis media with effusion (lasting longer than three months) should be reexamined periodically (every three to six months) by their doctors. Often, though, even these kids won't require treatment.

Whether or not the choice is made to treat with antibiotics, you can help to reduce the discomfort of an ear infection by using acetaminophen or ibuprofen for pain and fever as needed. Your doctor may also recommend using pain-relieving eardrops as long as the eardrum hasn't ruptured.

But certain children, such as those with persistent hearing loss or speech delay, may require ear tube surgery. In some cases, an ear, nose, and throat doctor will suggest surgically inserting tubes (called tympanostomy tubes) in the tympanic membrane. This allows fluid to drain from the middle ear and helps equalize the pressure in the ear because the eustachian tube is unable to.

Prevention

Some factors associated with the development of ear infections can't be changed (such as family history of frequent ear infections), but certain lifestyle choices can minimize the risk for kids:

- Breastfeed infants for at least six months to help to prevent the development of early episodes of ear infections. If a child is bottle-fed, hold the infant at an angle rather than allowing the child to lie down with the bottle.

- Prevent exposure to secondhand smoke, which can increase the frequency and severity of ear infections.

- Reduce exposure, if possible, to large groups of other kids, such as in child-care centers. Because multiple upper respiratory infections may also lead to frequent ear infections, limiting exposure may result in less frequent colds early on and, therefore, fewer ear infections.

- Both parents and kids should practice good hand washing. This is one of the most important ways to decrease person-to-person transmission of the germs that can cause colds and, therefore, ear infections.

- Keep children's immunizations up-to-date, because certain vaccines can help prevent ear infections.

Also be aware that research has shown that cold and allergy medications, such as antihistamines and decongestants, aren't helpful in preventing ear infections.

When to Call the Doctor

Although quite rare, ear infections that don't go away or severe repeated middle ear infections can lead to complications, including spread of the infection to nearby bones. So kids with an earache or a sense of fullness in the ear, especially when combined with fever, should be evaluated by their doctors if they aren't improving.

Other conditions can also result in earaches, such as teething, a foreign object in the ear, or hard earwax. Consult your doctor to help determine the cause of the discomfort and how to treat it.

Chapter 27

Gastrointestinal Pain

Chapter Contents

Section 27.1—Abdominal Adhesions 286

Section 27.2—Appendicitis 288

Section 27.3—Crohn Disease 291

Section 27.4—Diverticulosis and Diverticulitis 294

Section 27.5—Gallstones 297

Section 27.6—Gas in the Digestive Tract 299

Section 27.7—Gastroesophageal Reflux Disease
(Heartburn) 302

Section 27.8—Irritable Bowel Syndrome 305

Section 27.9—Pancreatitis 309

Section 27.1

Abdominal Adhesions

Excerpted from "Abdominal Adhesions," National Digestive
Diseases Information Clearinghouse (http://digestive.niddk.nih.gov),
NIH Pub. No. 09-5037, updated March 20, 2012.

What are abdominal adhesions?

Abdominal adhesions are bands of tissue that form between abdominal tissues and organs. Normally, internal tissues and organs have slippery surfaces, which allow them to shift easily as the body moves. Adhesions cause tissues and organs to stick together.

Although most adhesions cause no symptoms or problems, others cause chronic abdominal or pelvic pain. Adhesions are also a major cause of intestinal obstruction and female infertility.

Abdominal surgery is the most frequent cause of abdominal adhesions. Almost everyone who undergoes abdominal surgery develops adhesions; however, the risk is greater after operations on the lower abdomen and pelvis, including bowel and gynecological surgeries. Adhesions can become larger and tighter as time passes, causing problems years after surgery. Rarely, abdominal adhesions form without apparent cause.

What are the symptoms of abdominal adhesions?

Although most abdominal adhesions go unnoticed, the most common symptom is chronic abdominal or pelvic pain. The pain often mimics that of other conditions, including appendicitis, endometriosis, and diverticulitis.

Symptoms of an intestinal obstruction include severe abdominal pain or cramping, vomiting, bloating, loud bowel sounds, swelling of the abdomen, inability to pass gas, and constipation. A person with these symptoms should seek medical attention immediately.

How are abdominal adhesions and intestinal obstructions treated?

Treatment for abdominal adhesions is usually not necessary, as most do not cause problems. Surgery is currently the only way to break adhesions that cause pain, intestinal obstruction, or fertility problems.

More surgery, however, carries the risk of additional adhesions and is avoided when possible.

A complete intestinal obstruction usually requires immediate surgery. A partial obstruction can sometimes be relieved with a liquid or low-residue diet. A low-residue diet is high in dairy products, low in fiber, and more easily broken down into smaller particles by the digestive system.

Can abdominal adhesions be prevented?

Abdominal adhesions are difficult to prevent; however, surgical technique can minimize adhesions.

Laparoscopic surgery avoids opening up the abdomen with a large incision. Instead, the abdomen is inflated with gas while special surgical tools and a video camera are threaded through a few, small abdominal incisions. Inflating the abdomen gives the surgeon room to operate.

If a large abdominal incision is required, a special film-like material (Seprafilm) can be inserted between organs or between the organs and the abdominal incision at the end of surgery. The film-like material, which looks similar to wax paper, is absorbed by the body in about a week.

Other steps during surgery to reduce adhesion formation include using starch- and latex-free gloves, handling tissues and organs gently, shortening surgery time, and not allowing tissues to dry out.

Section 27.2

Appendicitis

Excerpted from "Appendicitis," National Digestive Diseases
Information Clearinghouse (http://digestive.niddk.nih.gov),
NIH Pub. No. 09-4547, updated February 16, 2012.

What is appendicitis?

Appendicitis is a painful swelling and infection of the appendix.
The appendix is a fingerlike pouch attached to the large intestine and
located in the lower right area of the abdomen. Scientists are not sure
what the appendix does, if anything, but removing it does not appear
to affect a person's health. The inside of the appendix is called the appendiceal lumen. Mucus created by the appendix travels through the
appendiceal lumen and empties into the large intestine.

What causes appendicitis?

Obstruction of the appendiceal lumen causes appendicitis. Mucus
backs up in the appendiceal lumen, causing bacteria that normally live
inside the appendix to multiply. As a result, the appendix swells and becomes infected. Sources of obstruction include feces, parasites, or growths
that clog the appendiceal lumen; enlarged lymph tissue in the wall of the
appendix, caused by infection in the gastrointestinal tract or elsewhere
in the body; inflammatory bowel disease, including Crohn disease and
ulcerative colitis; and trauma to the abdomen. An inflamed appendix will
likely burst if not removed. Bursting spreads infection throughout the
abdomen—a potentially dangerous condition called peritonitis.

What are the symptoms of appendicitis?

Most people with appendicitis have classic symptoms that a doctor
can easily identify. The main symptom of appendicitis is abdominal pain.
The abdominal pain usually has these characteristics:

• Occurs suddenly, often causing a person to wake up at night

• Occurs before other symptoms

- Begins near the belly button and then moves lower and to the right

- Is new and unlike any pain felt before

- Gets worse in a matter of hours

- Gets worse when moving around, taking deep breaths, coughing, or sneezing

Other symptoms of appendicitis may include loss of appetite, nausea, vomiting, constipation or diarrhea, inability to pass gas, a low-grade fever that follows other symptoms, abdominal swelling, and the feeling that passing stool will relieve discomfort.

Symptoms vary and can mimic other sources of abdominal pain, including intestinal obstruction, inflammatory bowel disease, pelvic inflammatory disease and other gynecological disorders, intestinal adhesions, and constipation.

What signs indicate that pain may be related to appendicitis?

Details about the abdominal pain are key to diagnosing appendicitis. The doctor will assess pain by touching or applying pressure to specific areas of the abdomen.

Responses that may indicate appendicitis include the following:

- **Guarding:** Guarding occurs when a person subconsciously tenses the abdominal muscles during an examination. Voluntary guarding occurs the moment the doctor's hand touches the abdomen. Involuntary guarding occurs before the doctor actually makes contact.

- **Rebound tenderness:** A doctor tests for rebound tenderness by applying hand pressure to a patient's abdomen and then letting go. Pain felt upon the release of the pressure indicates rebound tenderness. A person may also experience rebound tenderness as pain when the abdomen is jarred—for example, when a person bumps into something or goes over a bump in a car.

- **Rovsing's sign:** A doctor tests for Rovsing's sign by applying hand pressure to the lower left side of the abdomen. Pain felt on the lower right side of the abdomen upon the release of pressure on the left side indicates the presence of Rovsing's sign.

- **Psoas sign:** The right psoas muscle runs over the pelvis near the appendix. Flexing this muscle will cause abdominal pain if the appendix is inflamed. A doctor can check for the psoas sign by applying resistance to the right knee as the patient tries to lift the right thigh while lying down.

- **Obturator sign:** The right obturator muscle also runs near the appendix. A doctor tests for the obturator sign by asking the patient to lie down with the right leg bent at the knee. Moving the bent knee left and right requires flexing the obturator muscle and will cause abdominal pain if the appendix is inflamed.

Women of childbearing age may be asked to undergo a pelvic exam to rule out gynecological conditions, which sometimes cause abdominal pain similar to appendicitis.

The doctor may also examine the rectum, which can be tender from appendicitis.

How is appendicitis treated?

Typically, appendicitis is treated by removing the appendix. If appendicitis is suspected, a doctor will often suggest surgery without conducting extensive diagnostic testing. Prompt surgery decreases the likelihood the appendix will burst.

Surgery to remove the appendix is called appendectomy and can be done two ways. The older method, called laparotomy, removes the appendix through a single incision in the lower right area of the abdomen. The newer method, called laparoscopic surgery, uses several smaller incisions and special surgical tools fed through the incisions to remove the appendix. Laparoscopic surgery leads to fewer complications, such as hospital-related infections, and has a shorter recovery time.

Surgery occasionally reveals a normal appendix. In such cases, many surgeons will remove the healthy appendix to eliminate the future possibility of appendicitis. Occasionally, surgery reveals a different problem, which may also be corrected during surgery.

Sometimes an abscess forms around a burst appendix—called an appendiceal abscess. An abscess is a pus-filled mass that results from the body's attempt to keep an infection from spreading. An abscess may be addressed during surgery or, more commonly, drained before surgery. To drain an abscess, a tube is placed in the abscess through the abdominal wall. CT is used to help find the abscess. The drainage tube is left in place for about two weeks while antibiotics are given to treat infection. Six to eight weeks later, when infection and inflammation are under control, surgery is performed to remove what remains of the burst appendix.

Nonsurgical treatment may be used if surgery is not available, if a person is not well enough to undergo surgery, or if the diagnosis is unclear. Some research suggests that appendicitis can get better without surgery. Nonsurgical treatment includes antibiotics to treat infection and a liquid or soft diet until the infection subsides. A soft diet is low in fiber and easily breaks down in the gastrointestinal tract.

With adequate care, most people recover from appendicitis and do not need to make changes to diet, exercise, or lifestyle. Full recovery from surgery takes about four to six weeks. Limiting physical activity during this time allows tissues to heal.

What should people do if they think they have appendicitis?

Appendicitis is a medical emergency that requires immediate care. People who think they have appendicitis should see a doctor or go to the emergency room right away. Swift diagnosis and treatment reduce the chances the appendix will burst and improve recovery time.

Section 27.3

Crohn Disease

Excerpted from "Crohn's Disease," National Digestive Diseases Information Clearinghouse (http://digestive.niddk.nih.gov), NIH Pub. No. 12-3410, December 2011.

What is Crohn disease?

Crohn disease is a disease that causes inflammation, or swelling, and irritation of any part of the digestive tract—also called the gastrointestinal (GI) tract. The part most commonly affected is the end part of the small intestine, called the ileum.

The GI tract is a series of hollow organs joined in a long, twisting tube from the mouth to the anus. The movement of muscles in the GI tract, along with the release of hormones and enzymes, allows for the digestion of food.

Crohn disease is an inflammatory bowel disease (IBD), the general name for diseases that cause inflammation and irritation in the intestines. Crohn disease can be difficult to diagnose because its symptoms are similar to other intestinal disorders, such as ulcerative colitis and other IBDs, and irritable bowel syndrome. For example, ulcerative colitis and Crohn disease both cause abdominal pain and diarrhea. Crohn disease may also be called ileitis or enteritis.

In Crohn disease, inflammation extends deep into the lining of the affected part of the GI tract. Swelling can cause pain and can make the intestine—also called the bowel—empty frequently, resulting in diarrhea. Chronic—or long-lasting—inflammation may produce scar tissue that builds up inside the intestine to create a stricture. A stricture is a narrowed passageway that can slow the movement of food through the intestine, causing pain or cramps.

What are the symptoms of Crohn disease?

The most common symptoms of Crohn disease are abdominal pain, often in the lower right area, and diarrhea. Rectal bleeding, weight loss, and fever may also occur. Bleeding may be serious and persistent, leading to anemia—a condition in which red blood cells are fewer or smaller than normal, which means less oxygen is carried to the body's cells. The range and severity of symptoms varies.

What is the treatment for Crohn disease?

Treatment may include medications, surgery, nutrition supplementation, or a combination of these options. The goals of treatment are to control inflammation, correct nutritional deficiencies, and relieve symptoms such as abdominal pain, diarrhea, and rectal bleeding. Treatment for Crohn disease depends on its location, severity, and complications.

Treatment can help control Crohn disease and make recurrences less frequent, but no cure exists. Someone with Crohn disease may need long-lasting medical care and regular doctor visits to monitor the condition. Some people have long periods—sometimes years—of remission when they are free of symptoms, and predicting when a remission may occur or when symptoms will return is not possible. This changing pattern of the disease makes it difficult to be certain a treatment has helped.

Despite possible hospitalizations and the need to take medication for long periods of time, most people with Crohn disease have full lives—balancing families, careers, and activities.

What medications are used to treat Crohn disease?

Most people are first treated with medications containing mesalamine, a substance that helps control inflammation. Sulfasalazine is the most commonly used of these medications. People who do not benefit from sulfasalazine or who cannot tolerate it may be put on other mesalamine-containing medications, known as 5-aminosalicylic acid (5-ASA) agents, such as Asacol, Dipentum, or Pentasa. Possible side effects of mesalamine-containing medications include nausea, vomiting, heartburn, diarrhea, and headache.

Other medications that may be used in the treatment of Crohn disease include the following:

- Cortisone or steroids

- Immune system suppressors

- Biological therapies

- Antibiotics

- Antidiarrheal medications and fluid replacements

Is surgery used to treat Crohn disease?

About two-thirds of people with Crohn disease will require surgery at some point in their lives. Surgery becomes necessary to relieve symptoms that do not respond to medical therapy or to correct complications such as intestinal blockage, perforation, bleeding, or abscess—a painful, swollen, pus-filled area caused by infection. Surgery to remove part of the intestine can help people with Crohn disease, but it does not eliminate the disease. People with Crohn disease commonly need more than one operation because inflammation tends to return to the area next to where the diseased intestine was removed.

Because Crohn disease often recurs after surgery, people considering surgery should carefully weigh its benefits and risks compared with other treatments. People faced with this decision should get information from health care providers who routinely work with GI patients, including those who have had intestinal surgery. Patient advocacy organizations can suggest support groups and other information resources.

Section 27.4

Diverticulosis and Diverticulitis

Excerpted from "Diverticulosis and Diverticulitis," National Digestive Diseases Information Clearinghouse (http://digestive.niddk .nih.gov), NIH Pub. No. 08-1163, updated February 21, 2012.

What are diverticulosis and diverticulitis?

Many people have small pouches in the lining of the colon (large intestine) that bulge outward through weak spots. Each pouch is called a diverticulum. Multiple pouches are called diverticula. The condition of having diverticula is called diverticulosis. About 10 percent of Americans older than 40 have diverticulosis. The condition becomes more common as people age. About half of all people older than 60 have diverticulosis.

Diverticula are most common in the lower portion of the large intestine, called the sigmoid colon. When the pouches become inflamed, the condition is called diverticulitis. Ten to 25 percent of people with diverticulosis get diverticulitis. Diverticulosis and diverticulitis together are called diverticular disease.

What are the symptoms of diverticulosis and diverticulitis?

Diverticulosis: Most people with diverticulosis do not have any discomfort or symptoms. However, some people may experience crampy pain or discomfort in the lower abdomen, bloating, and constipation. Other conditions such as irritable bowel syndrome and stomach ulcers cause similar problems, so the symptoms do not always mean a person has diverticulosis. People with chronic symptoms should visit their doctor or health care provider.

Diverticulitis: The most common symptom of diverticulitis is abdominal pain. The most common sign on examination is tenderness in the lower left side of the abdomen. Usually, the pain is severe and comes on suddenly, but it can also be mild and become worse over several days. The intensity of the pain can fluctuate. A person may experience cramping, nausea, vomiting, fever, chills, or a change in bowel habits.

How is diverticular disease treated?

A high-fiber diet and pain medications help relieve symptoms in most cases of diverticulosis. Uncomplicated diverticulitis with mild symptoms usually requires the person to rest, take oral antibiotics, and be on a liquid diet for a period of time. Sometimes an attack of diverticulitis is serious enough to require a hospital stay, intravenous (IV) antibiotics, and possibly surgery.

Diverticulosis: Increasing the amount of fiber in the diet may reduce symptoms of diverticulosis and prevent complications such as diverticulitis. Fiber keeps stool soft and lowers pressure inside the colon so that bowel contents can move through easily. The American Dietetic Association recommends consuming 20 to 35 grams of fiber each day.

The doctor may also recommend taking a fiber product such as methylcellulose (Citrucel) or psyllium (Metamucil) one to three times a day. These products are available in powder, pills, or wafers, and provide 2.0 to 3.5 grams of fiber per dose. Fiber products should be taken with at least eight ounces of water.

Avoidance of nuts, popcorn, and sunflower, pumpkin, caraway, and sesame seeds has been recommended by physicians out of fear that food particles could enter, block, or irritate the diverticula. However, no scientific data support this treatment measure. Eating a high-fiber diet is the only requirement highly emphasized across the medical literature. Eliminating specific foods is not necessary. The seeds in tomatoes, zucchini, cucumbers, strawberries, and raspberries, as well as poppy seeds, are generally considered harmless. People differ in the amounts and types of foods they can eat. Decisions about diet should be made based on what works best for each person. Keeping a food diary may help identify what foods may cause symptoms.

If cramps, bloating, and constipation are problems, the doctor may prescribe a short course of pain medication. However, some pain medications actually cause constipation.

Diverticulitis: Treatment for diverticulitis focuses on clearing up the inflammation and infection, resting the colon, and preventing or minimizing complications.

Depending on the severity of symptoms, the doctor may recommend bed rest, oral antibiotics, a pain reliever, and a liquid diet. If symptoms ease after a few days, the doctor will recommend gradually increasing the amount of high-fiber foods in the diet.

Severe cases of diverticulitis with acute pain and complications will likely require a hospital stay. Most cases of severe diverticulitis are treated with IV antibiotics and a few days without food or drink to help the colon rest. In some cases, surgery may be necessary.

When is surgery necessary for diverticulitis?

If symptoms of diverticulitis are frequent, or the patient does not respond to antibiotics and resting the colon, the doctor may advise surgery. The surgeon removes the affected part of the colon and joins the remaining sections. This type of surgery—called colon resection—aims to prevent complications and future diverticulitis. The doctor may also recommend surgery for complications such as a fistula or partial intestinal obstruction.

Immediate surgery may be necessary when the patient has other complications, such as perforation, a large abscess, peritonitis, complete intestinal obstruction, or severe bleeding. In these cases, two surgeries may be needed because it is not safe to rejoin the colon right away. During the first surgery, the surgeon cleans the infected abdominal cavity, removes the portion of the affected colon, and performs a temporary colostomy, creating an opening, or stoma, in the abdomen. The end of the colon is connected to the opening to allow normal eating while healing occurs. Stool is collected in a pouch attached to the stoma. In the second surgery several months later, the surgeon rejoins the ends of the colon and closes the stoma.

Section 27.5

Gallstones

Excerpted from "Gallstones," National Digestive Diseases Information Clearinghouse (http://digestive.niddk.nih.gov), NIH Pub. No. 07-2897, updated February 23, 2010.

What are gallstones?

Gallstones are small, pebble-like substances that develop in the gallbladder. The gallbladder is a small, pear-shaped sac located below your liver in the right upper abdomen. Gallstones form when liquid stored in the gallbladder hardens into pieces of stone-like material. The liquid—called bile—helps the body digest fats. Bile is made in the liver, then stored in the gallbladder until the body needs it. The gallbladder contracts and pushes the bile into a tube—called the common bile duct—that carries it to the small intestine, where it helps with digestion.

The two types of gallstones are cholesterol stones and pigment stones. Cholesterol stones are usually yellow-green and are made primarily of hardened cholesterol. They account for about 80 percent of gallstones. Pigment stones are small, dark stones made of bilirubin. Gallstones can be as small as a grain of sand or as large as a golf ball. The gallbladder can develop just one large stone, hundreds of tiny stones, or a combination of the two.

Gallstones can block the normal flow of bile if they move from the gallbladder and lodge in any of the ducts that carry bile from the liver to the small intestine. The ducts include the hepatic ducts, which carry bile out of the liver, the cystic duct, which takes bile to and from the gallbladder, and the common bile duct, which takes bile from the cystic and hepatic ducts to the small intestine.

Bile trapped in these ducts can cause inflammation in the gallbladder, the ducts, or in rare cases, the liver. Other ducts open into the common bile duct, including the pancreatic duct, which carries digestive enzymes out of the pancreas. Sometimes gallstones passing through the common bile duct provoke inflammation in the pancreas—called gallstone pancreatitis—an extremely painful and potentially dangerous condition.

If any of the bile ducts remain blocked for a significant period of time, severe damage or infection can occur in the gallbladder, liver, or pancreas. Left untreated, the condition can be fatal. Warning signs of a serious problem are fever, jaundice, and persistent pain.

What are the symptoms of gallstones?

As gallstones move into the bile ducts and create blockage, pressure increases in the gallbladder and one or more symptoms may occur. Symptoms of blocked bile ducts are often called a gallbladder "attack" because they occur suddenly. Gallbladder attacks often follow fatty meals, and they may occur during the night. A typical attack can cause steady pain in the right upper abdomen that increases rapidly and lasts from 30 minutes to several hours, pain in the back between the shoulder blades, and pain under the right shoulder.

Notify your doctor if you think you have experienced a gallbladder attack. Although these attacks often pass as gallstones move, your gallbladder can become infected and rupture if a blockage remains.

People with any of the following symptoms should see a doctor immediately:

- Prolonged pain—more than five hours
- Nausea and vomiting
- Fever—even low-grade—or chills
- Yellowish color of the skin or whites of the eyes
- Clay-colored stools

Many people with gallstones have no symptoms; these gallstones are called "silent stones." They do not interfere with gallbladder, liver, or pancreas function and do not need treatment.

How are gallstones treated?

If you have gallstones without symptoms, you do not require treatment. If you are having frequent gallbladder attacks, your doctor will likely recommend you have your gallbladder removed—an operation called a cholecystectomy. Surgery to remove the gallbladder—a nonessential organ—is one of the most common surgeries performed on adults in the United States.

The most common complication in gallbladder surgery is injury to the bile ducts. An injured common bile duct can leak bile and cause a painful and potentially dangerous infection. Mild injuries can sometimes be treated nonsurgically. Major injury, however, is more serious and requires additional surgery.

If gallstones are present in the bile ducts, the physician—usually a gastroenterologist—may use endoscopic retrograde cholangiopancreatography (ERCP) to locate and remove them before or during gallbladder surgery. Occasionally, a person who has had a cholecystectomy is diagnosed with a gallstone in the bile ducts weeks, months, or even years after the surgery. The ERCP procedure is usually successful in removing the stone in these cases.

Nonsurgical approaches (such as oral dissolution therapy and the experimental procedure, contact dissolution therapy) are used only in special situations—such as when a patient has a serious medical condition preventing surgery—and only for cholesterol stones. Stones commonly recur within five years in patients treated nonsurgically.

Section 27.6

Gas in the Digestive Tract

Excerpted from "Gas in the Digestive Tract," National Digestive Diseases Information Clearinghouse (http://digestive.niddk.nih.gov), NIH Pub. No. 13-883, updated January 2, 2013.

What is gas in the digestive tract?

Gas is air in the digestive tract—the large, muscular tube that extends from the mouth to the anus, where the movement of muscles, along with the release of hormones and enzymes, allows for the digestion of food. Gas leaves the body when people burp through the mouth or pass gas through the anus.

Gas is primarily composed of carbon dioxide, oxygen, nitrogen, hydrogen, and sometimes methane. Flatus, gas passed through the anus, may also contain small amounts of gasses that contain sulfur. Flatus that contains more sulfur gasses has more odor.

Everyone has gas. However, many people think they burp or pass gas too often and that they have too much gas. Having too much gas is rare.

Gas in the digestive tract is usually caused by swallowing air and by the breakdown of certain foods in the large intestine by bacteria. Everyone swallows a small amount of air when eating and drinking. The amount of air swallowed increases when people eat or drink too fast, smoke, chew gum, suck on hard candy, drink carbonated or "fizzy" drinks, or wear loose-fitting dentures.

Disorders such as irritable bowel syndrome (IBS) can affect how gas moves through the intestines or increase pain sensitivity in the intestines. IBS is a functional GI disorder, meaning that the symptoms are caused by changes in how the digestive tract works. The most common symptoms of IBS are abdominal pain or discomfort, often reported as cramping, along with diarrhea, constipation, or both. IBS may give a sensation of bloating because of increased sensitivity to normal amounts of gas.

Eating a lot of fatty food can delay stomach emptying and cause bloating and discomfort, but not necessarily too much gas.

What are the symptoms of gas?

The most common symptoms of gas are burping, passing gas, bloating, and abdominal pain or discomfort. However, not everyone experiences these symptoms.

Burping: Burping, or belching, once in a while, especially during and after meals, is normal. However, people who burp frequently may be swallowing too much air and releasing it before the air enters the stomach.

Some people who burp frequently may have an upper GI disorder, such as gastroesophageal reflux disease—a chronic condition in which stomach contents flow back up into the esophagus. People may believe that swallowing air and releasing it will relieve the discomfort, and they may intentionally or unintentionally develop a habit of burping to relieve discomfort.

Passing gas: Passing gas around 13 to 21 times a day is normal. Flatulence is excessive gas in the stomach or intestine that can cause bloating and flatus. Flatulence may be the result of problems digesting certain carbohydrates.

Bloating: Bloating is a feeling of fullness and swelling in the abdomen, the area between the chest and hips. Problems digesting carbohydrates may cause increased gas and bloating. However, bloating is not always caused by too much gas. Bloating may result from diseases that affect how gas moves through the intestines, such as rapid gastric emptying, or from diseases that cause intestinal obstruction, such as colon cancer. People who have had many operations, internal hernias, or bands of internal scar tissue called adhesions may experience bloating.

Abdominal pain and discomfort: People may feel abdominal pain or discomfort when gas does not move through the intestines normally. People with IBS may be more sensitive to gas and feel pain when gas is present in the intestines.

How is gas treated?

Gas can be treated by reducing swallowed air, making dietary changes, or taking over-the-counter or prescription medications. People who think they have too much gas can try to treat gas on their own before seeing a health care provider. Health care providers can provide advice about reducing gas and prescribe medications that may help.

People may be able to reduce gas by eating less of the foods that cause gas. However, many healthy foods may cause gas, such as fruits and vegetables, whole grains, and milk products. The amount of gas caused by certain foods varies from person to person. Effective dietary changes depend on learning through trial and error which foods cause a person to have gas and how much of the offending foods one can handle.

While fat does not cause gas, limiting high-fat foods can help reduce bloating and discomfort. Less fat in the diet helps the stomach empty faster, allowing gases to move more quickly into the small intestine.

Some over-the-counter medications can help reduce gas or the symptoms associated with gas:

* Alpha-galactosidase (Beano), an over-the-counter digestive aid, contains the sugar-digesting enzyme that the body lacks to digest the sugar in beans and many vegetables. The enzyme comes in liquid and tablet form. Five drops are added per serving or one tablet is swallowed just before eating to break down the gas-producing sugars. Beano has no effect on gas caused by lactose or fiber.

* Simethicone (Gas-X, Mylanta Gas) can relieve bloating and abdominal pain or discomfort caused by gas.

* Lactase tablets or drops can help people with lactose intolerance digest milk and milk products to reduce gas. Lactase tablets are taken just before eating foods that contain lactose; lactase drops can be added to liquid milk products. Lactose-free and lactose-reduced milk and milk products are available at most grocery stores.

Health care providers may prescribe medications to help reduce symptoms, especially for people with small intestinal bacterial overgrowth or IBS.

Section 27.7

Gastroesophageal Reflux Disease (Heartburn)

Excerpted from "Heartburn, Gastroesophageal Reflux (GER), and Gastroesophageal Reflux Disease (GERD)," National Digestive Diseases Information Clearinghouse (http://digestive.niddk.nih.gov), NIH Pub. No. 07-882, updated April 30, 2012.

What is gastroesophageal reflux disease?

Gastroesophageal reflux disease (GERD) is a more serious form of gastroesophageal reflux (GER), which is common. GER occurs when the lower esophageal sphincter (LES) opens spontaneously, for varying periods of time, or does not close properly and stomach contents rise up into the esophagus. GER is also called acid reflux or acid regurgitation, because digestive juices—called acids—rise up with the food. The esophagus is the tube that carries food from the mouth to the stomach. The LES is a ring of muscle at the bottom of the esophagus that acts like a valve between the esophagus and stomach.

When acid reflux occurs, food or fluid can be tasted in the back of the mouth. When refluxed stomach acid touches the lining of the esophagus it may cause a burning sensation in the chest or throat called heartburn or acid indigestion. Occasional GER is common and does not necessarily mean one has GERD. Persistent reflux that occurs more than twice a week is considered GERD, and it can eventually lead to more serious health problems. People of all ages can have GERD.

What are the symptoms of GERD?

The main symptom of GERD in adults is frequent heartburn, also called acid indigestion—burning-type pain in the lower part of the mid-chest, behind the breast bone, and in the mid-abdomen. Most children under 12 years with GERD, and some adults, have GERD without heartburn. Instead, they may experience a dry cough, asthma symptoms, or trouble swallowing.

How is GERD treated?

See your health care provider if you have had symptoms of GERD and have been using antacids or other over-the-counter reflux medications for more than two weeks. Your health care provider may refer you to a gastroenterologist, a doctor who treats diseases of the stomach and intestines. Depending on the severity of your GERD, treatment may involve one or more of the following lifestyle changes, medications, or surgery.

These lifestyle changes may be involved in treating GERD:

- If you smoke, stop.

- Avoid foods and beverages that worsen symptoms.

- Lose weight if needed.

- Eat small, frequent meals.

- Wear loose-fitting clothes.

- Avoid lying down for three hours after a meal.

- Raise the head of your bed six to eight inches by securing wood blocks under the bedposts. Just using extra pillows will not help.

Your health care provider may recommend over-the-counter antacids or medications that stop acid production or help the muscles that empty your stomach. You can buy many of these medications without a prescription. However, see your health care provider before starting or adding a medication.

Antacids, such as Alka-Seltzer, Maalox, Mylanta, Rolaids, and Riopan, are usually the first drugs recommended to relieve heartburn and other mild GERD symptoms. Many brands on the market use different combinations of three basic salts— magnesium, calcium, and aluminum—with hydroxide or bicarbonate ions to neutralize the acid in your stomach. Antacids, however, can have side effects. Magnesium salt can lead to diarrhea, and aluminum salt may cause constipation. Aluminum and magnesium salts are often combined in a single product to balance these effects.

Calcium carbonate antacids, such as Tums, Titralac, and Alka-2, can also be a supplemental source of calcium. They can cause constipation as well.

Foaming agents, such as Gaviscon, work by covering your stomach contents with foam to prevent reflux.

H2 blockers, such as cimetidine (Tagamet HB), famotidine (Pepcid AC), nizatidine (Axid AR), and ranitidine (Zantac 75), decrease acid production. They are available in prescription strength and over-the-counter strength. These drugs provide short-term relief and are effective for about half of those who have GERD symptoms.

Proton pump inhibitors include omeprazole (Prilosec, Zegerid), lansoprazole (Prevacid), pantoprazole (Protonix), rabeprazole (AcipHex), and esomeprazole (Nexium), which are available by prescription. Prilosec is also available in over-the-counter strength. Proton pump inhibitors are more effective than H2 blockers and can relieve symptoms and heal the esophageal lining in almost everyone who has GERD.

Prokinetics help strengthen the LES and make the stomach empty faster. This group includes bethanechol (Urecholine) and metoclopramide (Reglan). Metoclopramide also improves muscle action in the digestive tract. Prokinetics have frequent side effects that limit their usefulness— fatigue, sleepiness, depression, anxiety, and problems with physical movement.

Because drugs work in different ways, combinations of medications may help control symptoms. People who get heartburn after eating may take both antacids and H2 blockers. The antacids work first to neutralize the acid in the stomach, and then the H2 blockers act on acid production. By the time the antacid stops working, the H2 blocker will have stopped acid production. Your health care provider is the best source of information about how to use medications for GERD.

If your symptoms do not improve with lifestyle changes or medications, you may need additional tests. A completely accurate diagnostic test for GERD does not exist, and tests have not consistently shown that acid exposure to the lower esophagus directly correlates with damage to the lining.

Surgery is an option when medicine and lifestyle changes do not help to manage GERD symptoms. Surgery may also be a reasonable alternative to a lifetime of drugs and discomfort.

Fundoplication is the standard surgical treatment for GERD. Usually a specific type of this procedure, called Nissen fundoplication, is performed. During the Nissen fundoplication, the upper part of the stomach is wrapped around the LES to strengthen the sphincter, prevent acid reflux, and repair a hiatal hernia.

The Nissen fundoplication may be performed using a laparoscope, an instrument that is inserted through tiny incisions in the abdomen. The doctor then uses small instruments that hold a camera to look at the abdomen and pelvis. When performed by experienced surgeons, laparoscopic fundoplication is safe and effective in people of all ages, including infants. The procedure is reported to have the same results as the standard fundoplication, and people can leave the hospital in one to three days and return to work in two to three weeks.

Endoscopic techniques used to treat chronic heartburn include the Bard EndoCinch system, NDO Plicator, and the Stretta system. These techniques require the use of an endoscope to perform the antireflux operation. The EndoCinch and NDO Plicator systems involve putting stitches in the LES to create pleats that help strengthen the muscle. The Stretta system uses electrodes to create tiny burns on the LES. When the burns heal, the scar tissue helps toughen the muscle. The long-term effects of these three procedures are unknown.

Section 27.8

Irritable Bowel Syndrome

Excerpted from "Irritable Bowel Syndrome," National Digestive Diseases Information Clearinghouse (http://digestive.niddk.nih.gov), NIH Pub. No. 12-693, updated July 2, 2012.

What is irritable bowel syndrome (IBS)?

Irritable bowel syndrome is a functional gastrointestinal (GI) disorder, meaning it is a problem caused by changes in how the GI tract works. People with a functional GI disorder have frequent symptoms, but the GI tract does not become damaged. IBS is not a disease; it is a group of symptoms that occur together. The most common symptoms of IBS are abdominal pain or discomfort, often reported as cramping, along with diarrhea, constipation, or both. In the past, IBS was called colitis, mucous colitis, spastic colon, nervous colon, and spastic bowel. The name was changed to reflect the understanding that the disorder has both physical and mental causes and is not a product of a person's imagination.

IBS is diagnosed when a person has abdominal pain or discomfort at least three times per month for the last three months without other disease or injury that could explain the pain. The pain or discomfort of IBS may occur with a change in stool frequency or consistency or may be relieved by a bowel movement.

IBS is often classified into four subtypes based on a person's usual stool consistency. These subtypes are important because they affect the types of treatment that are most likely to improve the person's symptoms. These are the four subtypes of IBS:

- IBS with constipation (IBS-C): hard or lumpy stools at least 25 percent of the time; loose or watery stools less than 25 percent of the time

- IBS with diarrhea (IBS-D): loose or watery stools at least 25 percent of the time; hard or lumpy stools less than 25 percent of the time

- Mixed IBS (IBS-M): hard or lumpy stools at least 25 percent of the time; loose or watery stools at least 25 percent of the time

- Unsubtyped IBS (IBS-U): hard or lumpy stools less than 25 percent of the time; loose or watery stools less than 25 percent of the time

What are the symptoms of IBS?

The symptoms of IBS include abdominal pain or discomfort and changes in bowel habits. To meet the definition of IBS, the pain or discomfort should be associated with two of the following three symptoms:

- Start with bowel movements that occur more or less often than usual

- Start with stool that appears looser and more watery or harder and more lumpy than usual

- Improve with a bowel movement

Other symptoms of IBS may include the following:

- Diarrhea—having loose, watery stools three or more times a day and feeling urgency to have a bowel movement

- Constipation—having hard, dry stools; three or fewer bowel movements in a week; or straining to have a bowel movement

- Feeling that a bowel movement is incomplete

- Passing mucus, a clear liquid made by the intestines that coats and protects tissues in the GI tract

- Abdominal bloating

Symptoms may often occur after eating a meal. To meet the definition of IBS, symptoms must occur at least three days a month.

How is IBS treated?

Though there is no cure for IBS, the symptoms can be treated with a combination of the following:

- Changes in eating, diet, and nutrition

- Medications

- Probiotics

- Therapies for mental health problems

Large meals can cause cramping and diarrhea, so eating smaller meals more often, or eating smaller portions, may help IBS symptoms. Eating meals that are low in fat and high in carbohydrates, such as pasta, rice, whole-grain breads and cereals, fruits, and vegetables, may help.

Certain foods and drinks may cause IBS symptoms in some people, such as foods high in fat, milk products, drinks with alcohol or caffeine, drinks with large amounts of artificial sweeteners, and foods that may cause gas, such as beans and cabbage. People with IBS may want to limit or avoid these foods. Keeping a food diary is a good way to track which foods cause symptoms so they can be excluded from or reduced in the diet.

Dietary fiber may lessen constipation in people with IBS, but it may not help with lowering pain. Fiber helps keep stool soft so it moves smoothly through the colon. The Academy of Nutrition and Dietetics recommends consuming 20 to 35 grams of fiber a day for adults.

When medications are used for treating IBS, the health care provider will select medications based on the person's symptoms.

- **Fiber supplements:** Fiber supplements may be recommended to relieve constipation when increasing dietary fiber is ineffective.

- **Laxatives:** Constipation can be treated with laxative medications. Laxatives work in different ways, and a health care provider can provide information about which type is best for each person.

- **Antidiarrheals:** Loperamide has been found to reduce diarrhea in people with IBS, though it does not reduce pain, bloating, or other symptoms. Loperamide reduces stool frequency and improves stool consistency by slowing the movement of stool through the colon.

- **Antispasmodics:** Antispasmodics, such as hyoscine, cimetropium, and pinaverium, help to control colon muscle spasms and reduce abdominal pain.

- **Antidepressants:** Tricyclic antidepressants (TCAs) and selective serotonin reuptake inhibitors (SSRIs) in low doses can help relieve IBS symptoms including abdominal pain. In theory, TCAs should be better for people with IBS-D and SSRIs should be better for people with IBS-C due to the effect on colon transit, but this has not been confirmed in clinical studies. TCAs work in people with IBS by reducing sensitivity to pain in the GI tract as well as normalizing GI motility and secretion.

- **Lubiprostone (Amitiza):** Lubiprostone is prescribed for people who have IBS-C. The medication has been found to improve symptoms of abdominal pain or discomfort, stool consistency, straining, and constipation severity.

- **Rifaximin:** The antibiotic rifaximin can reduce abdominal bloating by treating small intestinal bacterial overgrowth (SIBO). But scientists are still debating the use of antibiotics to treat IBS, and more research is needed.

Probiotics are live microorganisms, usually bacteria, that are similar to microorganisms normally found in the GI tract. Studies have found that probiotics, specifically *Bifidobacteria* and certain probiotic combinations, improve symptoms of IBS when taken in large enough amounts. But more research is needed. Probiotics can be found in dietary supplements, such as capsules, tablets, and powders, and in some foods, such as yogurt. A health care provider can give information about the right kind and right amount of probiotics to take to improve IBS symptoms.

The following therapies can help improve IBS symptoms due to mental health problems:

- **Talk therapy:** Talking with a therapist may reduce stress and improve IBS symptoms. Two types of talk therapy used to treat IBS are cognitive behavioral therapy and psychodynamic, or interpersonal, therapy. Cognitive behavioral therapy focuses on the person's thoughts and actions. Psychodynamic therapy focuses on how emotions affect IBS symptoms. This type of therapy often involves relaxation and stress management techniques.

- **Hypnotherapy:** In hypnotherapy, the therapist uses hypnosis to help the person relax into a trancelike state. This type of therapy may help the person relax the muscles in the colon.

- **Mindfulness training:** People practicing this type of meditation are taught to focus their attention on sensations occurring at the moment and to avoid worrying about the meaning of those sensations, also called catastrophizing.

Section 27.9

Pancreatitis

Excerpted from "Pancreatitis," National Digestive Diseases
Information Clearinghouse (http://digestive.niddk.nih.gov),
NIH Pub. No. 08-1596, updated August 16, 2012.

What is pancreatitis?

Pancreatitis is inflammation of the pancreas. The pancreas is a
large gland behind the stomach and close to the duodenum—the first
part of the small intestine. The pancreas secretes digestive juices, or
enzymes, into the duodenum through a tube called the pancreatic duct.
Pancreatic enzymes join with bile—a liquid produced in the liver and
stored in the gallbladder—to digest food. The pancreas also releases
the hormones insulin and glucagon into the bloodstream. These hormones help the body regulate the glucose it takes from food for energy.

Normally, digestive enzymes secreted by the pancreas do not become
active until they reach the small intestine. But when the pancreas is
inflamed, the enzymes inside it attack and damage the tissues that
produce them.

Pancreatitis can be acute or chronic. Either form is serious and can
lead to complications. In severe cases, bleeding, infection, and permanent tissue damage may occur.

What are the symptoms of acute pancreatitis and how is it treated?

Acute pancreatitis is inflammation of the pancreas that occurs
suddenly and usually resolves in a few days with treatment. Acute
pancreatitis can be a life-threatening illness with severe complications. The most common cause of acute pancreatitis is the presence of
gallstones—small, pebble-like substances made of hardened bile—that
cause inflammation in the pancreas as they pass through the common
bile duct. Chronic, heavy alcohol use is also a common cause. Other
causes of acute pancreatitis include abdominal trauma, medications,
infections, tumors, and genetic abnormalities of the pancreas.

Acute pancreatitis usually begins with gradual or sudden pain in the upper abdomen that sometimes extends through the back. The pain may be mild at first and feel worse after eating. But the pain is often severe and may become constant and last for several days. A person with acute pancreatitis usually looks and feels very ill and needs immediate medical attention. Other symptoms may include a swollen and tender abdomen, nausea and vomiting, fever, and a rapid pulse. Severe acute pancreatitis may cause dehydration and low blood pressure. The heart, lungs, or kidneys can fail. If bleeding occurs in the pancreas, shock and even death may follow.

Treatment for acute pancreatitis requires a few days' stay in the hospital for intravenous (IV) fluids, antibiotics, and medication to relieve pain. The person cannot eat or drink so the pancreas can rest. If vomiting occurs, a tube may be placed through the nose and into the stomach to remove fluid and air.

Unless complications arise, acute pancreatitis usually resolves in a few days. In severe cases, the person may require nasogastric feeding—a special liquid given in a long, thin tube inserted through the nose and throat and into the stomach—for several weeks while the pancreas heals.

Before leaving the hospital, the person will be advised not to smoke, drink alcoholic beverages, or eat fatty meals. In some cases, the cause of the pancreatitis is clear, but in others, more tests are needed after the person is discharged and the pancreas is healed.

What are the symptoms of chronic pancreatitis and how is it treated?

Chronic pancreatitis is inflammation of the pancreas that does not heal or improve—it gets worse over time and leads to permanent damage. Chronic pancreatitis, like acute pancreatitis, occurs when digestive enzymes attack the pancreas and nearby tissues, causing episodes of pain. Chronic pancreatitis often develops in people who are between the ages of 30 and 40.

The most common cause of chronic pancreatitis is many years of heavy alcohol use. The chronic form of pancreatitis can be triggered by one acute attack that damages the pancreatic duct. The damaged duct causes the pancreas to become inflamed. Scar tissue develops and the pancreas is slowly destroyed.

Other causes of chronic pancreatitis are hereditary disorders of the pancreas; cystic fibrosis—the most common inherited disorder leading to chronic pancreatitis; hypercalcemia—high levels of calcium in the blood; hyperlipidemia or hypertriglyceridemia—high levels of blood fats; some medicines; certain autoimmune conditions; and unknown causes.

Hereditary pancreatitis can present in a person younger than age 30, but it might not be diagnosed for several years. Episodes of abdominal pain and diarrhea lasting several days come and go over time and can progress to chronic pancreatitis. A diagnosis of hereditary pancreatitis is likely if the person has two or more family members with pancreatitis in more than one generation.

Most people with chronic pancreatitis experience upper abdominal pain, although some people have no pain at all. The pain may spread to the back, feel worse when eating or drinking, and become constant and disabling. In some cases, abdominal pain goes away as the condition worsens, most likely because the pancreas is no longer making digestive enzymes. Other symptoms include nausea, vomiting, weight loss, diarrhea, and oily stools.

People with chronic pancreatitis often lose weight, even when their appetite and eating habits are normal. The weight loss occurs because the body does not secrete enough pancreatic enzymes to digest food, so nutrients are not absorbed normally. Poor digestion leads to malnutrition due to excretion of fat in the stool.

Treatment for chronic pancreatitis may require hospitalization for pain management, IV hydration, and nutritional support. Nasogastric feedings may be necessary for several weeks if the person continues to lose weight.

When a normal diet is resumed, the doctor may prescribe synthetic pancreatic enzymes if the pancreas does not secrete enough of its own. The enzymes should be taken with every meal to help the person digest food and regain some weight. The next step is to plan a nutritious diet that is low in fat and includes small, frequent meals. A dietitian can assist in developing a meal plan. Drinking plenty of fluids and limiting caffeinated beverages is also important.

People with chronic pancreatitis are strongly advised not to smoke or consume alcoholic beverages, even if the pancreatitis is mild or in the early stages.

What is therapeutic endoscopic retrograde cholangiopancreatography (ERCP)?

Therapeutic endoscopic retrograde cholangiopancreatography (ERCP) is a specialized technique used to view the pancreas, gallbladder, and bile ducts and treat complications of acute and chronic pancreatitis—gallstones, narrowing or blockage of the pancreatic duct or bile ducts, leaks in the bile ducts, and pseudocysts—accumulations of fluid, and tissue debris.

Soon after a person is admitted to the hospital with suspected narrowing of the pancreatic duct or bile ducts, a physician with specialized training performs ERCP.

After lightly sedating the patient and giving medication to numb the throat, the doctor inserts an endoscope—a long, flexible, lighted tube with a camera—through the mouth, throat, and stomach into the small intestine. The endoscope is connected to a computer and screen. The doctor guides the endoscope and injects a special dye into the pancreatic or bile ducts that helps the pancreas, gallbladder, and bile ducts appear on the screen while x-rays are taken.

The following procedures can be performed using ERCP:

- **Sphincterotomy:** Using a small wire on the endoscope, the doctor finds the muscle that surrounds the pancreatic duct or bile ducts and makes a tiny cut to enlarge the duct opening. When a pseudocyst is present, the duct is drained.

- **Gallstone removal:** The endoscope is used to remove pancreatic or bile duct stones with a tiny basket. Gallstone removal is sometimes performed along with a sphincterotomy.

- **Stent placement:** Using the endoscope, the doctor places a tiny piece of plastic or metal that looks like a straw in a narrowed pancreatic or bile duct to keep it open.

- **Balloon dilatation:** Some endoscopes have a small balloon that the doctor uses to dilate, or stretch, a narrowed pancreatic or bile duct. A temporary stent may be placed for a few months to keep the duct open.

People who undergo therapeutic ERCP are at slight risk for complications, including severe pancreatitis, infection, bowel perforation, or bleeding. Complications of ERCP are more common in people with acute or recurrent pancreatitis. A patient who experiences fever, trouble swallowing, or increased throat, chest, or abdominal pain after the procedure should notify a doctor immediately.

Chapter 28

Gynecological Pain

Chapter Contents

Section 28.1—Childbirth and Pain 314

Section 28.2—Chronic Pelvic Pain 318

Section 28.3—Dysmenorrhea 321

Section 28.4—Dyspareunia 324

Section 28.5—Endometriosis.. 328

Section 28.6—Uterine Fibroids 331

Section 28.7—Vulvodynia.. 335

Section 28.1

Childbirth and Pain

"Dealing with Pain during Childbirth," November 2011, reprinted with permission from www.kidshealth.org. This information was provided by KidsHealth®, one of the largest resources online for medically reviewed health information written for parents, kids, and teens. For more articles like this, visit www.KidsHealth.org, or www.TeensHealth.org. Copyright © 1995-2012 The Nemours Foundation. All rights reserved.

If you're like most women, the pain of labor and delivery is one of the things that worry you about having a baby. This is certainly understandable, because labor is painful for most women.

It's possible to have labor with relatively little pain, but it's wise to prepare yourself by planning some strategies for coping with pain. Planning for pain is one of the best ways to ensure that you'll stay calm and be able to deal with it when the time comes.

Pain during Labor and Delivery

Pain during labor is caused by contractions of the muscles of the uterus and by pressure on the cervix. This pain may be felt as strong cramping in the abdomen, groin, and back, as well as an achy feeling. Some women experience pain in their sides or thighs as well.

Other causes of pain during labor include pressure on the bladder and bowels by the baby's head and the stretching of the birth canal and vagina.

Pain during labor is different for every woman. Although labor is often thought of as one of the more painful events in human experience, it ranges widely from woman to woman and even from pregnancy to pregnancy. Women experience labor pain differently— for some, it resembles menstrual cramps; for others, severe pressure; and for others, extremely strong waves that feel like diarrheal cramps.

It's often not the pain of each contraction on its own that women find the hardest, but the fact that the contractions keep coming—and that as labor progresses, there is less and less time between contractions to relax.

Preparing for Pain

To help with pain during labor, here are some things you can start doing before or during your pregnancy:

Regular and reasonable exercise (that your doctor says is OK) can help strengthen your muscles and prepare your body for the stress of labor. Exercise also can increase your endurance, which will come in handy if you have a long labor. The important thing to remember with any exercise is not to overdo it—and this is especially true if you're pregnant. Talk to your doctor about what he or she considers to be a safe exercise plan for you.

If you and your partner attend childbirth classes, you'll learn different techniques for handling pain, from visualization to stretches designed to strengthen the muscles that support your uterus. The two most common childbirth philosophies in the United States are the Lamaze technique and the Bradley method.

The Lamaze technique is the most widely used method in the United States. The Lamaze philosophy teaches that birth is a normal, natural, and healthy process and that women should be empowered to approach it with confidence. Lamaze classes educate women about the ways they can decrease their perception of pain, such as through relaxation techniques, breathing exercises, distraction, or massage by a supportive coach. Lamaze approach takes a neutral position toward pain medication, encouraging women to make an informed decision about whether it's right for them.

The Bradley method (also called Husband-Coached Birth) emphasizes a natural approach to birth and the active participation of the baby's father as birth coach. A major goal of this method is the avoidance of medications unless absolutely necessary. The Bradley method also focuses on good nutrition and exercise during pregnancy and relaxation and deep-breathing techniques as a method of coping with labor. Although the Bradley method advocates a medication-free birth experience, the classes do discuss unexpected complications or situations, like emergency cesarean sections.

Some ways to handle pain during labor include:

- hypnosis
- yoga
- meditation
- walking
- massage or counterpressure

315

- changing position
- taking a bath or shower
- listening to music
- distracting yourself by counting or performing an activity that keeps your mind otherwise occupied

Pain Medications

A variety of pain medications can be used during labor and delivery, depending on the situation. Talk to your health care provider about the risks and benefits of each.

Analgesics: Pain medications can be given many ways. If they are given intravenously (into an IV) or through a shot into a muscle, the medications can affect the whole body. These medicines can cause side effects in the mother, including drowsiness and nausea. They can also have effects on the baby.

Regional anesthesia: This is what most women think of when they consider pain medication during labor. By blocking the feeling from specific regions of the body, these methods can be used for pain relief in both vaginal and cesarean section deliveries.

Epidurals, a form of local anesthesia, relieve most of the pain from the entire body below the belly button, including the vaginal walls, during labor and delivery. An epidural involves medication given by an anesthesiologist through a thin, tube-like catheter that's inserted in the woman's lower back. The amount of medication can be increased or decreased according to a woman's needs. Very little medication reaches the baby, so there are usually no effects on the baby from this method of pain relief.

Epidurals do have some drawbacks—they can cause a woman's blood pressure to drop and can make it difficult to urinate. They can also cause itching, nausea, and headaches in the mother. The risks to the baby are minimal, but include problems caused by low blood pressure in the mother.

Tranquilizers: These drugs don't relieve pain, but they may help to calm and relax women who are very anxious. Sometimes they are used along with analgesics. These drugs can have effects on both the mother and baby, and are not often used. They can also make it difficult for women to remember the details of the birth. You should discuss the risks of taking tranquilizers first with your doctor.

Natural Childbirth

Some women choose to give birth using no medication at all, relying instead on relaxation techniques and controlled breathing for pain. If you'd like to experience childbirth without pain medication, make your wishes known to your health care provider.

Things to Consider

Here are some things to think about when considering pain control during labor:

- Medications can relieve much of your pain, but probably won't relieve all of it.

- Labor may hurt more than you anticipated. Some women who have previously said they want no pain medicine whatsoever end up changing their minds once they're actually in labor.

- Certain medications can affect your baby, causing the baby to be drowsy or have changes in the heart rate.

Talking to Your Health Care Provider

You'll want to review your pain control options with the person who'll be delivering your baby. Find out what pain control methods are available, how effective they're likely to be, and when it's best not to use certain medications.

If you want to use pain-control methods other than medication, make sure your health care provider and the hospital staff know. You might want to also consider writing a birth plan that makes your preferences clear.

Remember, too, that many women make decisions about pain relief during labor that they abandon—often for very good reason—at the last minute. Your ability to endure the pain of childbirth has nothing to do with your worth as a mother. By preparing and educating yourself, you can be ready to decide what pain management works best for you.

Section 28.2

Chronic Pelvic Pain

Excerpted from "Treating Chronic Pelvic Pain: A Review of the
Research for Women," Agency for Healthcare Research and Quality
(www.ahrq.gov), April 2012.

What is chronic pelvic pain?

Chronic pelvic pain (CPP) is ongoing pain in your pelvic area (the
area between your hips and below your belly button) that lasts for
three or more months. The pain may be dull, or it may be sharp and
cramping. It may be constant, or it may come and go. The pain might
not be in one specific spot and could be felt in your entire pelvic area.
You may also feel pressure in your pelvic area. CPP can make it difficult to do daily activities or exercise.

What causes chronic pelvic pain?

CPP is a complex condition that can have many causes. It may be
connected to other conditions. Some of these conditions include:

- **Irritable bowel syndrome:** A condition that affects your large intestine that can cause bloating, cramping, constipation, or diarrhea.

- **Endometriosis:** The tissue from the lining of your uterus grows
on the outside of that organ.

- **Tense pelvic floor muscles:** The muscles at the bottom of your
pelvic area tense up or cramp.

- **Painful bladder syndrome:** Your bladder becomes sensitive
and easily irritated.

- **Scar tissue in the pelvic area:** You may have scar tissue from an
infection, an operation, or other treatment that now causes pain.

How is CPP treated?

Very little is known about effective ways to treat CPP. Your doctor
may try one or more ways to help relieve your pain or help you cope with
it, but there is very little research to tell doctors which therapies work.

When a cause cannot be found, doctors may recommend a medicine, hormonal therapy, or surgery to try to relieve your CPP symptoms. Your doctor may suggest a narcotic or nonnarcotic pain reliever such as aspirin, Tylenol, Advil, Demerol, or OxyContin to help manage your pain. In addition, your doctor may also suggest counseling, physical therapy, changes in your diet, or exercise to help with your CPP.

The information that follows tells what researchers have found out about how well medicines, hormonal therapies, and surgeries work to relieve CPP symptoms. Just because there is not enough research on many of the therapies listed does not mean that the therapies do not work for some people.

Medicines: Gabapentin (Fanatrex, Gabarone, Gralise, Horizant, and Neurontin), Amitriptyline (Elavil, Endep, and Vanatrip), and Botulinum A toxin (commonly known as Botox, which is given as a shot).

- There is not enough research to know if any of these medicines help relieve CPP symptoms.

Hormonal therapies: Hormonal contraceptives (birth control), hormone shots, and medicines that act like hormones.

- There is not enough research to know if any other hormonal therapies help relieve CPP symptoms.

- In one study, women with endometriosis who took a hormone-like medicine called raloxifene (Evista) after having a diagnostic laparoscopy had their pain return quicker than women who did not take any medicine.

- In one study, women who took a hormone-like medicine called depot leuprolide (Lupron Depot) felt less pain than women who did not take any medicine. Most of the women in the study had endometriosis.

Surgeries: Laparoscopic adhesiolysis (scar tissue is removed in and around your bowel); LUNA, which stands for laparoscopic uterosacral nerve ablation (some of the nerves in or around your uterus are destroyed); utero-sacral ligament resection (some of the nerves and tissue around the uterus are removed); and hysterectomy (a surgeon removes all or part of your uterus and ovaries).

- A few studies showed that removing scar tissue through a laparoscope (called laparoscopic adhesiolysis) had no effect on relieving pelvic pain or improving the quality of a woman's life.

319

- A few studies showed that LUNA did not help pelvic pain any more than having a diagnostic laparoscopy.

- There is not enough evidence to know how well utero-sacral ligament resection or hysterectomy work to help relieve CPP symptoms.

What should I think about when making a decision about treating CPP?

When there is not much evidence to guide the decision you and your doctor need to make, your own wishes and values have an important role. You and your doctor should discuss these issues:

- The possible side effects of medicines and which side effects you are willing to tolerate if a medicine may help your pain.

- If you should try non-surgery therapies before surgery, since there is not much evidence that surgery will help relieve your pain.

- How you feel about a hysterectomy, if your doctor suggests this. You should think about how important becoming pregnant or not beginning menopause (if your ovaries are removed) is to you.

- Other ways to keep CPP from affecting your work, relationships, and daily life.

All therapies for CPP may be covered differently by your health insurance plan, and you may have out-of-pocket costs.

It is important to find additional support from friends, family, counselors, and others while you and your doctor work to find the right treatment.

Talk with your doctor about how much pain you feel and which treatment best fits your specific needs, wishes, and values. Ask your doctor these questions:

- How will we decide which therapies to try?

- What are the side effects or risks of each therapy?

- How long will it take until I start to feel better?

- How will I know if surgery is really needed?

- What resources are available for me to get support while we try to find the right treatment?

Section 28.3

Dysmenorrhea

"Painful Periods (Dysmenorrhea)," reprinted with permission from the University of California San Diego Student Health Services (http://studenthealth.ucsd.edu). © 2013 Regents of the University of California. All rights reserved.

It's Not Your Imagination!

Over the years you may have read ... or been told .... that it was "all in your mind" ... that you were exaggerating the actual discomfort ... or that it was simply the price you had to pay for being female. Medical experts, however, have shown that painful menstruation is a physical problem and that most cases can be successfully treated.

Symptoms

Dysmenorrhea often includes one or more of such symptoms as mild to severe cramping in the lower abdomen, backache pain and pulling on the inside of the thighs, nausea, vomiting, diarrhea, dizziness, fainting, or headache. If you are like most women who suffer from dysmenorrhea, the symptoms are usually more severe on the first day of flow. They probably decrease as your period continues, and in most cases last no more than 12–16 hours. However, some women experience discomfort from the beginning to the end of the menstrual flow, which may be for as long as 5–6 days.

A Common Problem

Dysmenorrhea is the most common cause of lost work and school hours among women in the United States. In fact, 42 million women in the United States suffer from painful menstrual symptoms. Of these, about 3½ million are unable to function for one to two days each month because the condition is so severe.

An Important Cause Has Been Found

In a very small number of cases, the cause of dysmenorrhea is actual disease or some physical abnormality. These conditions are usually not

321

difficult to diagnose and they can often by corrected by medication or surgery. But the causes of dysmenorrhea in a normal, healthy woman are not so clear. It has long been believed that heredity, psychological well-being, and environment are important influences. However, the most up-to-date thinking indicates that a group of chemicals in your body called *prostaglandins* may be the most direct influence.

Understanding Your Menstrual Cycle

To have a better understanding of how painful periods occur, it is important to know what happens to your body at the various stages of your menstrual cycle. At the beginning of your period (Day 1 of your cycle), a complex chemical called a hormone travels through your bloodstream and causes one of the thousands of egg cells stored in your ovaries to begin to ripen. As the egg matures, between the fifth and fourteenth day, estrogen levels increase. The estrogen travels through the bloodstream to the uterus, where it causes the lining of the uterus to thicken so that it will be able to nourish a fertilized egg cell.

By about the 14th day after menstruation begins, ovulation takes place. This means that the mature egg cell leaves the ovary and begins its journey through the fallopian tube toward the uterus. Progesterone levels then begin to increase, causing the blood supply to the uterus to increase. If the egg is not fertilized, all this preparation is unnecessary. Thus, the thick, blood-rich lining of the uterus is shed. Along with the unfertilized egg and other cellular matter, it is discharged through the vagina on about the 28th day, and another menstrual cycle begins.

Understanding the Role of Prostaglandins

In addition to the hormones in your body there are the previously mentioned chemicals called prostaglandins. It has been found that prostaglandins are involved in controlling many functions in your body, including intestinal activity; the change in diameter of your blood vessels, and uterine contractions.

Scientists believe that when there is an excess of a certain prostaglandin, uterine contractions are greater, and this causes the severe pain and discomfort of dysmenorrhea. It is also thought that the excess prostaglandin travels through your bloodstream, constricting vessels in various parts of your body and activating your large intestine. Thus, this prostaglandin is responsible for the headaches, dizziness, hot and cold flashes, diarrhea, and nausea that can accompany painful periods.

Nothing to Worry About... Other Than the Discomfort

If you are worrying that dysmenorrhea may be a harmful condition, you'll be relieved to know that it is not. It will not affect your ability to become pregnant. In fact, a uterine lining that produces painful menstrual cramps can only do so as a result of a normal menstrual cycle. So you can be more certain than women without dysmenorrhea that your reproductive functions are working properly.

The Problem May Decrease With Age

Dysmenorrhea doesn't usually affect young girls who are just starting their periods, because ovulation does not occur in these early cycles. However, you may have started to experience discomfort within a few months or years after menstruation began. Although physicians do not yet understand why, the condition is most common between the ages of 15 and 25. For many women, the discomfort begins to fade as they reach their late twenties or early thirties.

Fortunately there are many remedies that may make your periods more comfortable. The application of a hot water bottle or a heating pad to the abdomen during the first few hours of your period may provide some relief. Adequate rest can also be helpful. You should pursue normal activities if possible, including usual types of physical exercise.

Medications That Slow Down Prostaglandin Production

Since an excess of prostaglandins in the lining of the uterus seems to be one of the major causes of dysmenorrhea, any medication that reduces the amount of prostaglandins will be helpful in relieving the pain. Aspirin, for example, reduces prostaglandin production slightly, and some women do in fact get relief by taking aspirin during their monthly period. Birth control pills have also been shown to help relieve dysmenorrhea. Since they prevent ovulation, they prevent the full development of the lining of the uterus, and thus the amount of prostaglandin present is reduced. The pain experienced by many women is very severe, and now medication is available. It does not interfere with the regular cycle and has only minimal side effects. And because it inhibits prostaglandin production, it greatly reduces and in many cases completely eliminates the pain and discomfort of dysmenorrhea.

Section 28.4

Dyspareunia

"Painful sex in women (dyspareunia)," is reprinted with permission from DermNet NZ, the web site of the New Zealand Dermatological Society. Visit www.dermnetnz.org for patient information about skin diseases, conditions, and treatment. © 2012 New Zealand Dermatological Society. All rights reserved.

Dyspareunia (painful sex) is defined as persistent or recurrent genital pain that occurs just before, during or after intercourse. There are two types:

- Entry (superficial) dyspareunia, where pain is felt at the entrance to, or within the vagina

- Deep (abdominal) dyspareunia, where pain is felt in the abdomen.

Dyspareunia is common and may cause considerable distress to women and their sexual partners. It may be caused by structural, infective, and inflammatory diseases of the vulva, vagina and internal organs. Psychosocial factors inevitably contribute to, and result from, dyspareunia.

- Dyspareunia may be primary, i.e., occurred with the first attempt at intercourse and ever since; or secondary, i.e., occurring later, having previously had no pain with intercourse.

- Pain can occur on every attempt at intercourse or only on certain occasions or in certain situations.

Entry Dyspareunia

The most common vulval skin diseases resulting in superficial or entry dyspareunia include:

- Dryness or eczema/dermatitis especially when due to contact irritant or, less often, contact allergic factors (e.g., latex allergy), or chronic rubbing/scratching leading to lichen simplex

- Primary fissuring of posterior fourchette
- Medications that dry the skin, particularly isotretinoin
- Genital herpes or other sexually transmitted infections
- Lichen sclerosus
- Lichen planus
- Plasma cell vulvitis

Dyspareunia associated with dry vagina or vaginal inflammation (vaginitis) may be due to:

- Insufficient lubrication due to lack of sexual arousal or inability to reach orgasm
- Hormonal changes such as birth control medication, lactation, cancer treatment, or menopause (atrophic vaginitis)
- Irritation from vaginal lubricants, creams, foams, douches, pessaries, condoms, or devices
- Medications that dry mucosal surfaces, such as antihistamines or antidepressant medications such as amitriptyline
- Dry mucosae due to Sjögren syndrome
- Vulvovaginal candidiasis
- Bacterial vaginosis
- Chlamydia infection
- Trichomoniasis
- Erosive vaginal lichen planus
- Desquamative inflammatory vaginitis
- Radiation induced vaginitis following treatment for uterine or cervical cancer.

Dyspareunia may also result from:

- Malformation of the genitalia, e.g., narrowed vagina, labial adhesion, vaginal septa, imperforate hymen
- Injury, e.g., during childbirth, genital mutilation or surgery
- Urinary tract infection

- Interstitial cystitis (painful bladder syndrome)
- Any pain affecting the vestibule (if cause is unknown, this is called vestibulodynia)
- Any pain affecting the vulva (if cause is unknown, this is called vulvodynia)
- Tense pelvic floor muscles and/or vaginismus (involuntary pelvic muscle contractions during attempted intercourse)
- Low libido related to fear, anxiety and relationship problems including sexual abuse.

Deep Dyspareunia

Deep dyspareunia means sexual pain that is felt in the abdomen, rather than in the vagina. Causes may include:

- Recent pregnancy/childbirth
- Retroverted uterus (this refers to the position of the womb)
- Uterine prolapse
- Pelvic inflammatory disease or infection
- Endometriosis
- Ovarian cysts
- Uterine fibroids
- Bowel disease especially irritable bowel syndrome (IBS)
- Lumbosacral arthritis
- Adhesions following previous surgery or radiation
- Genital tract cancer.

Diagnosis of Dyspareunia

Correct diagnosis requires careful history and clinical examination of the whole body including external genitalia, and pelvic examination by a medical expert (e.g., gynecologist, sexual health physician, or general practitioner). Colposcopy (pelvic examination using magnification and a bright light) may be performed. The site of pain should be carefully identified. Examination under anaesthetic may be required if discomfort is too great to allow a normal internal examination.

Investigations may include:

• Bacterial and viral swabs

• Skin biopsy

• Ultrasound examination

• Radiographic examination

In many cases, no physical reason is found for dyspareunia and it is considered a pain syndrome.

Treatment of Dyspareunia

Intercourse should not be painful. It's important to feel relaxed before attempting intercourse. Foreplay leading to sexual excitement relaxes the pelvic muscles, widens the vagina, and releases vaginal fluids. Use liberal amounts of water-based lubricants and apply these to the penis and vaginal opening. Penetration from behind or woman-on-top may be better tolerated.

If a cause for the dyspareunia has been found, then appropriate treatment should help. General measures may also assist:

• Don't use scented bath oils or shower gels, soaps or douches.

• Emollients help vulval dryness and water-based lubricants or moisturizers are used for vaginal dryness.

• Estrogen cream, pessaries, or rings reduce hormone-associated vaginal dryness, and are often prescribed to post-menopausal women.

• Local anaesthetic cream or gel may allow pain-free penetration.

• Tricyclic medicines such as amitriptyline can reduce pain.

• Botulinum toxin has been used to relax hypertonic pelvic floor muscles (experimental).

An experienced pelvic floor physiotherapist can help in retraining the pelvic floor to relax using special exercises. Counselling or behavioral therapy is appropriate for some women or couples.

If vaginal intercourse remains painful, consider other sexual options including massage and mutual masturbation.

Section 28.5

Endometriosis

Excerpted from "Endometriosis Fact Sheet," Office on Women's Health, U.S. Department of Health and Human Services (www.womenshealth.gov), November 16, 2009.

What is endometriosis?

Endometriosis is a common health problem in women. It gets its name from the word, endometrium, the tissue that lines the uterus or womb. Endometriosis occurs when this tissue grows outside of the uterus on other organs or structures in the body. Most often, endometriosis is found on the ovaries, Fallopian tubes, tissues that hold the uterus in place, outer surface of the uterus, and the lining of the pelvic cavity. Other sites for growths can include the vagina, cervix, vulva, bowel, bladder, or rectum. In rare cases, endometriosis has been found in other parts of the body, such as the lungs, brain, and skin.

What are the symptoms of endometriosis?

The most common symptom of endometriosis is pain in the lower abdomen or pelvis, or the lower back, mainly during menstrual periods. The amount of pain a woman feels does not depend on how much endometriosis she has. Some women have no pain, even though their disease affects large areas. Other women with endometriosis have severe pain even though they have only a few small growths.

Symptoms of endometriosis can include the following:

- Very painful menstrual cramps; pain may get worse over time
- Chronic pain in the lower back and pelvis
- Pain during or after sex
- Intestinal pain
- Painful bowel movements or painful urination during menstrual periods
- Spotting or bleeding between menstrual periods
- Infertility or not being able to get pregnant

- Fatigue

- Diarrhea, constipation, bloating, or nausea, especially during menstrual periods

Recent research shows a link between other health problems in women with endometriosis and their families. Some of these include allergies, asthma, and chemical sensitivities and autoimmune diseases, in which the body's system that fights illness attacks itself instead. These can include hypothyroidism, multiple sclerosis, and lupus. Other links include chronic fatigue syndrome (CFS) and fibromyalgia, being more likely to get infections and mononucleosis, mitral valve prolapse (a condition in which one of the heart's valves does not close as tightly as normal), frequent yeast infections, and certain cancers, such as ovarian, breast, endocrine, kidney, thyroid, brain, and colon cancers, and melanoma and non-Hodgkin's lymphoma.

Why does endometriosis cause pain and health problems?

Growths of endometriosis are benign (not cancerous). But they still can cause many problems. To see why, it helps to understand a woman's menstrual cycle. Every month, hormones cause the lining of a woman's uterus to build up with tissue and blood vessels. If a woman does not get pregnant, the uterus sheds this tissue and blood. It comes out of the body through the vagina as her menstrual period.

Patches of endometriosis also respond to the hormones produced during the menstrual cycle. With the passage of time, the growths of endometriosis may expand by adding extra tissue and blood. The symptoms of endometriosis often get worse.

Tissue and blood that is shed into the body can cause inflammation, scar tissue, and pain. As endometrial tissue grows, it can cover or grow into the ovaries and block the fallopian tubes. Trapped blood in the ovaries can form cysts, or closed sacs. It also can cause inflammation and cause the body to form scar tissue and adhesions, tissue that sometimes binds organs together. This scar tissue may cause pelvic pain and make it hard for women to get pregnant. The growths can also cause problems in the intestines and bladder.

How is endometriosis treated?

There is no cure for endometriosis, but there are many treatments for the pain and infertility that it causes. Talk with your doctor about what option is best for you. The treatment you choose will depend on your symptoms, age, and plans for getting pregnant.

Pain medication: For some women with mild symptoms, doctors may suggest taking over-the-counter medicines for pain. These include ibuprofen (Advil and Motrin) or naproxen (Aleve). When these medicines don't help, doctors may prescribe stronger pain relievers.

Hormone treatment: When pain medicine is not enough, doctors often recommend hormone medicines to treat endometriosis. Only women who do not wish to become pregnant can use these drugs. Hormone treatment is best for women with small growths who do not have bad pain. Hormones come in many forms including pills, shots, and nasal sprays. Common hormones used for endometriosis include the following:

• Birth control pills to decrease the amount of menstrual flow and prevent overgrowth of tissue that lines the uterus

• GnRH agonists and antagonists greatly reduce the amount of estrogen in a woman's body, which stops the menstrual cycle

• Progestins. The hormone progestin can shrink spots of endometriosis by working against the effects of estrogen on the tissue.

• Danazol is a weak male hormone that lowers the levels of estrogen and progesterone in a woman's body.

Surgery: Surgery is usually the best choice for women with severe endometriosis—many growths, a great deal of pain, or fertility problems. There are both minor and more complex surgeries that can help. Your doctor might suggest one of the following:

• Laparoscopy can be used to diagnose and treat endometriosis. During this surgery, doctors remove growths and scar tissue or burn them away. The goal is to treat the endometriosis without harming the healthy tissue around it. Women recover from laparoscopy much faster than from major abdominal surgery.

• Laparotomy or major abdominal surgery that involves a much larger cut in the abdomen than with laparoscopy. This allows the doctor to reach and remove growths of endometriosis in the pelvis or abdomen.

• Hysterectomy is a surgery in which the doctor removes the uterus. Removing the ovaries as well can help ensure that endometriosis will not return. This is done when the endometriosis has severely damaged these organs. A woman cannot get pregnant after this surgery, so it should only be considered as a last resort.

Section 28.6

Uterine Fibroids

Excerpted from "Uterine Fibroids Fact Sheet," Office on Women's Health, U.S. Department of Health and Human Services (www.womenshealth.gov), May 13, 2008. Reviewed by David A. Cooke, MD, FACP, March 2013.

What are uterine fibroids?

Uterine fibroids are muscular tumors that grow in the wall of the uterus (womb). Another medical term for fibroids is *leiomyoma* or just *myoma*. Fibroids are almost always benign (not cancerous). Fibroids can grow as a single tumor, or there can be many of them in the uterus. They can be as small as an apple seed or as big as a grapefruit. In unusual cases they can become very large.

About 20 percent to 80 percent of women develop fibroids by the time they reach age 50. Fibroids are most common in women in their 40s and early 50s. Not all women with fibroids have symptoms. Women who do have symptoms often find fibroids hard to live with. Some have pain and heavy menstrual bleeding. Fibroids also can put pressure on the bladder, causing frequent urination, or the rectum, causing rectal pressure. Should the fibroids get very large, they can cause the abdomen (stomach area) to enlarge, making a woman look pregnant.

Most fibroids grow in the wall of the uterus. Doctors put them into three groups based on where they grow:

- Submucosal fibroids grow into the uterine cavity.

- Intramural fibroids grow within the wall of the uterus.

- Subserosal fibroids grow on the outside of the uterus.

Some fibroids grow on stalks that grow out from the surface of the uterus or into the cavity of the uterus. They might look like mushrooms. These are called pedunculated fibroids.

What are the symptoms of fibroids?

Most fibroids do not cause any symptoms, but some women with fibroids can have these symptoms:

- Heavy bleeding (which can be heavy enough to cause anemia) or painful periods

- Feeling of fullness in the pelvic area (lower stomach area)

- Enlargement of the lower abdomen

- Frequent urination

- Pain during sex

- Lower back pain

- Complications during pregnancy and labor, including a six-time greater risk of cesarean section

- Reproductive problems, such as infertility, which is very rare

How are fibroids treated?

Most women with fibroids do not have any symptoms. For women who do have symptoms, there are treatments that can help. Talk with your doctor about the best way to treat your fibroids. She or he will consider many things before helping you choose a treatment. Some of these things include the following:

- Whether or not you are having symptoms from the fibroids

- If you might want to become pregnant in the future

- The size of the fibroids

- The location of the fibroids

- Your age and how close to menopause you might be

If you have fibroids but do not have any symptoms, you may not need treatment. Your doctor will check during your regular exams to see if they have grown.

When are medications used to treat fibroids?

If you have fibroids and have mild symptoms, your doctor may suggest taking medication. Over-the-counter drugs such as ibuprofen or acetaminophen can be used for mild pain. If you have heavy bleeding during your period, taking an iron supplement can keep you from getting anemia or correct it if you already are anemic.

Several drugs commonly used for birth control can be prescribed to help control symptoms of fibroids. Low-dose birth control pills do not make fibroids grow and can help control heavy bleeding. The same is true of progesterone-like injections (for example, Depo-Provera). An IUD (intrauterine device) called Mirena contains a small amount of progesterone-like medication, which can be used to control heavy bleeding as well as for birth control.

Other drugs used to treat fibroids are *gonadotropin releasing hormone agonists* (GnRHa). The one most commonly used is Lupron. These drugs, given by injection, nasal spray, or implanted, can shrink your fibroids. Sometimes they are used before surgery to make fibroids easier to remove. Side effects of GnRHas can include hot flashes, depression, not being able to sleep, decreased sex drive, and joint pain. Most women tolerate GnRHas quite well. Most women do not get a period when taking GnRHas. This can be a big relief to women who have heavy bleeding. It also allows women with anemia to recover to a normal blood count. GnRHas can cause bone thinning, so their use is generally limited to six months or less. These drugs also are very expensive, and some insurance companies will cover only some or none of the cost. GnRHas offer temporary relief from the symptoms of fibroids; once you stop taking the drugs, the fibroids often grow back quickly.

When is surgery used to treat fibroids?

If you have fibroids with moderate or severe symptoms, surgery may be the best way to treat them. Here are the options:

Myomectomy: Surgery to remove fibroids without taking out the healthy tissue of the uterus. It is best for women who wish to have children after treatment for their fibroids or who wish to keep their uterus for other reasons. You can become pregnant after myomectomy. But if your fibroids were imbedded deeply in the uterus, you might need a cesarean section to deliver. Myomectomy can be performed in many ways. It can be major surgery (involving cutting into the abdomen) or performed with laparoscopy or hysteroscopy. The type of surgery that can be done depends on the type, size, and location of the fibroids. After myomectomy new fibroids can grow and cause trouble later. All of the possible risks of surgery are true for myomectomy. The risks depend on how extensive the surgery is.

Hysterectomy: Surgery to remove the uterus. This surgery is the only sure way to cure uterine fibroids. Fibroids are the most common reason that hysterectomy is performed. This surgery is used when a woman's fibroids are large, if she has heavy bleeding, is either near or past menopause, or does not want children. If the fibroids are large, a woman may need a hysterectomy that involves cutting into the abdomen to remove the uterus. If the fibroids are smaller, the doctor may be able to reach the uterus through the vagina, instead of making a cut in the abdomen. In some cases hysterectomy can be performed through the laparoscope. Removal of the ovaries and the cervix at the time of hysterectomy is usually optional. Women whose ovaries are not removed do not go into menopause at the time of hysterectomy. Hysterectomy is a major surgery. Although hysterectomy is usually quite safe, it does carry a significant risk of complications. Recovery from hysterectomy usually takes several weeks.

Endometrial ablation: The lining of the uterus is removed or destroyed to control very heavy bleeding. This can be done with laser, wire loops, boiling water, electric current, microwaves, freezing, and other methods. This procedure usually is considered minor surgery. It can be done on an outpatient basis or even in a doctor's office. Complications can occur, but are uncommon with most of the methods. Most people recover quickly. About half of women who have this procedure have no more menstrual bleeding. About three in 10 women have much lighter bleeding. But, a woman cannot have children after this surgery.

Myolysis: A needle is inserted into the fibroids, usually guided by laparoscopy, and electric current or freezing is used to destroy the fibroids.

Uterine fibroid embolization (UFE) or uterine artery embolization (UAE): A thin tube is threaded into the blood vessels that supply blood to the fibroid. Then, tiny plastic or gel particles are injected into the blood vessels. This blocks the blood supply to the fibroid, causing it to shrink. UFE can be an outpatient or inpatient procedure. Complications, including early menopause, are uncommon but can occur. Studies suggest fibroids are not likely to grow back after UFE, but more long-term research is needed. Not all fibroids can be treated with UFE. The best candidates for UFE are women who have fibroids that are causing heavy bleeding, have fibroids that are causing pain or pressing on the bladder or rectum, don't want to have a hysterectomy, and don't want to have children in the future.

Section 28.7

Vulvodynia

Excerpted from "NIH Research Plan on Vulvodynia,"
National Institute of Child Health and Human Development
(www.nichd.nih.gov), April 2012.

Vulvodynia is a term used to describe chronic pain or discomfort of the vulva. The nature of the pain may vary from woman to woman; vulvodynia can cause burning, stinging, irritation, or rawness. The pain may move around or always be in the same place; it can be constant, sporadic, or severe. Although it is difficult to determine how many women are affected by vulvodynia, studies suggest that many women may suffer from the condition. Researchers have estimated that 9 percent to 18 percent of women between the ages of 18 and 64 years may experience vulvar pain during their lifetime.

Vulvodynia can have a significant impact on a woman's quality-of-life. Women who suffer from vulvodynia report that sex and many routine or daily activities such as tampon insertion, sitting, or even wearing underclothing can become difficult or impossible.

Obtaining a diagnosis of vulvodynia can be difficult and time consuming. Vulvodynia tends to be diagnosed only when other causes of vulvar pain, such as infection or skin diseases, have been ruled out. To diagnose vulvodynia, a health care provider may recommend that a woman have blood drawn to assess levels of estrogen, progesterone, and testosterone. The provider may also perform a cotton-swab test, applying gentle pressure to various vulvar sites and asking the patient to rate the severity of the pain. If any areas of skin appear suspicious, these areas may be magnified or biopsied for further examination.

Because vulvodynia is often a diagnosis of exclusion, it can be difficult and time consuming to arrive at an actual diagnosis. The diagnostic process can be especially problematic for women who lack health insurance because they may not have the resources to continue excluding possible causes of pain before a provider can arrive at a diagnosis of vulvodynia. Moreover, some women may be reluctant to discuss their pain or seek treatment.

A definitive root cause of vulvodynia remains unknown. Researchers speculate that one or more of the following may cause, or contribute to, vulvodynia:

- An injury to, or irritation of, the nerves that transmit pain and other sensations from the vulva

- An increase in nerve fiber density in the vulvar vestibule

- Elevated levels of inflammatory substances in the vulvar tissue

- An abnormal response of vulvar cells to environmental factors

- Altered hormone receptor expression in the vulvar tissue

- Genetic susceptibility to chronic vestibular inflammation

- Genetic susceptibility to chronic widespread pain

- Genetic factors associated with an inability to combat vulvovaginal infection

- A localized hypersensitivity to *Candida* or other vulvovaginal organisms

- Pelvic floor muscle dysfunction, weakness, or spasm

The general lack of awareness of vulvodynia among clinicians and women across the age spectrum presents a particular challenge in the diagnosis and treatment of vulvodynia in teenage girls. Many health care providers may be reluctant to bring up the subject of vulvovaginal pain with teenage girls because of its perceived association with sexual activity, although vulvovaginal pain is not limited to sexually active females. Like adult women, teen girls may also be reticent to bring up issues of vulvovaginal pain with their health care providers or with their parents/caregivers. As a result, many teenage girls and adult women suffer vulvar pain in silence, with neither diagnoses nor treatments.

Although some treatments are successful for some women, there is currently no cure that works for all women, nor is there a standard panel of therapeutics known to reliably treat vulvodynia. A variety of treatment options may be presented to patients, including the following:

- Oral medications, such as pain medications, tricyclic antidepressants, anticonvulsants, or antihistamines

- Biofeedback therapy, intended to help patients decrease pain sensation

- Topical medications, such as lidocaine ointment or hormonal creams

- Nerve block injections
- Physical therapy to strengthen pelvic floor muscles
- Surgery to remove the affected skin and tissue in localized vulvodynia
- Diet modification
- Neurostimulation and spinal infusion pump
- Complementary or alternative medicine

Chapter 29

Headaches

Chapter Contents

Section 29.1—Primary and Secondary Headache
　　　　Disorders... 340
Section 29.2—Hormones and Migraine 352
Section 29.3—Analgesic Rebound 354
Section 29.4—Giant Cell Arteritis 355

Section 29.1

Primary and Secondary Headache Disorders

Excerpted from "Headache: Hope Through Research," National Institute of Neurological Disorders and Stroke (www.ninds.nih.gov), NIH Pub. No. 09-158, updated February 11, 2013.

Introduction

Anyone can experience a headache. Nearly two out of three children will have a headache by age 15. More than nine in ten adults will experience a headache sometime in their life. Headache is our most common form of pain and a major reason cited for days missed at work or school as well as visits to the doctor. Without proper treatment, headaches can be severe and interfere with daily activities.

Certain types of headache run in families. Episodes of headache may ease or even disappear for a time and recur later in life. It's possible to have more than one type of headache at the same time.

Primary headaches occur independently and are not caused by another medical condition. It's uncertain what sets the process of a primary headache in motion. A cascade of events that affect blood vessels and nerves inside and outside the head causes pain signals to be sent to the brain. Brain chemicals called neurotransmitters are involved in creating head pain, as are changes in nerve cell activity (called cortical spreading depression). Migraine, cluster, and tension-type headache are the more familiar types of primary headache.

Secondary headaches are symptoms of another health disorder that causes pain-sensitive nerve endings to be pressed on or pulled or pushed out of place. They may result from underlying conditions including fever, infection, medication overuse, stress or emotional conflict, high blood pressure, psychiatric disorders, head injury or trauma, stroke, tumors, and nerve disorders (particularly trigeminal neuralgia, a chronic pain condition that typically affects a major nerve on one side of the jaw or cheek).

Headaches can range in frequency and severity of pain. Some individuals may experience headaches once or twice a year, while others may experience headaches more than 15 days a month. Some headaches may recur or last for weeks at a time. Pain can range from mild to disabling and may be accompanied by symptoms such as nausea or increased sensitivity to noise or light, depending on the type of headache.

Why Headaches Hurt

Information about touch, pain, temperature, and vibration in the head and neck is sent to the brain by the trigeminal nerve, one of 12 pairs of cranial nerves that start at the base of the brain.

The nerve has three branches that conduct sensations from the scalp, the blood vessels inside and outside of the skull, the lining around the brain (the meninges), and the face, mouth, neck, ears, eyes, and throat.

Brain tissue itself lacks pain-sensitive nerves and does not feel pain. Headaches occur when pain-sensitive nerve endings called nociceptors react to headache triggers (such as stress, certain foods or odors, or use of medicines) and send messages through the trigeminal nerve to the thalamus, the brain's "relay station" for pain sensation from all over the body. The thalamus controls the body's sensitivity to light and noise and sends messages to parts of the brain that manage awareness of pain and emotional response to it. Other parts of the brain may also be part of the process, causing nausea, vomiting, diarrhea, trouble concentrating, and other neurological symptoms.

When to See a Doctor

Not all headaches require a physician's attention. But headaches can signal a more serious disorder that requires prompt medical care. Immediately call or see a physician if you or someone you're with experience any of these symptoms:

- Sudden, severe headache that may be accompanied by a stiff neck

- Severe headache accompanied by fever, nausea, or vomiting that is not related to another illness

- "First" or "worst" headache, often accompanied by confusion, weakness, double vision, or loss of consciousness

- Headache that worsens over days or weeks or has changed in pattern or behavior

- Recurring headache in children

- Headache following a head injury

- Headache and a loss of sensation or weakness in any part of the body, which could be a sign of a stroke

- Headache associated with convulsions

- Headache associated with shortness of breath

- Two or more headaches a week

- Persistent headache in someone who has been previously headache-free, particularly in someone over age 50

- New headaches in someone with a history of cancer or HIV/ AIDS

Diagnosing Your Headache

How and under what circumstances a person experiences a headache can be key to diagnosing its cause. Keeping a headache journal can help a physician better diagnose your type of headache and determine the best treatment. After each headache, note the time of day when it occurred; its intensity and duration; any sensitivity to light, odors, or sound; activity immediately prior to the headache; use of prescription and nonprescription medicines; amount of sleep the previous night; any stressful or emotional conditions; any influence from weather or daily activity; foods and fluids consumed in the past 24 hours; and any known health conditions at that time. Women should record the days of their menstrual cycles. Include notes about other family members who have a history of headache or other disorder. A pattern may emerge that can be helpful to reducing or preventing headaches.

Once your doctor has reviewed your medical and headache history and conducted a physical and neurological exam, lab screening and diagnostic tests may be ordered to either rule out or identify conditions that might be the cause of your headaches. Blood tests and urinalysis can help diagnose brain or spinal cord infections, blood vessel damage, and toxins that affect the nervous system. Testing a sample of the fluid that surrounds the brain and spinal cord can detect infections, bleeding in the brain (called a brain hemorrhage), and measure any buildup of pressure within the skull. Diagnostic imaging, such as with computed tomography (CT) and magnetic resonance imaging (MRI), can detect irregularities in blood vessels and bones, certain brain tumors and cysts, brain damage from head injury, brain hemorrhage, inflammation, infection, and other disorders. Neuroimaging also gives doctors a way to see what's happening in the brain during headache attacks.

An electroencephalogram (EEG) measures brain wave activity and can help diagnose brain tumors, seizures, head injury, and inflammation that may lead to headaches.

Primary Headache Disorders

Primary headache disorders are divided into four main groups: migraine, tension-type headache, trigeminal autonomic cephalgias (a group of short-lasting but severe headaches), and a miscellaneous group.

Migraine

Migraines involve recurrent attacks of moderate to severe pain that is throbbing or pulsing and often strikes one side of the head. Untreated attacks last from 4 to 72 hours. Other common symptoms are increased sensitivity to light, noise, and odors; and nausea and vomiting. Routine physical activity, movement, or even coughing or sneezing can worsen the headache pain.

Migraines occur most frequently in the morning, especially upon waking. Some people have migraines at predictable times, such as before menstruation or on weekends following a stressful week of work. Many people feel exhausted or weak following a migraine but are usually symptom-free between attacks.

Migraine is divided into four phases, all of which may be present during the attack:

- Premonitory symptoms occur up to 24 hours prior to developing a migraine. These include food cravings, unexplained mood changes (depression or euphoria), uncontrollable yawning, fluid retention, or increased urination.

- Aura. Some people will see flashing or bright lights or what looks like heat waves immediately prior to or during the migraine, while others may experience muscle weakness or the sensation of being touched or grabbed.

- Headache. A migraine usually starts gradually and builds in intensity. It is possible to have migraine without a headache.

- Postdrome (following the headache). Individuals are often exhausted or confused following a migraine. The postdrome period may last up to a day before people feel healthy.

The two major types of migraine are migraine with aura and migraine without aura.

Migraine with aura, previously called classic migraine, includes visual disturbances and other neurological symptoms that appear about 10 to 60 minutes before the actual headache and usually last no more than an hour. Individuals may temporarily lose part or all of their vision. The aura may occur without headache pain, which can strike at any time. Other classic symptoms include trouble speaking; an abnormal sensation, numbness, or muscle weakness on one side of the body; a tingling sensation in the hands or face, and confusion. Nausea, loss of appetite, and increased sensitivity to light, sound, or noise may precede the headache.

Migraine without aura, or common migraine, is the more frequent form of migraine. Symptoms include headache pain that occurs without warning and is usually felt on one side of the head, along with nausea, confusion, blurred vision, mood changes, fatigue, and increased sensitivity to light, sound, or noise.

Other types of migraine include abdominal, basilar-type, and hemiplegic migraine. Abdominal migraine involves moderate to severe pain in the middle of the abdomen lasting one to 72 hours, with little or no headache. Additional symptoms include nausea, vomiting, and loss of appetite. Basilar-type migraine symptoms include partial or total loss of vision or double vision, dizziness and loss of balance, poor muscle coordination, slurred speech, a ringing in the ears, and fainting. Hemiplegic migraine is a rare but severe form of migraine that causes temporary paralysis.

Menstrually related migraine affects women around the time of their period, although most women with menstrually related migraine also have migraines at other times of the month. Symptoms may include migraine without aura (which is much more common during menses than migraine with aura), pulsing pain on one side of the head, nausea, vomiting, and increased sensitivity to sound and light.

Ophthalmoplegic migraine is an uncommon form of migraine with head pain, along with a droopy eyelid, large pupil, and double vision that may last for weeks, long after the pain is gone.

Retinal migraine is a condition characterized by attacks of visual loss or disturbances in one eye. These attacks, like the more common visual auras, are usually associated with migraine headaches.

Status migrainosus is a rare and severe type of acute migraine in which disabling pain and nausea can last 72 hours or longer. The pain and nausea may be so intense that sufferers need to be hospitalized.

Migraine treatment: Migraine treatment is aimed at relieving symptoms and preventing additional attacks. Quick steps to ease symptoms may include napping or resting with eyes closed in a quiet, darkened room; placing a cool cloth or ice pack on the forehead, and drinking lots of fluid, particularly if the migraine is accompanied by vomiting. Small amounts of caffeine may help relieve symptoms during a migraine's early stages.

Drug therapy for migraine is divided into acute and preventive treatment. Acute or "abortive" medications are taken as soon as symptoms occur to relieve pain and restore function. Preventive treatment involves taking medicines daily to reduce the severity of future attacks or keep them from happening. The U.S. Food and Drug Administration (FDA) has approved a variety of drugs for these treatment methods. Headache drug use should be monitored by a physician, since some drugs may cause side effects.

Acute treatment for migraine may include any of the following drugs.

- Triptan drugs increase levels of the neurotransmitter serotonin in the brain. Serotonin causes blood vessels to constrict and lowers the pain threshold. Triptans—the preferred treatment for migraine—ease moderate to severe migraine pain and are available as tablets, nasal sprays, and injections.

- Ergot derivative drugs bind to serotonin receptors on nerve cells and decrease the transmission of pain messages along nerve fibers. They are most effective during the early stages of migraine and are available as nasal sprays and injections.

- Non-prescription analgesics or over-the-counter drugs such as ibuprofen, aspirin, or acetaminophen can ease the pain of less severe migraine headache.

- Combination analgesics involve a mix of drugs such as acetaminophen plus caffeine and/or a narcotic for migraine that may be resistant to simple analgesics.

- Nonsteroidal anti-inflammatory drugs can reduce inflammation and alleviate pain.

- Nausea relief drugs can ease queasiness brought on by various types of headache.

- Narcotics are prescribed briefly to relieve pain. These drugs should not be used to treat chronic headaches.

Taking headache relief drugs more than three times a week may lead to medication overuse headache (previously called rebound headache), in which the initial headache is relieved temporarily but reappears as the drug wears off. Taking more of the drug to treat the new headache leads to progressively shorter periods of pain relief and results in a pattern of recurrent chronic headache. Headache pain ranges from moderate to severe and may occur with nausea or irritability. It may take weeks for these headaches to end once the drug is stopped.

Everyone with migraine needs effective treatment at the time of the headaches. Some people with frequent and severe migraine need preventive medications. In general, prevention should be considered if migraines occur one or more times weekly, or if migraines are less frequent but disabling. Preventive medicines are also recommended for individuals who take symptomatic headache treatment more than three times a week. Physicians will also recommend that a migraine sufferer take one or more preventive medications two to three months to assess drug effectiveness, unless intolerable side effects occur.

Non-drug therapy for migraine includes biofeedback and relaxation training, both of which help individuals cope with or control the development of pain and the body's response to stress.

Lifestyle changes that reduce or prevent migraine attacks in some individuals include exercising, avoiding food and beverages that trigger headaches, eating regularly scheduled meals with adequate hydration, stopping certain medications, and establishing a consistent sleep schedule. Obesity increases the risk of developing chronic daily headache, so a weight loss program is recommended for obese individuals.

Tension-Type Headache

Tension-type headache, previously called muscle contraction headache, is the most common type of headache. Its name indicates the role of stress and mental or emotional conflict in triggering the pain and contracting muscles in the neck, face, scalp, and jaw. Tension-type headaches may also be caused by jaw clenching, intense work, missed meals, depression, anxiety, or too little sleep. Sleep apnea may also cause tension-type headaches, especially in the morning. The pain is usually mild to moderate and feels as if constant pressure is being applied to the front of the face or to the head or neck. It also may feel as if a belt is being tightened around the head. Most often the pain is felt on both sides of the head. People who suffer tension-type headaches may also feel overly sensitive to light and sound but there is no pre-headache aura as with migraine. Typically, tension-type headaches usually disappear once the period of stress or related cause has ended.

There are two forms of tension-type headache: Episodic tension-type headaches occur between 10 and 15 days per month, with each attack lasting from 30 minutes to several days. Although the pain is not disabling, the severity of pain typically increases with the frequency of attacks. Chronic tension-type attacks usually occur more than 15 days per month over a three-month period. The pain, which can be constant over a period of days or months, strikes both sides of the head and is more severe and disabling than episodic headache pain. Chronic tension headaches can cause sore scalps—even combing your hair can be painful. Most individuals will have had some form of episodic tension-type headache prior to onset of chronic tension-type headache.

Depression and anxiety can cause tension-type headaches. Headaches may appear in the early morning or evening, when conflicts in the office or at home are anticipated. Other causes include physical postures that strain head and neck muscles (such as holding your chin down while reading or holding a phone between your shoulder and ear), degenerative arthritis of the neck, and temporomandibular joint dysfunction (a disorder of the joints between the temporal bone located above the ear and the mandible, or lower jaw bone).

The first step in caring for a tension-type headache involves treating any specific disorder or disease that may be causing it. For example, arthritis of the neck is treated with anti-inflammatory medication and temporomandibular joint dysfunction may be helped by corrective devices for the mouth and jaw. A sleep study may be needed to detect sleep apnea and should be considered when there is a history of snoring, daytime sleepiness, or obesity.

A physician may suggest using analgesics, nonsteroidal anti-inflammatory drugs, or antidepressants to treat a tension-type headache that is not associated with a disease. Triptan drugs, barbiturates (drugs that have a relaxing or sedative effect), and ergot derivatives may provide relief to people who suffer from both migraine and tension-type headache.

Alternative therapies for chronic tension-type headaches include biofeedback, relaxation training, meditation, and cognitive-behavioral therapy to reduce stress. A hot shower or moist heat applied to the back of the neck may ease symptoms of infrequent tension headaches. Physical therapy, massage, and gentle exercise of the neck may also be helpful.

Trigeminal Autonomic Cephalgias

Some primary headaches are characterized by severe pain in or around the eye on one side of the face and autonomic (or involuntary) features on the same side, such as red and teary eye, drooping eyelid, and runny nose. These disorders, called trigeminal autonomic cephalgias (cephalgia meaning head pain), differ in attack duration and frequency, and have episodic and chronic forms. Episodic attacks occur on a daily or near-daily basis for weeks or months with pain-free remissions. Chronic attacks occur on a daily or near-daily basis for a year or more with only brief remissions.

Cluster headache—the most severe form of primary headache—involves sudden, extremely painful headaches that occur in "clusters," usually at the same time of the day and night for several weeks. They strike one side of the head, often behind or around one eye, and may be preceded by a migraine-like aura and nausea. The pain usually peaks five to ten minutes after onset and continues at that intensity for up to three hours. The nose and the eye on the affected side of the face may get red, swollen, and teary. Some people will experience restlessness and agitation, changes in heart rate and blood pressure, and sensitivity to light, sound, or smell. Cluster headaches often wake people from sleep.

Treatment options include oxygen therapy—in which pure oxygen is breathed through a mask to reduce blood flow to the brain—and triptan drugs. Certain antipsychotic drugs, calcium-channel blockers, and anticonvulsants can reduce pain severity and frequency of attacks. In extreme cases, electrical stimulation of the occipital nerve to prevent nerve signaling or surgical procedures that destroy or cut certain facial nerves may provide relief.

Miscellaneous Primary Headaches

Other headaches that are not caused by other disorders include the following:

- Chronic daily headache refers to a group of headache disorders that occur at least 15 days a month during a three-month period. Individuals feel constant, mostly moderate pain throughout the day on the sides or top of the head. They may also experience other types of headache.

  - Hemicrania continua is marked by continuous, fluctuating pain that always occurs on the same side of the face and head. The headache may last from minutes to days and is associated with symptoms including tearing, red and irritated eyes, sweating, stuffy or runny nose, and swollen and drooping eyelids. The pain may get worse as the headache progresses. The nonsteroidal anti-inflammatory drug indomethacin usually provides rapid relief from symptoms.

Corticosteroids may also provide temporary relief from some symptoms.

- New daily persistent headache (NDPH), previously called chronic benign daily headache, is known for its constant daily pain that ranges from mild to severe. Individuals can often recount the exact date and time that the headache began. The disorder has two forms: one that usually ends on its own within several months and does not require treatment, and a longer-lasting form that is difficult to treat. Muscle relaxants, antidepressants, and anticonvulsants may provide some relief.

- Primary stabbing headache, also known as "ice pick" or "jabs and jolts" headache, is characterized by intense piercing pain that strikes without warning and generally lasts one to 10 seconds. The disorder is hard to treat, because each attack is extremely short.

- Primary exertional headache may be brought on by fits of coughing or sneezing or intense physical activity such as running, basketball, lifting weights, or sexual activity. Warm-up exercises prior to the physical activity can help prevent the headache and indomethacin can relieve the headache pain.

- Hypnic headache, previously called "alarm-clock" headache, awakens people mostly at night. Both men and women are affected by this disorder, which is usually treated with caffeine, indomethacin, or lithium.

- Ice cream headache (sometimes called "brain freeze") happens when cold materials such as cold drinks or ice cream hit the warm roof of your mouth. Local blood vessels constrict to reduce the loss of body heat and then relax and allow the blood flow to increase. The resulting burst of pain lasts for about five minutes. The pain stops once the body adapts to the temperature change.

Secondary Headache Disorders

Secondary headache disorders are caused by an underlying illness or condition that affects the brain. Secondary headaches are usually diagnosed based on other symptoms that occur concurrently and the characteristics of the headaches. The list that follows includes some of the more serious causes of secondary headache:

- **Brain tumor:** A tumor that is growing in the brain can press against nerve tissue and pain-sensitive blood vessel walls, disrupting communication between the brain and the nerves or restricting the supply of blood to the brain.

- **Disorders of blood vessels in the brain, including stroke:** Several disorders associated with blood vessel formation and activity can cause headache. Most notable among these conditions is stroke. Headache itself can cause stroke or accompany a series of blood vessel disorders that can cause a stroke. There are two forms of stroke. A hemorrhagic stroke occurs when an artery in the brain bursts, spilling blood into the surrounding tissue. An ischemic stroke occurs when an artery supplying the brain with blood becomes blocked, suddenly decreasing or stopping blood flow and causing brain cells to die.

- **Exposure to a substance or its withdrawal:** Headaches may result from toxic states such as drinking alcohol, following carbon monoxide poisoning, or from exposure to toxic chemicals and metals, cleaning products or solvents, and pesticides. The withdrawal from certain medicines or caffeine after frequent or excessive use can also cause headaches.

- **Head injury:** Headaches are often a symptom of a concussion or other head injury. The headache may develop either immediately or months after a blow to the head, with pain felt at the injury site or throughout the head.

- **Increased intracranial pressure:** A growing tumor, infection, or hydrocephalus (an extensive buildup of cerebrospinal fluid in the brain) can raise pressure in the brain and compress nerves and blood vessels, causing headaches.

- **Inflammation from meningitis, encephalitis, and other infections:** Inflammation from infections can harm or destroy nerve cells and cause dull to severe headache pain, brain damage, or stroke, among other conditions. Inflammation of the brain and spinal cord (meningitis and encephalitis) requires urgent medical attention. Headaches may also occur with a fever or a flu-like infection. A headache may accompany a bacterial infection of the upper respiratory tract that spreads to and inflames the lining of the sinus cavities.

- **Seizures:** Migraine-like headache pain may occur during or after a seizure. Moderate to severe headache pain may last for several hours and worsen with sudden movements of the head or when sneezing, coughing, or bending.

- **Spinal fluid leak:** About one-fourth of people who undergo a lumbar puncture (which involves a small sampling of the spinal fluid being removed for testing) develop a headache due to a leak of cerebrospinal fluid following the procedure.

- **Structural abnormalities of the head, neck and spine:** Headache pain and loss of function may be triggered by structural abnormalities in the head or spine, restricted blood flow through the neck, irritation to nerves anywhere along the path from the spinal cord to the brain, or stressful or awkward positions of the head and neck. Cervicogenic headaches are caused by structural irregularities in either the head or neck. In a Chiari malformation, the back of the skull is too small for the brain. Syringomyelia, a fluid-filled cyst within the spinal cord, can cause pain, numbness, weakness, and headaches.

- **Trigeminal neuralgia:** The trigeminal nerve conducts sensations to the brain from the upper, middle, and lower portions of the face, as well as inside the mouth. The presumed cause of trigeminal neuralgia is a blood vessel pressing on the nerve as it exits the brain stem, but other causes have been described.

Headache and Sleep Disorders

Headaches are often a secondary symptom of a sleep disorder. For example, tension-type headache is regularly seen in persons with insomnia or sleep-wake cycle disorders. Nearly three-fourths of individuals who suffer from narcolepsy complain of either migraine or cluster headache. Migraines and cluster headaches appear to be related to the number of and transition between rapid eye movement (REM) and other sleep periods an individual has during sleep. Hypnic headache awakens individuals mainly at night but may also interrupt daytime naps. Reduced oxygen levels in people with sleep apnea may trigger early morning headaches.

Getting the proper amount of sleep can ease headache pain. Generally, too little or too much sleep can worsen headaches, as can overuse of sleep medicines. Daytime naps often reduce deep sleep at night and can produce headaches in some adults. Some sleep disorders and secondary headache are treated using antidepressants. Check with a doctor before using over-the-counter medicines to ease sleep-associated headaches.

Coping with Headache

Headache treatment is a partnership between you and your doctor, and honest communication is essential. Finding a quick fix to your headache may not be possible. It may take some time for your doctor or specialist to determine the best course of treatment. Avoid using over-the-counter medicines more than twice a week, as they may actually worsen headache pain and the frequency of attacks. Visit a local headache support group meeting (if available) to learn how others with headache cope with their pain and discomfort. Relax whenever possible to ease stress and related symptoms, get enough sleep, regularly perform aerobic exercises, and eat a regularly scheduled and healthy diet that avoids food triggers. Gaining more control over your headache, stress, and emotions will make you feel better and let you embrace daily activities as much as possible.

Section 29.2

Hormones and Migraine

"Hormones and Migraine," © 2012 National Headache Foundation (www.headaches.org); reprinted with permission.

Migraine occurs more often in women than in men. Although migraine headaches are equally common in young girls and boys, the number of girls affected increases sharply after the onset of menstruation. It seems clear that certain hormonal changes that occur during puberty in girls, and remain throughout adulthood, are implicated in the triggering and frequency of migraine attacks in women.

The finding that 60% of women sufferers related attacks to their menstrual cycle supports this link between female hormone changes and migraine headaches. Attacks may occur several days before or during the woman's menstrual period. There are women who also get the headache mid-cycle, at the time of ovulation. Estrogen levels fluctuate throughout the menstrual cycle. The headaches typically occur in association with drops in the estrogen level. Few women (less than

10%) have headaches only with menses. Therefore, in most women, hormones are just one of many migraine triggers.

Triptans are the first line acute treatment for menstrually related migraine. These medications should be taken early in the attack and repeated if necessary. If the attacks are predictable, short-term preventive therapy can be started one to two days before the anticipated headache. The nonsteroidal anti-inflammatory agents can be used for 5–7 days around the period and help reduce headache frequency as well as relieve menstrual cramps. Stabilization of hormones may also benefit the migraines. This may include an estrogen patch or estrogen pills taken the week of the period. Daily triptans taken around the period may also reduce the headaches. Daily preventive treatment throughout the month may be necessary if the headaches continue to be frequent.

Oral contraceptives may affect the incidence of migraine. This was more common a decade or more ago because of the higher estrogen content in birth control pills. Some of the current triphasic pill products may also exacerbate migraine. There are variable effects today with the availability of contraceptive pills, transdermal patch, or vaginal ring. Some women benefit, some do not, and others have worsening of their migraines. For some women the use of the pill, patch, or ring for three or four consecutive cycles, without taking any days off, may help to reduce the number of menstrual migraines from 12 per year to three or four.

Pregnancy also influences migraine. Some women with migraine find their attacks disappear completely, occur less often, or are milder during pregnancy. Attacks either worsen or remain unchanged in others.

As women near menopause, the estrogen levels may fluctuate more and trigger an increase in migraines. Daily preventive therapy may again be necessary if the headaches are frequent and the periods are unpredictable. Women who go through natural menopause may have fewer headache problems than women having hysterectomies. In menopause, the use of continuous estrogen replacement without any days off helps to minimize migraine for many women. The dose should be the lowest effective dose. Synthetic estrogens (made in the lab) and skin patches may be better tolerated than products containing Premarin. Natural hormone products have not been carefully studied for their effect on headache. Progesterone agents rarely have an effect on migraine.

The use of the birth control pill or hormone replacement needs to be considered within the light of the type of migraine, smoking history, and other medical factors such as high blood pressure. For some women the use of hormonal therapies may put them at increased risk for serious medical consequences. Discussion with your physician is of importance to weigh the benefits and risks.

Section 29.3

Analgesic Rebound

"Analgesic Rebound," © 2012 National Headache Foundation
(www.headaches.org); reprinted with permission.

Analgesic rebound is also known as "medication overuse headache." Analgesic agents are prescription or over-the-counter medications used to control pain including migraine and other types of headaches. When used on a daily or near daily basis, these analgesics can perpetuate the headache process. They may decrease the intensity of the pain for a few hours; however, they appear to feed into the pain system in such a way that chronic headaches may result. The medication overuse headache (MOH) may feel like a dull, tension-type headache or may be a more severe migraine-like headache. Other medication taken to prevent or treat the headaches may not be effective while analgesics are being overused. MOH can occur with most analgesics but are more likely with products containing caffeine or butalbital.

Unless the overused analgesics are completely discontinued, the chronic headache is likely to continue unabated. Usually when analgesics are discontinued the headache may get worse for several days and the sufferer may experience nausea or vomiting. However, after a period of three to five days, sometimes longer, these symptoms begin to improve. Preventive medication will be needed to reduce the need for analgesics. For those patients willing to persevere, the headaches will gradually improve as response to more appropriate medication occurs. Most patients are able to stop the use of analgesics at home under physician supervision, but some find it difficult and may require hospitalization.

If you have overused analgesics, you are at high risk of relapsing and using too many analgesics again in the future. Medications such as ergots, triptans, opioids and barbiturates should not be used more than ten days per month. Simple analgesics should not be used for more than 15 days per month. By observing these limits patients will reduce the risk of MOH.

Section 29.4

Giant Cell Arteritis

"Giant Cell Arteritis," © 2012 American College of Rheumatology (www.rheumatology.org). All rights reserved. Reprinted with permission.

In an older adult, a new, persisting headache—especially if together with flu-like symptoms, unexplained fatigue (tiredness) or fevers—can be due to an illness called giant cell arteritis or GCA. A disease of blood vessels, GCA can occur together with polymyalgia rheumatica (also called PMR).

Fast Facts

- GCA generally occurs in older adults, usually those over the age of 60.

- If GCA affects blood flow to the eye, loss of vision can occur.

- Loss of vision can be prevented by prompt diagnosis and treatment.

What is giant cell arteritis?

GCA is a type of vasculitis or arteritis, a group of diseases whose main feature is inflammation of blood vessels. In GCA, the vessels most often involved are the arteries of the scalp and head, especially the arteries over the temples, which is why another term for GCA is *temporal arteritis*.

Giant cell arteritis can cause swelling and thickening of the small artery under the skin, called the temporal artery.

GCA can overlap with PMR. At some point, 5%–15% of patients with PMR will have a diagnosis of GCA. Looked at another way, about 50% of patients with GCA have symptoms of PMR. The two conditions may occur at the same time or on their own.

The most common symptom (what you feel) of GCA is a new headache, usually around the temples, but headache due to GCA can occur anywhere, including the front, top and back of the skull. Almost as common are more widespread symptoms, such as fatigue, loss of appetite, weight loss, or a flu-like feeling. There may be pain in the jaw with chewing. Sometimes the only sign of GCA is unexplained fever. Less common symptoms include pains in the face, tongue, or throat.

If GCA spreads to the blood supply of the eye, eyesight can be affected. Problems with vision can include temporary blurring, double vision, or blindness. Permanent loss of vision in GCA can occur suddenly, but proper treatment can prevent this complication. In fact, if vision is intact at the time the patient starts treatment, the risk of later loss of sight is one in 100 or less.

It is vital that patients who have PMR, either active or inactive, report any symptoms of new headache, changes in vision, or jaw pain right away to their doctors.

What causes giant cell arteritis?

As with PMR, the cause of GCA is not known.

Who gets giant cell arteritis?

GCA affects the same types of patients as does PMR. It occurs only in adults usually over age 50, in women more than men, and in whites more than nonwhites.

How is giant cell arteritis diagnosed?

There is no simple blood test or noninvasive way to confirm the diagnosis of GCA. The erythrocyte sedimentation rate, or "sed rate," a blood test that measures inflammation, is high in most people with GCA. But because other diseases can cause high sedimentation rates, doctors cannot rely on this finding as proof of GCA.

It is common to do a biopsy—or surgical removal—of a small piece of the temporal artery and study it under a microscope for signs of inflammation. This biopsy is an outpatient procedure, done under local anesthesia (numbing of that site while you are awake). It leaves just a small scar—which usually cannot be seen—at the hairline in front of the ear. In GCA, the biopsy shows inflammation of the artery. If there is doubt about the diagnosis based on the first biopsy, your doctor may do a biopsy of the temporal artery on the other side of your head.

How is giant cell arteritis treated?

The treatment for GCA should begin as soon as possible because of the risk of loss of vision. If your doctor strongly suspects GCA, treatment can start before you get the results of a temporal artery biopsy.

Unlike the treatment for PMR, which requires only low-dose corticosteroids (also called glucocorticoids), GCA treatment usually involves high doses of corticosteroids. Typically, the dose is 40–60 milligrams (mg) per day of prednisone (Deltasone, Orasone, etc.). Headaches and other symptoms quickly decrease with treatment, and the sedimentation rate declines to a normal range.

The high dose of corticosteroids usually continues for a month, and then slowly the dose is decreased (*tapered*). The speed at which your doctor lowers the dose may change if you have recurring symptoms of GCA or large increases in the sedimentation rate. In most cases, though, the prednisone dose can be reduced to about 5–10 mg per day over a few months. Patients are usually tapered off this medicine by 1–2 years. GCA rarely returns after treatment.

Living with Giant Cell Arteritis

As would be expected, side effects are more common with higher doses of corticosteroids. For instance, corticosteroid treatment can cause bone loss. Therefore, your doctor may want you to get a bone density test. To protect against osteoporosis and the risk of fractures (broken bones), take supplements of calcium and vitamin D. Your doctor also may suggest you take a prescription medicine to protect your bones. These include the bisphosphonates: risedronate (Actonel), alendronate (Fosamax), ibandronate (Boniva) or zoledronic acid (Reclast).

Some of the other side effects from high-dose corticosteroids—for instance, jitteriness, poor sleep, and weight gain—can be unpleasant, but are reversible. They get better as you take smaller doses. Muscle weakness, cataracts and skin bruising also can occur with corticosteroid use. See your doctor often to check for side effects.

Points to Remember

- GCA, a disease of blood vessels, may occur together with PMR.

- A new, persisting headache is a common symptom of GCA.

- Symptoms of GCA promptly improve with corticosteroids, and the risk of loss of vision is prevented.

The Rheumatologist's Role in the Treatment of Giant Cell Arteritis

Giant cell arteritis can be hard to detect and requires prompt treatment to prevent complications, especially loss of vision. Rheumatologists are experts in inflammatory diseases of blood vessels and are skilled in the detection and management of these uncommon illnesses.

Chapter 30

Multiple Sclerosis Pain

Nagging, burning, aching, sharp, and excruciating are words that are used to describe pain experienced by people with multiple sclerosis (MS). About two thirds of people with MS experience some level of pain at some time in their life. Pain should always be addressed as it impacts function and is often associated with depression, anxiety, and fatigue.

Causes of MS Pain

Pain in MS is directly related to either an MS lesion or plaque in the nervous system (nerve pain), or the effects of disability. When MS makes moving about difficult, stress on muscles, bones, and joints can cause pain (musculoskeletal pain). Pain in MS can be caused or worsened by infection or pressure ulcers.

Nerve pain can be continuous and steady or sudden and irregular. Nerve pain is reported in varying degrees of severity. Fifty percent of those who report MS pain say their pain is constant and severe. Intermittent, sudden pain is described as shooting, stabbing, electric shock-like, or searing and is often caused by sensations that normally do not cause pain like the weight of bed covers, chewing, or a cold

"Multiple Sclerosis Pain," by Heidi Maloni PhD, ANP-BC, National Clinical Nursing Director, VA Medical Center, U.S. Department of Veterans Affairs (www.va.gov), November 2009.

breeze. Other examples of intermittent pain include the feelings of tightness, cramping, clawing, and sudden spasms of a limb.

Tightness or band-like feelings, nagging, numbness, tingling in legs or arms, burning, aching, and throbbing pain is termed constant or steady nerve pain. Steady nerve pain is often worse at night or during changes in temperature and can be worsened with exercise. The most common pain syndromes experienced by people with MS include: headache (seen more in MS than the general population), continuous burning pain in the legs and/or arms, back pain, and painful spasms.

Treatment of MS Pain

Pain is not easily measured. Pain is what the person with pain says it is. Pain affects sleep, mood, relationships, and the ability to play and work. A clue to good pain management is improvement in these functions. Keeping a pain journal, recording when, where, and how long pain lasts, describing the pain (aching, pulling, sharp, cramping, burning, stabbing etc), recording what makes pain better or worse and what treatments are used is a valuable tool.

Assessing the type and the cause of pain is important to appropriate pain treatment. Pain management is approached medically, behaviorally, physically, and in some cases, surgically. Pain is complex and often requires a team approach and the skills of pain management experts.

Medication Management

There are many proven medications used to manage pain in MS. Your provider will know of the most up-to-date medications and combination medications. The use of medications to manage pain in MS is always a balance of risk versus benefit. In other words, medication side effects vs. the effects of pain are considered and continually evaluated in terms of their impact on quality of life.

Behavioral Management

Relaxation, meditation, imagery, hypnosis, distraction, and biofeedback are strategies that increase the tolerance to pain. Getting involved in work or social activities, joining a support group or even having a good laugh are techniques that can minimize pain. Interesting to note, higher pain severity is reported by people with MS who are unemployed or homebound.

Physical Management

Physical agents that minimize pain include the application of heat, cold, or pressure, physical therapy, exercise, massage, acupuncture, yoga, tai chi, and transcutaneous nerve stimulation (TENS). These techniques and therapies are often overlooked but should be considered from the start of pain symptoms.

Surgical Management

Surgical pain management interventions are sought when medical, physical, and behavioral options fail. Surgical procedures to relieve pain may be short lived and carry risks of having worse pain or nerve damage that result in numbness and tingling.

Summary

Pain is recognized as a common symptom of MS directly related to the disease and its consequences. Pain is a symptom that demands serious attention, as it has such persistent impact on role, mood, capacity to work and rest, and interpersonal relationships. Untreated pain causes isolation, anger, and depression. The management of pain in MS should include medications and behavioral and physical modalities that work together to relieve pain. The goal of MS pain management is achievable and functional, to improve mood, sleep, and quality of life.

Chapter 31

Neuralgia and Neurological Pain

Chapter Contents

Section 31.1—Understanding Nerve Pain 364

Section 31.2—Arachnoiditis 367

Section 31.3—Central Pain Syndrome 368

Section 31.4—Complex Regional Pain Syndrome 370

Section 31.5—Glossopharyngeal Neuralgia 371

Section 31.6—Meralgia Paresthetica 372

Section 31.7—Paresthesia 373

Section 31.8—Pinched Nerve 374

Section 31.9—Piriformis Syndrome 375

Section 31.10–Shingles and Postherpetic Neuralgia 376

Section 31.11–Tabes Dorsalis 380

Section 31.12–Tarlov Cysts 381

Section 31.1

Understanding Nerve Pain

"Understanding Nerve Pain," © 2004 American Chronic Pain Association. All rights reserved. Reprinted with permission. For additional information, visit www.theacpa.org. Reviewed by David A. Cooke, MD, FACP, March 2013.

You Are Not Alone

We've all experienced pain—whether it's a leg cramp from running or achy arms from lifting a heavy box. But there is a different type of pain that affects the nerves in our bodies. And it can cause unbearable pain that never seems to go away.

More than fifteen million people in the U.S. and Europe have what is called neuropathic pain or nerve pain. This is a puzzling and frustrating condition that can make even the simplest act, such as walking or putting on socks, agonizing.

Many people don't know what it is they are feeling. And they don't know how to describe it to their doctor. Because of this, they are not getting the care necessary to help ease their suffering.

We are here to help. This section of this chapter provides a brief explanation of nerve pain—how it happens, what it feels like, and steps you can take to begin your recovery. You also can find more information about nerve pain, pain support groups, and resources for finding a doctor by visiting the American Chronic Pain Association on the web at www.theacpa.org.

How Nerve Pain Happens

There are millions of nerves linked to one another throughout your body. These nerves make up your central nervous system. Think of it as a series of electrical wires or telephone lines connecting your brain and body, allowing them to communicate.

For example, when you step on the beach in the summertime, nerves in your feet send a message to your brain that you are stepping on something hot. As a result, your feet may feel like they are burning. Or, if you accidentally touch a live electrical outlet, nerves in your hand will send a signal that you're being shocked.

But like wires that short circuit, nerves can become injured and stop working the way they should. If the nerve isn't working properly, it may begin sending the wrong signals to the brain. So, injured nerves might tell your brain that your foot is burning or your hand is being shocked by electricity even when you aren't stepping on something hot or touching an electrical socket.

Nerves can become injured or damaged in a number of ways, such as an injury to the spine or from a medical illnesses like diabetes, shingles, a stroke, HIV infection, or cancer and its treatments.

Nerve Pain Feels Like

Many people with nerve pain often don't describe this feeling as "painful." Instead, they may describe it as being pricked with pins and needles or shocked by electricity. Often, pain can be caused by something that is not painful, such as the light touch of bed sheets.

Other Common Symptoms Include

- Numbness

- Burning

- Tingling

- A stabbing sensation

- Pins and needles

- Electric-shock pain

Pain Can Interfere with Your Daily Life

When nerve pain is not properly managed, it can end up controlling the way you live. Simply walking to the market can be agonizing. Even wearing clothing, like socks, or the touch of a bed sheet can cause an unbearable burning pain.

Many pain sufferers cannot get a good night's sleep or go to work because of their pain. They don't think they will ever get relief and often begin feeling hopeless and depressed. They might stay at home more often and stop seeing their friends or family.

Take Control of Your Pain

There are ways to take control and manage your nerve pain. But you need to get involved in your care and take on a share of the responsibility for your wellbeing. Half the battle is won when you take an active role and begin to help yourself.

You can do this by:

- Talking to your doctor about your pain and about how best to manage it.

- Asking about medicines that are developed specifically to treat nerve pain.

- Learning how to relax and set realistic goals.

- Exercising. Identify a moderate program you can do safely.

- Getting your family and friends involved.

- Contacting the American Chronic Pain Association (ACPA) at 800-533-3231. ACPA can help you find a support group in your area or start a group with information and support from the national office.

How Can You Tell If It's Nerve Pain or Muscle Pain?

Nerve Pain

- Doesn't seem to be caused by an event or trauma

- Constant and/or recurring pain that doesn't seem to go away

- Burning, stabbing, pins and needles; even wearing clothing is painful

- Feel depressed, helpless; normal pain medicine like aspirin does not stop the pain

Muscle Pain

- Caused by a physical injury, such as a fall

- Pain that stops once an injury heals

- Sore and achy muscles

- Feel distressed but hopeful because more pain medicine relieves the pain

Section 31.2

Arachnoiditis

"Arachnoiditis Information Page,"
National Institute of Neurological Disorders and Stroke
(www.ninds.nih.gov), January 13, 2011.

What is arachnoiditis?

Arachnoiditis describes a pain disorder caused by the inflammation of the arachnoid, one of the membranes that surround and protect the nerves of the spinal cord. The arachnoid can become inflamed because of an irritation from chemicals, infection from bacteria or viruses, as the result of direct injury to the spine, chronic compression of spinal nerves, or complications from spinal surgery or other invasive spinal procedures. Inflammation can sometimes lead to the formation of scar tissue and adhesions, which cause the spinal nerves to "stick" together. If arachnoiditis begins to interfere with the function of one or more of these nerves, it can cause a number of symptoms, including numbness, tingling, and a characteristic stinging and burning pain in the lower back or legs. Some people with arachnoiditis will have debilitating muscle cramps, twitches, or spasms. It may also affect bladder, bowel, and sexual function. In severe cases, arachnoiditis may cause paralysis of the lower limbs.

Is there any treatment?

Arachnoiditis remains a difficult condition to treat, and long-term outcomes are unpredictable. Most treatments for arachnoiditis are focused on pain relief and the improvement of symptoms that impair daily function. A regimen of pain management, physiotherapy, exercise, and psychotherapy is often recommended. Surgical intervention is controversial since the outcomes are generally poor and provide only short-term relief. Clinical trials of steroid injections and electrical stimulation are needed to evaluate the efficacy of these treatments.

What is the prognosis?

Arachnoiditis is a disorder that causes chronic pain and neurological deficits and does not improve significantly with treatment. Surgery may only provide temporary relief. The outlook for someone with arachnoiditis is complicated by the fact that the disorder has no predictable pattern or severity of symptoms.

Section 31.3

Central Pain Syndrome

"Central Pain Syndrome Information Page,"
National Institute of Neurological Disorders and Stroke
(www.ninds.nih.gov), January 13, 2011.

What is central pain syndrome?

Central pain syndrome is a neurological condition caused by damage to or dysfunction of the central nervous system (CNS), which includes the brain, brainstem, and spinal cord. This syndrome can be caused by stroke, multiple sclerosis, tumors, epilepsy, brain or spinal cord trauma, or Parkinson disease. The character of the pain associated with this syndrome differs widely among individuals partly because of the variety of potential causes. Central pain syndrome may affect a large portion of the body or may be more restricted to specific areas, such as hands or feet. The extent of pain is usually related to the cause of the CNS injury or damage. Pain is typically constant, may be moderate to severe in intensity, and is often made worse by touch, movement, emotions, and temperature changes, usually cold temperatures. Individuals experience one or more types of pain sensations, the most prominent being burning. Mingled with the burning may be sensations of "pins and needles;" pressing, lacerating, or aching pain; and brief, intolerable bursts of sharp pain similar to the pain caused by a dental probe on an exposed nerve. Individuals may have numbness in the areas affected by the pain. The burning and loss of touch sensations are usually most severe on the distant parts of the body, such as the feet or hands. Central pain syndrome often begins shortly after the causative injury or damage, but may be delayed by months or even years, especially if it is related to post-stroke pain.

Is there any treatment?

Pain medications often provide some reduction of pain, but not complete relief of pain, for those affected by central pain syndrome. Tricyclic antidepressants such as nortriptyline or anticonvulsants such as Neurontin (gabapentin) can be useful. Lowering stress levels appears to reduce pain.

What is the prognosis?

Central pain syndrome is not a fatal disorder, but the syndrome causes disabling chronic pain and suffering among the majority of individuals who have it.

Section 31.4

Complex Regional Pain Syndrome

"Complex Regional Pain Syndrome Information Page,"
National Institute of Neurological Disorders and Stroke
(www.ninds.nih.gov), September 19, 2012.

What is complex regional pain syndrome?

Complex regional pain syndrome (CRPS) is a chronic pain condition. The key symptom of CRPS is continuous, intense pain out of proportion to the severity of the injury, which gets worse rather than better over time. CRPS most often affects one of the arms, legs, hands, or feet. Often the pain spreads to include the entire arm or leg. Typical features include dramatic changes in the color and temperature of the skin over the affected limb or body part, accompanied by intense burning pain, skin sensitivity, sweating, and swelling.

Doctors aren't sure what causes CRPS. In some cases the sympathetic nervous system plays an important role in sustaining the pain. Another theory is that CRPS is caused by a triggering of the immune response, which leads to the characteristic inflammatory symptoms of redness, warmth, and swelling in the affected area.

Is there any treatment?

Because there is no cure for CRPS, treatment is aimed at relieving painful symptoms. Doctors may prescribe topical analgesics, antidepressants, corticosteroids, and opioids to relieve pain. However, no single drug or combination of drugs has produced consistent long-lasting improvement in symptoms. Other treatments may include physical therapy, sympathetic nerve block, spinal cord stimulation, and intrathecal drug pumps to deliver opioids and local anesthetic agents via the spinal cord.

What is the prognosis?

The prognosis for CRPS varies from person to person. Spontaneous remission from symptoms occurs in certain individuals. Others can have unremitting pain and crippling, irreversible changes in spite of treatment.

Section 31.5

Glossopharyngeal Neuralgia

"Glossopharyngeal Neuralgia Information Page," National Institute of
Neurological Disorders and Stroke (www.ninds.nih.gov), September 19, 2012.

What is glossopharyngeal neuralgia?

Glossopharyngeal neuralgia (GN) is a rare pain syndrome that
affects the glossopharyngeal nerve (the ninth cranial nerve that lies
deep within the neck) and causes sharp, stabbing pulses of pain in
the back of the throat and tongue, the tonsils, and the middle ear. The
excruciating pain of GN can last for a few seconds to a few minutes,
and may return multiple times in a day or once every few weeks. Many
individuals with GN relate the attacks of pain to specific trigger factors
such as swallowing, drinking cold liquids, sneezing, coughing, talking,
clearing the throat, and touching the gums or inside the mouth. GN can
be caused by compression of the glossopharyngeal nerve, but in some
cases, no cause is evident. Like trigeminal neuralgia, it is associated
with multiple sclerosis. GN primarily affects the elderly.

Is there any treatment?

Most doctors will attempt to treat the pain first with drugs. Some
individuals respond well to anticonvulsant drugs, such as carbamazepine and gabapentin. Surgical options, including nerve resection,
tractotomy, or microvascular decompression, should be considered
when individuals either don't respond to, or stop responding to, drug
therapy. Surgery is usually successful at ending the cycles of pain,
although there may be some sensory loss in the mouth, throat, or
tongue.

What is the prognosis?

Some individuals recover from an initial attack and never have
another. Others will experience clusters of attacks followed by periods
of short or long remission. Individuals may lose weight if they fear that
chewing, drinking, or eating will cause an attack.

371

Section 31.6

Meralgia Paresthetica

"Meralgia Paresthetica Information Page," National Institute of Neurological Disorders and Stroke (www.ninds.nih.gov), March 16, 2009.

What is meralgia paresthetica?

Meralgia paresthetica is a disorder characterized by tingling, numbness, and burning pain in the outer side of the thigh. The disorder is caused by compression of the lateral femoral cutaneous nerve, a sensory nerve to the skin, as it exits the pelvis. People with the disorder often notice a patch of skin that is sensitive to touch and sometimes painful. Meralgia paresthetica should not be associated with weakness or radiating pain from the back.

Is there any treatment?

Treatment for meralgia paresthetica is symptomatic and supportive. The majority of cases improve with conservative treatment by wearing looser clothing and losing weight. Medications used to treat neurogenic pain, such as antiseizure or antidepressant medications, may alleviate symptoms of pain. In a few cases, in which pain is persistent or severe, surgical intervention may be indicated.

What is the prognosis?

Meralgia paresthetica usually has a good prognosis. In most cases, meralgia paresthetica will improve with conservative treatment or may even spontaneously resolve. Surgical intervention is not always fully successful.

Section 31.7

Paresthesia

"Paresthesia Information Page," National Institute
of Neurological Disorders and Stroke (www.ninds.nih.gov), May 6, 2010.

What is paresthesia?

Paresthesia refers to a burning or prickling sensation that is usually
felt in the hands, arms, legs, or feet, but can also occur in other parts
of the body. The sensation, which happens without warning, is usually
painless and described as tingling or numbness, skin crawling, or itching.

Most people have experienced temporary paresthesia—a feeling of
"pins and needles"—at some time in their lives when they have sat
with legs crossed for too long, or fallen asleep with an arm crooked
under their head. It happens when sustained pressure is placed on
a nerve. The feeling quickly goes away once the pressure is relieved.

Chronic paresthesia is often a symptom of an underlying neurological
disease or traumatic nerve damage. Paresthesia can be caused by disorders affecting the central nervous system, such as stroke and transient
ischemic attacks (mini-strokes), multiple sclerosis, transverse myelitis,
and encephalitis. A tumor or vascular lesion pressed up against the
brain or spinal cord can also cause paresthesia. Nerve entrapment syndromes, such as carpal tunnel syndrome, can damage peripheral nerves
and cause paresthesia accompanied by pain. Diagnostic evaluation is
based on determining the underlying condition causing the paresthetic
sensations. An individual's medical history, physical examination, and
laboratory tests are essential for the diagnosis. Physicians may order
additional tests depending on the suspected cause of the paresthesia.

Is there any treatment?

The appropriate treatment for paresthesia depends on accurate
diagnosis of the underlying cause.

What is the prognosis?

The prognosis for those with paresthesia depends on the severity
of the sensations and the associated disorders.

Section 31.8

Pinched Nerve

"Pinched Nerve Information Page,"
National Institute of Neurological Disorders and Stroke
(www.ninds.nih.gov), September 27, 2011.

What is pinched nerve?

The term "pinched nerve" is a colloquial term and not a true medical term. It is used to describe one type of damage or injury to a nerve or set of nerves. The injury may result from compression, constriction, or stretching. Symptoms include numbness, "pins and needles," or burning sensations, and pain radiating outward from the injured area. One of the most common examples of a single compressed nerve is the feeling of having a foot or hand "fall asleep."

A "pinched nerve" frequently is associated with pain in the neck or lower back. This type of pain can be caused by inflammation or pressure on the nerve root as it exits the spine. If the pain is severe or lasts a long time, you may need to have further evaluation from your physician.

Several problems can lead to similar symptoms of numbness, pain, and tingling in the hands or feet but without pain in the neck or back. These can include peripheral neuropathy, carpal tunnel syndrome, and tennis elbow. The extent of such injuries may vary from minor, temporary damage to a more permanent condition. Early diagnosis is important to prevent further damage or complications. Pinched nerve is a common cause of on-the-job injury.

Is there any treatment?

The most frequently recommended treatment for pinched nerve is rest for the affected area. Nonsteroidal anti-inflammatory drugs (NSAIDs) or corticosteroids may be recommended to help alleviate pain. Physical therapy is often useful, and splints or collars may be used to relieve symptoms. Depending on the cause and severity of the pinched nerve, surgery may be needed.

What is the prognosis?

With treatment, most people recover from pinched nerve. However, in some cases, the damage is irreversible.

Section 31.9

Piriformis Syndrome

"Piriformis Syndrome Information Page," National Institute of Neurological Disorders and Stroke (www.ninds.nih.gov), February 14, 2007. Reviewed by David A. Cooke, MD, FACP, March 2013.

What is piriformis syndrome?

Piriformis syndrome is a rare neuromuscular disorder that occurs when the piriformis muscle compresses or irritates the sciatic nerve—the largest nerve in the body. The piriformis muscle is a narrow muscle located in the buttocks. Compression of the sciatic nerve causes pain—frequently described as tingling or numbness—in the buttocks and along the nerve, often down to the leg. The pain may worsen as a result of sitting for a long period of time, climbing stairs, walking, or running.

Is there any treatment?

Generally, treatment for the disorder begins with stretching exercises and massage. Anti-inflammatory drugs may be prescribed. Cessation of running, bicycling, or similar activities may be advised. A corticosteroid injection near where the piriformis muscle and the sciatic nerve meet may provide temporary relief. In some cases, surgery is recommended.

What is the prognosis?

The prognosis for most individuals with piriformis syndrome is good. Once symptoms of the disorder are addressed, individuals can usually resume their normal activities. In some cases, exercise regimens may need to be modified in order to reduce the likelihood of recurrence or worsening.

Section 31.10

Shingles and Postherpetic Neuralgia

Excerpted from "Shingles: Hope through Research," National Institute of Neurological Disorders and Stroke (www.ninds.nih.gov), January 10, 2013.

What is shingles?

Scientists call the virus that causes chickenpox and shingles varicella-zoster virus or VZV. VZV belongs to a group of viruses called herpesviruses. This group includes the herpes simplex virus that causes cold sores, fever blisters, mononucleosis, genital herpes (a sexually transmitted disease), and Epstein-Barr virus involved in infectious mononucleosis. Like VZV, other herpesviruses can hide in the nervous system after an initial infection and then travel down nerve cell fibers to cause a renewed infection. Repeated episodes of cold sores on the lips are the most common example.

As early as 1909, scientists suspected that the viruses causing chickenpox and shingles were one and the same. In the 1920s and 1930s, the case was strengthened by an experiment in which children were inoculated with fluid from shingles blisters. Within two weeks, about half of the children developed chickenpox. Finally, in 1958, detailed analyses of the viruses taken from patients with either chickenpox or shingles confirmed that the viruses were identical.

Virtually all adults in the United States have had chickenpox, even if it was so mild as to pass unnoticed, and thus may develop shingles later in life. In the original exposure to VZV (chickenpox), some of the virus particles leave the blood and settle into clusters of nerve cells (neurons) called sensory ganglia, where they remain for many years in an inactive (latent) form. The sensory ganglia, which are adjacent to the spinal cord and brain, relay information to the brain about what the body is sensing—heat, cold, touch, pain.

When the VZV reactivates, it spreads down the long nerve fibers (axons) that extend from the sensory cell bodies to the skin. The viruses multiply, the telltale rash erupts, and the person now has herpes-zoster, or shingles. With shingles, the nervous system is more deeply involved than it was during the bout with chickenpox, and the symptoms are often more complex and severe.

What are the symptoms of shingles?

The first sign of shingles is often burning or tingling pain, or itch, in one particular location on only one side of the body. After several days or a week, a rash of fluid-filled blisters appears. These are similar to chickenpox but appear in a cluster rather than scattered over the body. The cluster typically appears in one area on one side of the body. Recent studies have shown that subtle cases of shingles with only a few blisters, or none, are more common than previously thought. These cases may remain unrecognized. Cases without any known lesions are known as zoster sine herpete.

Shingles pain can be mild or intense. Some people have mostly itching; some feel pain from the gentlest touch or breeze. The most common location for shingles is a band, called a dermatome, spanning one side of the trunk around the waistline. The second most common location is on one side of the face around the eye and on the forehead. However, shingles can involve any part of the body. The number of blisters or lesions is variable. Some rashes merge and produce an area that looks like a severe burn. Other patients may have just a few scattered lesions that don't cause severe symptoms.

For most healthy people, shingles rashes heal within a few weeks, the pain and itch that accompany the lesions subside, and the blisters leave no scars. Other people may have sensory symptoms that linger for a few months.

How should shingles be treated?

Currently there is no cure for shingles, but attacks can be made less severe and shorter by using prescription antiviral drugs such as acyclovir, valacyclovir, or famciclovir as soon as possible after symptoms begin. Early treatment can reduce or prevent severe pain and help blisters dry faster. Antiviral drugs can reduce by about half the risk of being left with postherpetic neuralgia, which is chronic pain that can last for months or years after the shingles rash clears. Doctors recommend starting antiviral drugs at the first sign of the shingles rash, or even if the telltale symptoms indicate that a rash is about to erupt. Even if a patient is not seen by a doctor at the beginning of the illness, it may still be useful to start antiviral medications if new lesions are forming. It is important not to miss any doses or stop taking the medication early. Other treatments to consider are anti-inflammatory corticosteroids such as prednisone. These are routinely used when the eye or other facial nerves are affected.

Most people with shingles can be treated at home.

People with shingles should also try to relax and reduce stress (stress can make pain worse and lead to depression); eat regular, well-balanced meals; and perform gentle exercises, such as walking or stretching to keep active and stop thinking about the pain (but check with your doctor first). Placing a cool, damp washcloth on the blisters—but not when wearing a topical cream or patch—can help blisters dry faster and relieve pain.

Can shingles be prevented?

Immunization with the varicella vaccine (or chickenpox vaccine)—now recommended in the United States for all children between 18 months and adolescence—can protect children from getting chickenpox. People who have been vaccinated against chickenpox are less likely to get shingles because the weak, "attenuated" strain of virus used in the chickenpox vaccine is less likely to survive in the body over decades. Not enough data currently exists to indicate whether shingles can occur later in life in a person who was vaccinated against chickenpox

In May 2006, the U.S. Food and Drug Administration (FDA) approved a VZV vaccine (Zostavax) for use in people 60 and older who have had chickenpox. In March 2011, the FDA extended the approval to include adults 50–59 as well.

The shingles vaccine is a preventive therapy and not a treatment for those who already have shingles or postherpetic neuralgia.

What is postherpetic neuralgia?

Sometimes, particularly in older people, shingles pain persists long after the rash has healed. This postherpetic neuralgia can be mild or severe—the most severe cases can lead to insomnia, weight loss, depression, and disability. Postherpetic neuralgia is not directly life-threatening. About a dozen medications in four categories have been shown in clinical trials to provide some pain relief. These include the following:

- **Tricyclic antidepressants (TCAs):** TCAs are often the first type of drug given to patients suffering from postherpetic neuralgia. The TCA amitriptyline was commonly prescribed in the past, but although effective, it has a high rate of side effects. Desipramine and nortriptyline have fewer side effects and are better choices for older adults, the most likely group to have postherpetic neuralgia. Common side effects of TCAs include dry eyes and mouth, constipation, and grogginess. People with heart arrhythmias, previous heart attacks, or narrow angle glaucoma should usually use a different class of drugs.

- **Anticonvulsants:** Some drugs that reduce seizures can also treat postherpetic neuralgia because seizures and pain both involve abnormally increased firing of nerve cells. The antiseizure medication gabapentin is most often prescribed; carbamazepine is effective for postherpetic neuralgia but has rare, potentially dangerous side effects, including drowsiness or confusion, dizziness, and sometimes ankle swelling.

- **Opioids:** Opioids are strong pain medications used for all types of pain. They include oxycodone, morphine, tramadol, and methadone. Opioids can have side effects—including drowsiness, mental dulling, and constipation—and can be addictive, so their use must be monitored carefully in those with a history of addiction.

- **Topical local anesthetics:** Local anesthetics applied directly to the skin of the painful area affected by postherpetic neuralgia are also effective. Lidocaine, the most commonly prescribed, is available in cream, gel, or spray form. It is also available in a patch that has been approved by the Food and Drug Administration for use specifically in postherpetic neuralgia. Topical local anesthetics stay in the skin and therefore do not cause problems such as drowsiness or constipation. Capsaicin cream may be somewhat effective and is available over the counter, but most people find that it causes severe burning pain during application.

What is postherpetic itch?

The itch that sometimes occurs during or after shingles can be quite severe and painful. Clinical experience suggests that postherpetic itch is harder to treat than postherpetic neuralgia. Topical local anesthetics provide substantial relief to some patients. Since postherpetic itch typically develops in skin that has severe sensory loss, it is particularly important to avoid scratching. Scratching numb skin too long or too hard can cause injury.

Section 31.11

Tabes Dorsalis

"Tabes Dorsalis Information Page," National Institute of Neurological Disorders and Stroke (www.ninds.nih.gov), February 14, 2007. Reviewed by David A. Cooke, MD, FACP, March 2013.

What is tabes dorsalis?

Tabes dorsalis is a slow degeneration of the nerve cells and nerve fibers that carry sensory information to the brain. The degenerating nerves are in the dorsal columns of the spinal cord (the portion closest to the back of the body) and carry information that help maintain a person's sense of position. Tabes dorsalis is the result of an untreated syphilis infection. Symptoms may not appear for some decades after the initial infection and include weakness, diminished reflexes, unsteady gait, progressive degeneration of the joints, loss of coordination, episodes of intense pain and disturbed sensation, personality changes, dementia, deafness, visual impairment, and impaired response to light. The disease is more frequent in males than in females. Onset is commonly during mid-life. The incidence of tabes dorsalis is rising, in part due to co-associated HIV infection.

Is there any treatment?

Penicillin, administered intravenously, is the treatment of choice. Associated pain can be treated with opiates, valproate, or carbamazepine. Patients may also require physical or rehabilitative therapy to deal with muscle wasting and weakness. Preventive treatment for those who come into sexual contact with an individual with tabes dorsalis is important.

What is the prognosis?

If left untreated, tabes dorsalis can lead to paralysis, dementia, and blindness. Existing nerve damage cannot be reversed.

Section 31.12

Tarlov Cysts

"Tarlov Cysts Information Page," National Institute of Neurological
Disorders and Stroke (www.ninds.nih.gov), June 14, 2012.

What are Tarlov cysts?

Tarlov cysts are sacs filled with cerebrospinal fluid that most often
affect nerve roots in the sacrum, the group of bones at the base of the
spine. These cysts (also known as meningeal or perineural cysts) can
compress nerve roots, causing lower back pain, sciatica (shock-like or
burning pain in the lower back, buttocks, and down one leg to below
the knee), urinary incontinence, headaches (due to changes in cerebrospinal fluid pressure), constipation, sexual dysfunction, and some
loss of feeling or control of movement in the leg and/or foot. Pressure
on the nerves next to the cysts can also cause pain and deterioration
of surrounding bone. Tarlov cysts can be diagnosed using magnetic
resonance imaging (MRI); however, it is estimated that the majority
of the cysts observed by MRI cause no symptoms. Tarlov cysts may
become symptomatic following shock, trauma, or exertion that causes
the buildup of cerebrospinal fluid. Women are at much higher risk of
developing these cysts than are men.

Is there any treatment?

Tarlov cysts may be drained and shunted to relieve pressure and
pain, but relief is often only temporary and fluid build-up in the cysts
will recur. Corticosteroid injections may also temporarily relieve pain.
Other drugs may be prescribed to treat chronic pain and depression.
Injecting the cysts with fibrin glue (a combination of naturally occurring substances based on the clotting factor in blood) may provide
temporary relief of pain.

Some scientists believe the herpes simplex virus, which thrives in
an alkaline environment, can cause Tarlov cysts to become symptomatic. Making the body less alkaline, through diet or supplements, may
lessen symptoms. Microsurgical removal of the cyst may be an option in

select individuals who do not respond to conservative treatments and who continue to experience pain or progressive neurological damage.

What is the prognosis?

In some instances Tarlov cysts can cause nerve pain and other pain, weakness, or nerve root compression. Acute and chronic pain may require changes in lifestyle. If left untreated, nerve root compression can cause permanent neurological damage.

Chapter 32

Neuropathies

Chapter Contents

Section 32.1—Peripheral Neuropathy 384
Section 32.2—Diabetic Neuropathies 389

Section 32.1

Peripheral Neuropathy

Excerpted from "Peripheral Neuropathy Fact Sheet," National Institute of Neurological Disorders and Stroke (www.ninds.nih.gov), NIH Pub. No. 04-4853, updated September 19, 2012.

What is peripheral neuropathy?

Peripheral neuropathy describes damage to the peripheral nervous system, the vast communications network that transmits information from the brain and spinal cord (the central nervous system) to every other part of the body. Peripheral nerves also send sensory information back to the brain and spinal cord, such as a message that the feet are cold or a finger is burned. Damage to the peripheral nervous system interferes with these vital connections. Like static on a telephone line, peripheral neuropathy distorts and sometimes interrupts messages between the brain and the rest of the body.

Because every peripheral nerve has a highly specialized function in a specific part of the body, a wide array of symptoms can occur when nerves are damaged. Some people may experience temporary numbness, tingling, and pricking sensations (paresthesia), sensitivity to touch, or muscle weakness. Others may suffer more extreme symptoms, including burning pain (especially at night), muscle wasting, paralysis, or organ or gland dysfunction. People may become unable to digest food easily, maintain safe levels of blood pressure, sweat normally, or experience normal sexual function. In the most extreme cases, breathing may become difficult or organ failure may occur.

Some forms of neuropathy involve damage to only one nerve and are called mononeuropathies. More often though, multiple nerves affecting all limbs are affected-called polyneuropathy. Occasionally, two or more isolated nerves in separate areas of the body are affected—called mononeuritis multiplex.

In acute neuropathies, such as Guillain-Barré syndrome, symptoms appear suddenly, progress rapidly, and resolve slowly as damaged nerves heal. In chronic forms, symptoms begin subtly and progress slowly. Some people may have periods of relief followed by relapse.

Others may reach a plateau stage where symptoms stay the same for many months or years. Some chronic neuropathies worsen over time, but very few forms prove fatal unless complicated by other diseases. Occasionally the neuropathy is a symptom of another disorder.

In the most common forms of polyneuropathy, the nerve fibers (individual cells that make up the nerve) most distant from the brain and the spinal cord malfunction first. Pain and other symptoms often appear symmetrically, for example, in both feet followed by a gradual progression up both legs. Next, the fingers, hands, and arms may become affected, and symptoms can progress into the central part of the body. Many people with diabetic neuropathy experience this pattern of ascending nerve damage.

How are the peripheral neuropathies classified?

More than 100 types of peripheral neuropathy have been identified, each with its own characteristic set of symptoms, pattern of development, and prognosis. Impaired function and symptoms depend on the type of nerves—motor, sensory, or autonomic—that are damaged. Motor nerves control movements of all muscles under conscious control, such as those used for walking, grasping things, or talking. Sensory nerves transmit information about sensory experiences, such as the feeling of a light touch or the pain resulting from a cut. Autonomic nerves regulate biological activities that people do not control consciously, such as breathing, digesting food, and heart and gland functions. Although some neuropathies may affect all three types of nerves, others primarily affect one or two types. Therefore, doctors may use terms such as predominantly motor neuropathy, predominantly sensory neuropathy, sensory-motor neuropathy, or autonomic neuropathy to describe a patient's condition.

What are the symptoms of peripheral nerve damage?

Symptoms are related to the type of affected nerve and may be seen over a period of days, weeks, or years. Muscle weakness is the most common symptom of motor nerve damage. Other symptoms may include painful cramps and fasciculations (uncontrolled muscle twitching visible under the skin), muscle loss, bone degeneration, and changes in the skin, hair, and nails. These more general degenerative changes also can result from sensory or autonomic nerve fiber loss.

Sensory nerve damage causes a more complex range of symptoms because sensory nerves have a wider, more highly specialized range of functions. Larger sensory fibers enclosed in myelin (a fatty protein that coats and insulates many nerves) register vibration, light touch, and position sense. Damage to large sensory fibers lessens the ability to feel vibrations and touch, resulting in a general sense of numbness, especially in the hands and feet. People may feel as if they are wearing gloves and stockings even when they are not. Many patients cannot recognize by touch alone the shapes of small objects or distinguish between different shapes. This damage to sensory fibers may contribute to the loss of reflexes (as can motor nerve damage). Loss of position sense often makes people unable to coordinate complex movements like walking or fastening buttons, or to maintain their balance when their eyes are shut. Neuropathic pain is difficult to control and can seriously affect emotional well-being and overall quality of life. Neuropathic pain is often worse at night, seriously disrupting sleep and adding to the emotional burden of sensory nerve damage.

Smaller sensory fibers without myelin sheaths transmit pain and temperature sensations. Damage to these fibers can interfere with the ability to feel pain or changes in temperature. People may fail to sense that they have been injured from a cut or that a wound is becoming infected. Others may not detect pains that warn of impending heart attack or other acute conditions. (Loss of pain sensation is a particularly serious problem for people with diabetes, contributing to the high rate of lower limb amputations among this population.) Pain receptors in the skin can also become over-sensitized, so that people may feel severe pain (allodynia) from stimuli that are normally painless (for example, some may experience pain from bed sheets draped lightly over the body).

Symptoms of autonomic nerve damage are diverse and depend upon which organs or glands are affected. Autonomic nerve dysfunction can become life threatening and may require emergency medical care in cases when breathing becomes impaired or when the heart begins beating irregularly. Common symptoms of autonomic nerve damage include an inability to sweat normally, which may lead to heat intolerance; a loss of bladder control, which may cause infection or incontinence; and an inability to control muscles that expand or contract blood vessels to maintain safe blood pressure levels. A loss of control over blood pressure can cause dizziness, lightheadedness, or even fainting when a person moves suddenly from a seated to a standing position (a condition known as postural or orthostatic hypotension).

Gastrointestinal symptoms frequently accompany autonomic neuropathy. Nerves controlling intestinal muscle contractions often malfunction, leading to diarrhea, constipation, or incontinence. Many people also have problems eating or swallowing if certain autonomic nerves are affected.

What treatments are available?

No medical treatments now exist that can cure inherited peripheral neuropathy. However, there are therapies for many other forms. Any underlying condition is treated first, followed by symptomatic treatment. Peripheral nerves have the ability to regenerate, as long as the nerve cell itself has not been killed. Symptoms often can be controlled, and eliminating the causes of specific forms of neuropathy often can prevent new damage.

In general, adopting healthy habits—such as maintaining optimal weight, avoiding exposure to toxins, following a physician-supervised exercise program, eating a balanced diet, correcting vitamin deficiencies, and limiting or avoiding alcohol consumption—can reduce the physical and emotional effects of peripheral neuropathy. Active and passive forms of exercise can reduce cramps, improve muscle strength, and prevent muscle wasting in paralyzed limbs. Various dietary strategies can improve gastrointestinal symptoms. Timely treatment of injury can help prevent permanent damage. Quitting smoking is particularly important because smoking constricts the blood vessels that supply nutrients to the peripheral nerves and can worsen neuropathic symptoms. Self-care skills such as meticulous foot care and careful wound treatment in people with diabetes and others who have an impaired ability to feel pain can alleviate symptoms and improve quality of life. Such changes often create conditions that encourage nerve regeneration.

Systemic diseases frequently require more complex treatments. Strict control of blood glucose levels has been shown to reduce neuropathic symptoms and help people with diabetic neuropathy avoid further nerve damage. Inflammatory and autoimmune conditions leading to neuropathy can be controlled in several ways. Immunosuppressive drugs such as prednisone, cyclosporine, or azathioprine may be beneficial. Plasmapheresis—a procedure in which blood is removed, cleansed of immune system cells and antibodies, and then returned to the body—can limit inflammation or suppress immune system activity. High doses of immunoglobulins, proteins that function as antibodies, also can suppress abnormal immune system activity.

Neuropathic pain is often difficult to control. Mild pain may sometimes be alleviated by analgesics sold over the counter. Several classes of drugs have recently proved helpful to many patients suffering from more severe forms of chronic neuropathic pain. These include mexiletine, a drug developed to correct irregular heart rhythms (sometimes associated with severe side effects); several antiepileptic drugs, including gabapentin, phenytoin, and carbamazepine; and some classes of antidepressants, including tricyclics such as amitriptyline. Injections of local anesthetics such as lidocaine or topical patches containing lidocaine may relieve more intractable pain. In the most severe cases, doctors can surgically destroy nerves; however, the results are often temporary and the procedure can lead to complications.

Mechanical aids can help reduce pain and lessen the impact of physical disability. Hand or foot braces can compensate for muscle weakness or alleviate nerve compression. Orthopedic shoes can improve gait disturbances and help prevent foot injuries in people with a loss of pain sensation. If breathing becomes severely impaired, mechanical ventilation can provide essential life support.

Surgical intervention often can provide immediate relief from mononeuropathies caused by compression or entrapment injuries. Repair of a slipped disk can reduce pressure on nerves where they emerge from the spinal cord; the removal of benign or malignant tumors can also alleviate damaging pressure on nerves. Nerve entrapment often can be corrected by the surgical release of ligaments or tendons.

Section 32.2

Diabetic Neuropathies

Excerpted from "Diabetic Neuropathies: The Nerve Damage of Diabetes,"
National Diabetes Information Clearinghouse, a service of the National In-
stitute of Diabetes and Digestive and Kidney Diseases (www.niddk.nih.gov),
June 25, 2012.

What are diabetic neuropathies?

Diabetic neuropathies are a family of nerve disorders caused by
diabetes. People with diabetes can, over time, develop nerve damage throughout the body. Some people with nerve damage have no
symptoms. Others may have symptoms such as pain, tingling, or
numbness—loss of feeling—in the hands, arms, feet, and legs. Nerve
problems can occur in every organ system, including the digestive
tract, heart, and sex organs.

About 60 to 70 percent of people with diabetes have some form
of neuropathy. People with diabetes can develop nerve problems at
any time, but risk rises with age and longer duration of diabetes. The
highest rates of neuropathy are among people who have had diabetes
for at least 25 years. Diabetic neuropathies also appear to be more
common in people who have problems controlling their blood glucose,
also called blood sugar, as well as those with high levels of blood fat
and blood pressure and those who are overweight.

What causes diabetic neuropathies?

The causes are probably different for different types of diabetic
neuropathy. Researchers are studying how prolonged exposure to high
blood glucose causes nerve damage. Nerve damage is likely due to a
combination of factors:

* Metabolic factors, such as high blood glucose, long duration of diabetes, abnormal blood fat levels, and possibly low levels of insulin

* Neurovascular factors, leading to damage to the blood vessels
  that carry oxygen and nutrients to nerves

- Autoimmune factors that cause inflammation in nerves

- Mechanical injury to nerves, such as carpal tunnel syndrome

- Inherited traits that increase susceptibility to nerve disease

- Lifestyle factors, such as smoking or alcohol use

What are the symptoms of diabetic neuropathies?

Symptoms depend on the type of neuropathy and which nerves are affected. Some people with nerve damage have no symptoms at all. For others, the first symptom is often numbness, tingling, or pain in the feet. Symptoms are often minor at first, and because most nerve damage occurs over several years, mild cases may go unnoticed for a long time. Symptoms can involve the sensory, motor, and autonomic (or involuntary) nervous systems. In some people, mainly those with focal neuropathy, the onset of pain may be sudden and severe.

Symptoms of nerve damage may include the following:

- Numbness, tingling, or pain in the toes, feet, legs, hands, arms, and fingers

- Wasting of the muscles of the feet or hands

- Indigestion, nausea, or vomiting

- Diarrhea or constipation

- Dizziness or faintness due to a drop in blood pressure after standing or sitting up

- Problems with urination

- Erectile dysfunction in men or vaginal dryness in women

- Weakness

Symptoms that are not due to neuropathy, but often accompany it, include weight loss and depression.

What are the types of diabetic neuropathy?

Diabetic neuropathy can be classified as peripheral, autonomic, proximal, or focal. Each affects different parts of the body in various ways.

- Peripheral neuropathy, the most common type of diabetic neuropathy, causes pain or loss of feeling in the toes, feet, legs, hands, and arms.

- Autonomic neuropathy causes changes in digestion, bowel and bladder function, sexual response, and perspiration. It can also affect the nerves that serve the heart and control blood pressure, as well as nerves in the lungs and eyes. Autonomic neuropathy can also cause hypoglycemia unawareness, a condition in which people no longer experience the warning symptoms of low blood glucose levels.

- Proximal neuropathy causes pain in the thighs, hips, or buttocks and leads to weakness in the legs.

- Focal neuropathy results in the sudden weakness of one nerve or a group of nerves, causing muscle weakness or pain. Any nerve in the body can be affected.

How can I prevent diabetic neuropathies?

The best way to prevent neuropathy is to keep your blood glucose levels as close to the normal range as possible. Maintaining safe blood glucose levels protects nerves throughout your body. For additional information about preventing diabetes complications, including neuropathy, see the Prevent Diabetes Problems Series at www.diabetes .niddk.nih.gov/dm/pubs/complications.

How are diabetic neuropathies treated?

The first treatment step is to bring blood glucose levels within the normal range to help prevent further nerve damage. Blood glucose monitoring, meal planning, physical activity, and diabetes medicines or insulin will help control blood glucose levels. Symptoms may get worse when blood glucose is first brought under control, but over time, maintaining lower blood glucose levels helps lessen symptoms. Good blood glucose control may also help prevent or delay the onset of further problems. As scientists learn more about the underlying causes of neuropathy, new treatments may become available to help slow, prevent, or even reverse nerve damage.

As described in the following sections, additional treatment depends on the type of nerve problem and symptom. If you have problems with your feet, your doctor may refer you to a foot care specialist.

Pain relief: Doctors usually treat painful diabetic neuropathy with oral medications, although other types of treatments may help some people. People with severe nerve pain may benefit from a combination of medications or treatments. Talk with your health care provider about options for treating your neuropathy.

Medications used to help relieve diabetic nerve pain include the following:

- Tricyclic antidepressants, such as amitriptyline, imipramine, and desipramine (Norpramin, Pertofrane)

- Other types of antidepressants, such as duloxetine (Cymbalta), venlafaxine, bupropion (Wellbutrin), paroxetine (Paxil), and citalopram (Celexa)

- Anticonvulsants, such as pregabalin (Lyrica), gabapentin (Gabarone, Neurontin), carbamazepine, and lamotrigine (Lamictal)

- Opioids and opioid-like drugs, such as controlled-release oxycodone, an opioid; and tramadol (Ultram), an opioid that also acts as an antidepressant

Duloxetine and pregabalin are approved by the U.S. Food and Drug Administration specifically for treating painful diabetic peripheral neuropathy.

You do not have to be depressed for an antidepressant to help relieve your nerve pain. All medications have side effects, and some are not recommended for use in older adults or those with heart disease. Because over-the-counter pain medicines such as acetaminophen and ibuprofen may not work well for treating most nerve pain and can have serious side effects, some experts recommend avoiding these medications.

Treatments that are applied to the skin—typically to the feet—include capsaicin cream and lidocaine patches (Lidoderm). Studies suggest that nitrate sprays or patches for the feet may relieve pain. Studies of alpha-lipoic acid, an antioxidant, and evening primrose oil have shown that they can help relieve symptoms and may improve nerve function.

A device called a bed cradle can keep sheets and blankets from touching sensitive feet and legs. Acupuncture, biofeedback, or physical therapy may help relieve pain in some people. Treatments that involve electrical nerve stimulation, magnetic therapy, and laser or light therapy may be helpful but need further study. Researchers are also studying several new therapies in clinical trials.

Gastrointestinal problems: To relieve mild symptoms of gastroparesis—indigestion, belching, nausea, or vomiting—doctors suggest eating small, frequent meals; avoiding fats; and eating less fiber. When symptoms are severe, doctors may prescribe erythromycin to speed digestion, metoclopramide to speed digestion and help relieve nausea, or other medications to help regulate digestion or reduce stomach acid secretion.

To relieve diarrhea or other bowel problems, doctors may prescribe an antibiotic such as tetracycline, or other medications as appropriate.

Dizziness and weakness: Sitting or standing slowly may help prevent the light-headedness, dizziness, or fainting associated with blood pressure and circulation problems. Raising the head of the bed or wearing elastic stockings may also help. Some people benefit from increased salt in the diet and treatment with salt-retaining hormones. Others benefit from high blood pressure medications. Physical therapy can help when muscle weakness or loss of coordination is a problem.

Urinary and sexual problems: To clear up a urinary tract infection, the doctor will probably prescribe an antibiotic. Drinking plenty of fluids will help prevent another infection. People who have incontinence should try to urinate at regular intervals—every three hours, for example—since they may not be able to tell when the bladder is full.

To treat erectile dysfunction in men, the doctor will first do tests to rule out a hormonal cause. Several methods are available to treat erectile dysfunction caused by neuropathy. Medicines are available to help men have and maintain erections by increasing blood flow to the penis. Some are oral medications and others are injected into the penis or inserted into the urethra at the tip of the penis. Mechanical vacuum devices can also increase blood flow to the penis. Another option is to surgically implant an inflatable or semirigid device in the penis.

Vaginal lubricants may be useful for women when neuropathy causes vaginal dryness. To treat problems with arousal and orgasm, the doctor may refer women to a gynecologist.

Foot care: People with neuropathy need to take special care of their feet. The nerves to the feet are the longest in the body and are the ones most often affected by neuropathy. Loss of sensation in the feet means that sores or injuries may not be noticed and may become ulcerated or infected. Circulation problems also increase the risk of foot ulcers.

More than half of all lower-limb amputations in the United States occur in people with diabetes—86,000 amputations per year. Doctors estimate that nearly half of the amputations caused by neuropathy and poor circulation could have been prevented by careful foot care.

Follow these steps to take care of your feet:

- Clean your feet daily, using warm—not hot—water and a mild soap. Avoid soaking your feet. Dry them with a soft towel and dry carefully between your toes.

- Inspect your feet and toes every day for cuts, blisters, redness, swelling, calluses, or other problems. Use a mirror—laying a mirror on the floor works well—or get help from someone else if you cannot see the bottoms of your feet. Notify your health care provider of any problems.

- Moisturize your feet with lotion, but avoid getting the lotion between your toes.

- After a bath or shower, file corns and calluses gently with a pumice stone.

- Each week or when needed, cut your toenails to the shape of your toes and file the edges with an emery board.

- Always wear shoes or slippers to protect your feet from injuries. Prevent skin irritation by wearing thick, soft, seamless socks.

- Wear shoes that fit well and allow your toes to move. Break in new shoes gradually by first wearing them for only an hour at a time.

- Before putting your shoes on, look them over carefully and feel the insides with your hand to make sure they have no tears, sharp edges, or objects in them that might injure your feet.

- If you need help taking care of your feet, make an appointment to see a foot doctor, also called a podiatrist.

For additional information about foot care, contact the National Diabetes Information Clearinghouse at 800-860-8747. See the publication "Prevent Diabetes Problems: Keep Your Feet and Skin Healthy" at www.diabetes.niddk.nih.gov/dm/pubs/complications_feet. Materials are also available from the National Diabetes Education Program, including the fact sheet "Take Care of Your Feet for a Lifetime" at www.ndep.nih.gov/campaigns/Feet/Feet_overview.htm.

Chapter 33

Phantom and Stump Pain

After an amputation, a patient may feel abnormal sensations in a limb (or other amputated body part) which is no longer part of his/her body.

Unlike phantom pain, stump pain occurs in the body part that actually exists, in the stump that remains. It typically is described as a "sharp," "burning," "electric-like," or "skin-sensitive" pain.

Any patient who undergoes an amputation, whether it be traumatic from an unexpected injury or from planned surgery, can develop phantom pain, stump pain, or both. Some studies suggest if a patient has pain in the area about to be amputated before the amputation, there is a greater likelihood of developing phantom pain.

Phantom Pain

The patient's arms or legs are usually involved, but complex regional pain syndrome (CRPS) may affect any part of the body, such as the face or trunk. In some patients, many different areas of the body are affected. CRPS can be progressive (meaning that it gets worse at one site or spreads to other sites), or it can stay the same for a long time or even improve on its own.

"Phantom and Stump Pain," reprinted with permission from www.StopPain.org, the website of the Department of Pain Medicine and Palliative Care at Beth Israel Medical Center, New York, New York. © Continuum Health Partners, Inc., reviewed 2013.

Following an amputation, abnormal sensations can be felt from the amputated body part; that is, a patient may feel sensations in a limb (or any other amputated body part) which is no longer part of his/her body. In fact, these unusual phantom sensations occur in most people following amputation. The sensations can be changes in size or position, or actual feelings of heat, cold, or touch. In some patients, these abnormal sensations include pain. Because the pain is experienced in a part of the body that is no longer present, it is called phantom pain. Luckily, for most patients, both the phantom sensations and pain gradually resolve with time.

The actual cause of phantom pain is not known. Most authorities currently believe that both phantom pain and other phantom sensations are generated from the spinal cord and brain. It is believed that when a body part is amputated, the brain region responsible for perceiving sensation from that area begins to function abnormally, leading to the perception that the body part still exists.

Treatment of Phantom Pain

The treatment of phantom pain is difficult. No one treatment has shown to be effective in a majority of sufferers. Fortunately, there are treatment approaches that may be helpful in some patients.

Drug Therapy

Drugs used for phantom pain are:

- Antiseizure drugs (such as gabapentin, carbamazepine)
- Antidepressants (such as amitriptyline, nortriptyline)
- Local anesthetics (such as mexiletine)
- Alpha-2 adrenergic agonists (such as clonidine or tizanidine)
- Others, including calcitonin, baclofen, dextromethorphan; Opioids (such as morphine, oxycodone, methadone)

Other Therapies

Other approaches include:

- Nerve blocks
- Spinal cord stimulation
- Hypnosis, biofeedback, and other cognitive techniques (such as relaxation training and distraction)

Stump Pain

Stump pain is located at the end of an amputated limb's stump. Unlike phantom pain, it occurs in the body part that actually exists, in the stump that remains. It typically is described as a "sharp," "burning," "electric-like," or "skin-sensitive" pain.

Stump pain is due to a damaged nerve in the stump region. Nerves damaged in the amputation surgery try to heal and may form abnormally sensitive regions, called neuromas. A neuroma can cause pain and skin sensitivity.

Treatment of Stump Pain

No one treatment has been shown to be effective for stump pain. Because it is a pain due to an injured peripheral nerve, drugs used for nerve pain may be helpful (see Treatment of Phantom Pain). If the stump pain affects a limb, revision of the prosthesis is sometimes beneficial. Other approaches also are tried in selected cases, including:

- Nerve blocks

- Transcutaneous electrical nerve stimulation (TENS)

- Surgical revision of the stump or removal of the neuroma (This procedure may fail because the neuroma can grow back; some patients actually get worse after surgery.)

- Cognitive therapies

Phantom and Stump Pain Websites

Applied Neurology (Journal): Clinical Pearls on Phantom Limb Pain
http://appneurology.com/showArticle.jhtml?articleId=196500155

Article: What is the best way to manage phantom limb pain? (Journal of Family Practice)
http://www.jfponline.com/pdf%2F5803%2F5803JFP_Clininq2.pdf

Clinical Practice Guideline: Rehabilitation of Lower Limb Amputation (VA/DoD)
http://www.guideline.gov/summary/summary.aspx?doc_id=11758&nbr

Mayo Clinic: Phantom Pain
http://www.mayoclinic.com/invoke.cfm?id=DS00444

Amputee Coalition of America
http://www.amputee-coalition.org

National Amputation Foundation
http://www.nationalamputation.org

Chapter 34

Sickle Cell Pain

What is sickle cell pain?

Sickle cell disease is one of the most common inherited diseases worldwide, and pain is the most important symptom of the disease. The pain is often described as deep, gnawing, and throbbing. The skin may be tender, red, and warm in the painful areas. Kids with sickle cell disease may experience a wide variety of pain ranging from mild to severe, starting as early as six months old and continuing throughout their lives.

The pain of sickle cell anemia is very frustrating. You never know when it will strike and it is often difficult to get it under control.

How can you avoid triggering a pain crisis?

Most pain episodes do not have an obvious reason for their occurrence. But here are some possible causes and things that your child should avoid if possible:

- Swimming in cold water

- Being out in cold weather

Excerpted from "Pain in Sickle Cell Disease (Sickle Cell Anemia)," http://www.med.umich.edu/yourchild/topics/sicklecell.htm, written and compiled by Kyla Boyse, R.N. and Brendan P. Kelly, M.D, reviewed by Andrew D. Campbell, M.D, updated May 2009. Content provided by the University of Michigan Health System, © 2009. All rights reserved. Reprinted with permission.

- Getting too hot
- Getting dehydrated from not drinking enough fluids
- Colds and infections
- Overdoing it—not getting enough sleep and rest
- Drinking alcohol or smoking
- Menstruation (getting your period)
- Stress
- Being around second-hand smoke

What are the particular dangers of smoking around kids with sickle cell disease?

Research shows that kids with sickle cell disease who are exposed to environmental tobacco smoke (ETS) at home have more than twice as many pain episodes (pain crises) as sickle cell patients who were not exposed. Sickle cell crises involve serious symptoms and often require hospitalization. Researchers in one study estimate that ETS exposure increases the risk of crisis by 90% among children with sickle cell disease. If you smoke, either quit or don't smoke around your child.

When should my child see the doctor for sickle cell pain?

If your child has sickle cell disease, is under two years old, and has pain or fever, they should see a doctor right away. Other serious warning signs that signal a need for immediate medical treatment are:

- Pain that doesn't go away with home treatment
- Severe abdominal pain (stomachache) or swollen belly
- Chest pain
- Sudden vision problems
- Headache that's different from usual
- Feeling more and more tired
- Fever over 101° F—always check temperature with a thermometer if your child seems sick
- Vomiting
- Problems with breathing or lungs
- Not being able to move (paralysis)

- Sudden weakness

- Sudden loss of feeling (numbness)

- Swollen joints

- Painful erection of the penis that won't go away (priapism)

How can I recognize pain in my child? Why is describing pain so important?

Everyone can feel pain, even babies and young children. Sometimes children have a hard time expressing themselves and may find it hard to tell you where it hurts and what it feels like.

For this reason, doctors and nurses are using new tools to help define pain in the kids they care for. Pain charts and scales for children use pictures or numbers to describe their pain. Describing the pain can help parents, doctors, and nurses understand how bad the pain is, and how to best treat it. Talking to your child's doctors and nurses about pain is important. The more they know about your child's pain, the more they can help. Pay attention to how your child acts. For example, when your child is in pain, they may be restless or unable to sleep.

The first step in treating your child's pain is to tell your child's doctor or nurse about it. Your health care provider will ask several questions about the pain, including where it hurts, what it feels like, and how it has changed since it started.

Your child's doctor may ask you to keep a pain diary with your child, which keeps track of when your child has pain throughout the day. This diary can also document how the pain changes after taking pain medications. If medications do not seem to work, or if your child has a bad reaction, tell the doctor and keep a list of these problem medicines for future reference.

- Pain management for children (http://www.health-first.org/health_info/your_health_first/kids/pain.cfm) has an example of the faces pain scale, and general information about pain and non-drug pain relief.

- The Oucher (http://www.oucher.org/the_scales.html) is a pain measurement scale with photographs of children's faces that is especially helpful with younger kids who may have trouble using a number scale.

- All about how to know if your child is in pain (http://www.phoenix childrens.com/emily-center/child-health-topics/handouts/Pain

-472.pdf), measuring pain on pain scales, and using your child's behavior to tell how bad the pain is.

- Measuring pain in cognitively impaired children (http://www .apa.org/monitor/apr02/givingvoice.html).

How can we treat the pain at home?

Many pain crises can be managed at home. Your child will need to increase their fluid intake and should use the pain pills prescribed by their doctor. If you can't take care of the pain at home with these measures, or if the warning signs listed above occur, then get medical care right away.

In addition to drinking lots of water and taking pain pills, there are many other ways to help your child fight the pain of sickle cell disease. As with other kinds of pain, it's best to use many different approaches at once to get the best pain relief. Biofeedback, cognitive strategies, self-hypnosis, and progressive relaxation all show great promise as useful treatments to add in to the usual sickle cell pain treatment.

To find out more about all the different options in pain-control strategies, see "Your Child: Pain and Your Child or Teen" (http://www .med.umich.edu/yourchild/topics/pain.htm)

What kind of treatment is my child likely to receive in the hospital?

If treating the pain at home didn't work, you would bring your child to the hospital. At the hospital, your child will probably receive treatment similar to this:

- Morphine by IV [intravenous administration] in the ER [emergency room].

- Hydromorphone may also be used by IV.

- An anti-inflammatory medication like Toradol by mouth (pills) or by IV, or ibuprofen pills is added to help treat the inflammatory pain.

- Medical staff should assess your child's pain every 15–30 minutes at first. More morphine or hydromorphone will be given until your child has moderate pain relief.

- Pain medications should be scheduled at defined times and should not be given only once the pain is worse. It is much harder to get out-of-control pain back under control than it is to keep pain controlled.

- Intramuscular (IM) injections can scar or cause abscesses. They are also not a good, consistent way to get the pain medicines absorbed into the body. For these reasons, they are not used to deliver sickle cell pain medicines.

- If your child has complications or the pain can't be brought down to a level where the pain pills alone are working, your child may need a stay in the hospital. During a hospital stay, your child may use patient-controlled analgesia (PCA). Once pain pills alone keep the pain in check, your child is ready to go home from the hospital.

- Common side effects of pain medications used to treat sickle cell pain include constipation and retaining urine. Your child may need other medications to treat these problems and may have to have a urinary catheter to drain their bladder.

- If your child gets itching, hives, or bad reactions to the medicines, your doctors might have to switch the pain medications.

- In addition to the medication, you, the hospital staff, and your child should be teaching, practicing and using other pain control strategies, such as self-hypnosis, progressive relaxation, deep breathing, distraction, guided imagery, and play. Combining many strategies at once is much more effective than just using medication alone.

What are the challenges of pain treatment in the ER or hospital?

A fear of addiction, by patients, families, and health care workers can sometimes interfere with appropriate treatment of pain. However, there are detailed treatment guidelines that outline the right way to treat sickle cell pain.

What about meperidine (Demerol)?

Meperidine (Demerol) has been a controversial medicine. Meperidine should not be taken by mouth for chronic or acute pain in sickle cell disease. Intravenous (IV) meperidine should not be used as a first-line medication for sickle cell pain, because it can be toxic to the nervous system at higher doses. However, if your child has a morphine or hydromorphone allergy, or when they have improved in the past using meperidine briefly, meperidine may be a good choice.

What about hydroxyurea?

The medicine hydroxyurea has been used for over a decade to treat sickle cell disease in adults. It is not yet approved for use in children, but is showing promise in many studies. It looks like it may be both effective and safe for children, and is proven to help with pain and other complications in both children and adults. Continuing research looks at long-term effects and safety of hydroxyurea treatment in kids.

How does sickle cell pain affect my child's life?

Sickle cell disease is a hard condition to cope with. Controlling the pain can be very frustrating. Because there are no outward signs of the pain, sometimes people don't believe a child is suffering as much as they really are. In addition to the pain, there are many ways kids with sickle cell have to change the way they live. For example, they may not be able to go swimming with their friends if the pool is too cold, and frequent hospital stays interrupt their lives. These kinds of restrictions can really cramp a kid's style.

You may need to work with your child's school to be sure your child is getting the help and support needed. With proper supports in school, kids with sickle cell pain can participate in most activities. Find out how to work with the school system (http://www.choa.org/default.aspx?id=411) to get the help in school that your child needs. This information includes tips for parents, school nurses and teachers.

Sickle cell disease, like any chronic condition, challenges kids and their families in all kinds of ways. When they find helpful coping strategies, kids and their families can rise to the occasion.

See "Your Child: Chronic Conditions" (http://www.med.umich.edu/yourchild/topics/chronic.htm) for more information and ideas for helping your child and your family cope with this chronic condition.

Chapter 35

Sinus Pain

Chapter Contents

Section 35.1—Sinusitis 406
Section 35.2—Paranasal Sinus and Nasal Cavity
      Cancer 411

Section 35.1

Sinusitis

Excerpted from "Sinusitis," National Institute of Allergy
and Infectious Diseases (www.niaid.nih.gov), January 2012.

Your nose is stuffy. You have thick, yellowish mucus. You're coughing, and you feel tired and achy. You think that you have a cold. You take medicines to relieve your symptoms, but they don't help. When you also get a terrible headache, you finally drag yourself to the doctor. After listening to your history of symptoms and examining your face and forehead, the doctor says you have sinusitis.

What is sinusitis?

Sinusitis simply means your sinuses are inflamed—red and swollen—because of an infection or another problem. Your sinuses—specifically, paranasal sinuses—are four pairs of cavities (air-filled spaces) located within the skull or bones of your head surrounding the nose.

There are several types of sinusitis. Health experts usually identify them as follows:

- Acute, which lasts up to four weeks

- Subacute, which lasts four to 12 weeks

- Chronic, which lasts more than 12 weeks and can continue for months or even years

- Recurrent, with several attacks within a year

What are the symptoms of sinusitis?

One of the most common symptoms of any type of sinusitis is pain, and the location depends on which sinus is affected.

- If you have pain in your forehead, the problem lies in your frontal sinuses (over the eyes in the brow area).

- Experiencing pain between your eyes, sometimes with swelling of the eyelids and tissues around your eyes, and tenderness when you touch the sides of your nose may mean sinusitis has developed in your ethmoid sinuses (just behind the bridge of the nose, between the eyes).

- Pain in your upper jaw and teeth, with tender cheeks, may mean your maxillary sinuses (inside each cheekbone) are involved.

- Pain in your neck, with earaches, and deep achiness at the top of your head could be a sign that your sphenoid sinuses (behind the ethmoids in the upper region of the nose and behind the eyes) are involved (though these sinuses are affected less often).

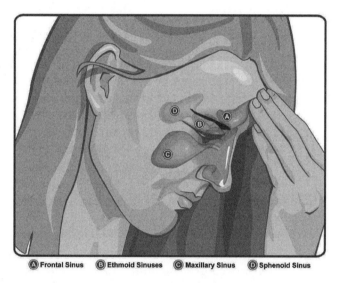

Ⓐ Frontal Sinus Ⓑ Ethmoid Sinuses Ⓒ Maxillary Sinus Ⓓ Sphenoid Sinus

Figure 35.1. *The sinuses are named for the bones that contain them.* *(Courtesy: National Institute of Allergy and Infectious Diseases)*

Most people with sinusitis have pain or tenderness in several places, and their symptoms usually do not clearly indicate which sinuses are inflamed. Pain is not as common in chronic sinusitis as it is in acute sinusitis.

In addition to the pain, people who have sinusitis (acute or chronic) often have thick nasal secretions that can be white, yellowish, greenish, or blood-tinged. Sometimes these secretions drain in the back of the throat and are difficult to clear. This is referred to as "post-nasal drip." Also, cases of acute and chronic sinusitis are usually accompanied by a stuffy nose, as well as by a general feeling of fullness over the entire face.

Less common symptoms of sinusitis (acute or chronic) can include tiredness, decreased sense of smell, cough that may be worse at night, sore throat, bad breath, and fever.

On very rare occasions, acute sinusitis can result in brain infection and other serious complications.

Because your nose can get stuffy or congested when you have a condition like the common cold, you may confuse simple nasal congestion with sinusitis. A cold usually lasts about seven to 14 days and goes away without treatment. Acute sinusitis often lasts longer and typically causes more symptoms than a cold.

How is sinusitis treated?

After diagnosing sinusitis and identifying a possible cause, your healthcare professional can suggest various treatments.

Acute sinusitis: If you have acute sinusitis, your healthcare professional may recommend the following:

- Antibiotics to control a bacterial infection, if present
- Pain relievers to reduce any pain
- Decongestants (medicines that shrink the swollen membranes in the nose and make it easier to breathe)

Even if you have acute sinusitis, your healthcare professional may choose not to use an antibiotic because many cases of acute sinusitis will end on their own. However, if you do not feel better after a few days, you should contact your healthcare professional again.

Follow your healthcare professional's instruction on how to use over-the-counter or prescription decongestant nose drops and sprays. You should use these medicines for only a few days, as longer term use can lead to even more congestion and swelling of your nasal passages.

If you suffer from sinusitis and nasal allergies, such as hay fever, your healthcare professional may recommend medicine to control your allergies. This may include a nasal steroid spray that reduces the swelling around the sinus passages and allows the sinuses to drain.

If you have asthma and then get sinusitis, your asthma may worsen. You should contact your healthcare professional, who may change your asthma treatment.

Chronic rhinosinusitis: Healthcare professionals often find it difficult to treat chronic rhinosinusitis successfully. They have two options to offer patients: medicine and surgery. Medicine options include the following:

- Nasal steroid sprays are helpful for many people, but most people still do not get full relief of symptoms with these medicines.

- A long course of antibiotics is occasionally recommended by physicians, but results from clinical research do not support this kind of antibiotic use.

- Saline (saltwater) washes or saline nasal sprays can be helpful in chronic rhinosinusitis because they remove thick secretions and allow the sinuses to drain.

- Oral steroids, such as prednisone, may be prescribed for severe chronic rhinosinusitis. However, oral steroids are powerful medicines with significant side effects, and these medicines typically are prescribed when other medicines have failed.

Research is needed to develop new, more effective treatments.

When medicine fails, surgery may be the only alternative for treating chronic rhinosinusitis. The goal of surgery is to improve sinus drainage and reduce blockage of the nasal passages. Nasal surgery usually is performed to accomplish the following:

- Enlarge the natural openings of the sinuses

- Remove nasal polyps

- Correct significant structural problems inside the nose and the sinuses if they contribute to sinus obstruction

Although most people have fewer symptoms and a better quality of life after surgery, problems can reoccur, sometimes even after a short period of time.

In children, problems can sometimes be eliminated by removing the adenoids. These gland-like tissues, located high in the throat behind and above the roof of the mouth, can obstruct the nasal passages.

Can sinusitis be prevented?

There are no methods that have been scientifically proven to prevent acute or chronic sinusitis. Your healthcare professional may recommend the following measures that can help:

- Keep your nose as moist as possible with frequent use of saline sprays or washes.

- Avoid very dry indoor environments and use a humidifier, if necessary. Be aware, however, that a humid environment also may increase the amount of mold, dust mite, or cockroach allergens in your home; this is important only if you are allergic to any of those organisms.

- Avoid exposure to irritants, such as cigarette and cigar smoke or strong odors from chemicals.

- Avoid exposure to substances to which you are allergic.

- If you haven't been tested for allergies and you are getting frequent sinus infections, ask your healthcare professional to give you an allergy evaluation or refer you to an allergy specialist.

- Avoid long periods of swimming in pools treated with chlorine, which can irritate the lining of the nose and sinuses.

- Avoid water diving, which forces water into the sinuses from the nasal passages.

Air travel may pose a problem if you suffer from acute or chronic sinusitis. When air pressure in a plane is reduced, pressure can build up in your head, blocking your sinuses or the eustachian tubes (the airways between the middle ear and the back of the throat that equalize air pressure on either side of the eardrum). As a result, you might feel discomfort in your sinuses or middle ear during the plane's ascent or descent. Some health experts recommend using decongestant nose drops or sprays before a flight to avoid this problem.

Section 35.2

Paranasal Sinus and Nasal Cavity Cancer

Excerpted from PDQ® Cancer Information Summary. National Cancer Institute; Bethesda, MD. Paranasal Sinus and Nasal Cavity Cancer Treatment (PDQ): Patient version. Updated 01/2013. Available at: www.cancer.gov. Accessed March 1, 2013.

Paranasal sinus and nasal cavity cancer is a disease in which malignant (cancer) cells form in the tissues of the paranasal sinuses and nasal cavity.

Paranasal Sinuses

Paranasal means near the nose. The paranasal sinuses are hollow, air-filled spaces in the bones around the nose. The sinuses are lined with cells that make mucus, which keeps the inside of the nose from drying out during breathing.

There are several paranasal sinuses named after the bones that surround them: the frontal sinuses are in the lower forehead above the nose; the maxillary sinuses are in the cheekbones on either side of the nose; the ethmoid sinuses are beside the upper nose, between the eyes; and the sphenoid sinuses are behind the nose, in the center of the skull.

Nasal Cavity

The nose opens into the nasal cavity, which is divided into two nasal passages. Air moves through these passages during breathing. The nasal cavity lies above the bone that forms the roof of the mouth and curves down at the back to join the throat. The area just inside the nostrils is called the nasal vestibule. A small area of special cells in the roof of each nasal passage sends signals to the brain to give the sense of smell.

Together the paranasal sinuses and the nasal cavity filter and warm the air, and make it moist before it goes into the lungs. The movement of air through the sinuses and other parts of the respiratory system help make sounds for talking.

Paranasal Sinus and Nasal Cavity Cancer

Paranasal sinus and nasal cavity cancer is a type of head and neck cancer.

Different types of cells in the paranasal sinus and nasal cavity may become malignant. The most common type of paranasal sinus and nasal cavity cancer is squamous cell carcinoma. This type of cancer forms in the squamous cells (thin, flat cells) lining the inside of the paranasal sinuses and the nasal cavity.

Other types of paranasal sinus and nasal cavity cancer include the following:

- **Melanoma:** Cancer that starts in cells called melanocytes, the cells that give skin its natural color.

- **Sarcoma:** Cancer that starts in muscle or connective tissue.

- **Inverting papilloma:** Benign tumors that form inside the nose. A small number of these change into cancer.

- **Midline granulomas:** Cancer of tissues in the middle part of the face.

Being exposed to certain chemicals or dust in the workplace can increase the risk of paranasal sinus and nasal cavity cancer.

Anything that increases your chance of getting a disease is called a risk factor. Having a risk factor does not mean that you will get cancer; not having risk factors doesn't mean that you will not get cancer. Talk with your doctor if you think you may be at risk. Risk factors for paranasal sinus and nasal cavity cancer include the following:

- Being exposed to certain workplace chemicals or dust, such as those found in the following jobs: furniture-making, sawmill work, woodworking (carpentry), shoemaking, metal-plating, and flour mill or bakery work.

- Being infected with human papillomavirus (HPV).

- Being male and older than 40 years.

- Smoking.

Possible signs of paranasal sinus and nasal cavity cancer include sinus problems and nosebleeds.

These and other symptoms may be caused by paranasal sinus and nasal cavity cancer. Other conditions may cause the same symptoms. There may be no symptoms in the early stages. Symptoms may appear as the tumor grows. Check with your doctor if you have any of the following problems:

- Blocked sinuses that do not clear, or sinus pressure
- Headaches or pain in the sinus areas
- A runny nose
- Nosebleeds
- A lump or sore inside the nose that does not heal
- A lump on the face or roof of the mouth
- Numbness or tingling in the face
- Swelling or other trouble with the eyes, such as double vision or the eyes pointing in different directions
- Pain in the upper teeth, loose teeth, or dentures that no longer fit well
- Pain or pressure in the ear

Certain factors affect prognosis (chance of recovery) and treatment options. The prognosis (chance of recovery) and treatment options depend on the following:

- Where the tumor is in the paranasal sinus or nasal cavity and whether it has spread
- The size of the tumor
- The type of cancer
- The patient's age and general health
- Whether the cancer has just been diagnosed or has recurred (come back)

Paranasal sinus and nasal cavity cancers often have spread by the time they are diagnosed and are hard to cure. After treatment, a lifetime of frequent and careful follow-up is important because there is an increased risk of developing a second kind of cancer in the head or neck.

Chapter 36

Somatoform Pain Disorder

Somatoform pain disorder is pain that is severe enough to disrupt a person's everyday life.

The pain is like that of a physical disorder, but no physical cause is found. The pain is thought to be due to psychological problems.

The pain that people with this disorder feel is real. It is not created or faked on purpose (malingering).

Causes

In the past, this disorder was thought to be related to emotional stress. The pain was often said to be "all in their head."

However, patients with somatoform pain disorder seem to experience painful sensations in a way that increases their pain level. Pain and worry create a cycle that is hard to break.

People who have a history of physical or sexual abuse are more likely to have this disorder. However, not every person with somatoform pain disorder has a history of abuse.

As researchers learn more about the connections between the brain and body, there is more evidence that emotional well-being affects the way in which pain is perceived.

"Somatoform Pain Disorder," © 2013 ADAM, Inc. Reprinted with permission.

Symptoms

The main symptom of somatoform pain disorder is chronic pain that lasts for several months and limits a person's work, relationships, and other activities.

Patients are often very worried or stressed about their pain.

Exams and Tests

A thorough medical evaluation, including laboratory work and radiologic scans (MRI, CT, ultrasound, x-ray), is done to determine possible causes of the pain.

Somatoform pain disorder is diagnosed when these tests do not reveal a clear source of the pain.

Treatment

Prescription and nonprescription pain medications often do not work very well. These medications also can have side effects, and may carry the risk for abuse.

Chronic pain syndromes of all types can often be treated with antidepressants and talk therapy.

Cognitive behavioral therapy (CBT), a kind of talk therapy, can help you deal with your pain. During therapy, you will learn:

- To recognize what seems to make the pain worse

- To develop ways of coping with the painful body sensations

- To keep yourself more active, even if you still have the pain

Antidepressant medications also often help with both the pain and the worry surrounding the pain. Commonly used antidepressants include:

- Selective serotonin reuptake inhibitors (SSRIs), such as fluoxetine (Prozac), sertraline (Zoloft), paroxetine (Paxil), fluvoxamine (Luvox), citalopram (Celexa), and escitalopram (Lexapro)

- Tricyclic antidepressants

Some patients may not believe that their pain is connected to emotional factors and may refuse these treatments.

Supportive measures that also can be helpful include:

- Distraction techniques

- Hot and cold packs

- Hypnosis
- Massage
- Physical therapy
- Stress reduction exercises
- Support groups

People with this disorder may benefit from treatment at pain centers.

Outlook (Prognosis)

The outlook is worse for patients who have had symptoms for a long time. Your outlook will improve if you can start doing your previous activities, even with the pain.

Seeking out a mental health professional who has experience treating people with chronic pain has been shown to improve outcomes.

Possible Complications

- Addiction to prescription pain medications (if they are not used correctly)
- Complications from surgery
- Depression and anxiety

When to Contact a Medical Professional

Call your health care provider if you or your child experiences chronic pain.

Chapter 37

Stroke and Pain

What Do You Need to Know?

Pain after a stroke is caused by many things. Your loved one can have one or more types of pain. The key is to find the cause of the pain so it can be treated.

Local Pain

Local pain results from physical problems. After a part of the body is paralyzed (unable to move) or weakened, the muscles may become tight and stiff. These changes in the muscles can cause pain. This pain is often felt in the joints, most often in the shoulders. Your loved one may also have sore muscles from learning new ways to walk or move. Pain may be caused by lying or sitting in one place too long. Other common causes are pressure sores or painful leg cramps at night.

Central Pain

Central pain is a direct result of damage to the brain from the stroke. Sensations like light touch are felt as pain when they should not be painful. This pain is described as burning or aching. The pain is usually on the side of the body affected by the stroke. It is often constant and may get worse over time. Changes in cold and hot temperatures may increase the pain. Movement or touching may increase the pain.

"Pain after Stroke," U.S. Department of Veterans Affairs (www.va.gov), May 10, 2011.

Why Is It Important to Get Help?

Talk to the healthcare team about your loved one's pain. Pain often leads to other problems. For instance, pain can cause depression and loss of sleep. Your loved one may stop moving a painful part of the body. Over time, the joint of this body part may "lock up" and your loved one will lose movement.

What Treatments Should You Discuss with Your Healthcare Team?

Pain usually lessens with treatment. There are many treatments to ask about.

Pain Medicines

Pain medicines are one of the most important treatments. Use pain medicines that your healthcare team suggests. Follow the directions on the label of the medicine. Give pain medicines on a regular basis. Do not wait until the pain gets bad to give pain medicines. Do not stop using medicines for fear of addiction. When pain medicines are used correctly, they do not cause addiction.

Over-the-counter (OTC) pain medicines, like Tylenol or Advil relieve mild pain. These OTC medicines may interact with other medicines your loved one takes. Check with your healthcare team before taking any OTC medicines. For more severe pain, stronger prescription pain medicines like narcotics are often needed. (Brand names and types of medicines are provided as examples only. Their inclusion does not mean that these products are endorsed by VA or any other government agency. Also, if a particular brand name is not mentioned, this does not mean or imply that the product is unsatisfactory.)

Medicines used to treat depression, spasticity (tightness and stiffness of muscles), or seizures may relieve central pain. Shots or injections of cortisone (steroids) into joints like the shoulder may help.

Exercises

Exercises to strengthen muscles can help your loved one move better. For example, stretching exercises decrease the tightness and soreness of the muscles. Talk with a physical therapist about the best exercise plan.

Heat Therapy

Heat therapy like heating pads and warm baths may soothe sore muscles and stiff joints.

Electrical Nerve Stimulation

Electrical nerve stimulation (often called TENS or TNS) improves the strength of the muscles and often reduces pain. Patches or electrodes are placed on the skin. A mild electrical current runs through these patches. This is not painful.

Complementary or Alternative Therapies

Complementary or alternative therapies like acupuncture, massage therapy, and yoga often relieve pain.

What If the Pain Continues?

Everyone has the right to good pain control. Ask your healthcare team to try different treatments to relieve the pain. If the pain continues, ask about other types of care.

Pain clinics are helpful for people whose pain is difficult to treat. Ask about pain clinics in your area.

Psychologists help stroke survivors find ways to live with pain that cannot be completely relieved. Psychologists also help survivors who are sad or depressed due to living with pain.

How Can You Help Your Loved One Describe the Pain?

Your healthcare team needs to know how your loved one feels. Ask your loved one to rate the pain. Use a pain scale of "0–10," with "0" being no pain and "10" being the worst pain your loved one has ever felt. If your loved one can't speak, use a pain scale, like the Wong-Baker Faces Pain Rating Scale described in Chapter 41—Diagnosing and Evaluating Pain.

Take note of where your loved one hurts. What things bring on the pain? What makes it worse? When does the pain occur? How does it feel? Report these symptoms to your healthcare team. My Health*e*Vet has a pain journal (available at http://www.myhealth.va.gov) you can use to track your loved one's pain. You must be registered to use this feature.

Remember that some stroke survivors have trouble speaking. Watch for signs of pain such as moaning or changes in behaviors. Some stroke survivors may not feel pain. They may not know when they are cut or burned by hot water. Watch for sores and other injuries.

Talk with Your Loved One about the Pain

- Pain almost always is a real problem. Believe your loved one's complaints.

- Allow time for your loved one to talk about the pain.

- Talk about feelings of sadness related to the pain. Watch for signs of depression. Report problems to your healthcare team. Learn more about depression after stroke.

Helpful Tips

- Help your loved one remain active to keep muscles strong and reduce pain.

- Talk with your healthcare team about correct ways to exercise. Also ask about how best to position paralyzed or weak arms and legs. Splints or other devices may be helpful.

- Support a weak or paralyzed arm to reduce pain in the shoulder. Ask your healthcare team about using an arm sling. Provide support for the arm on a lapboard or raised armrest. Use pillows while lying in bed.

- Have your loved one wear loose, comfortable clothing.

- Help your loved one relax. Find an activity that your loved one enjoys such as playing with the dog or watching television. Suggest activities like listening to music, reading a book, prayer or meditation.

- Use warm baths, showers, warm washcloths or heating pads. Be sure to check the temperature so as not to cause burns. Cool cloths and ice may also help. Talk with your healthcare team about the best plan.

Remember

- Pain is almost always a real problem. Believe your loved one. Get help for any signs or problems of pain.

- Pain can cause other problems like depression and loss of sleep.

- Treatment is based on what is causing the pain. Ask about the pain. Help your loved one describe the pain to the healthcare team.

- Everyone has the right to good pain control. Ask for different treatments if the pain is not relieved.

Chapter 38

Surgical Pain

Chapter Contents

Section 38.1—What You Need to Know about Pain
Control after Surgery.. 424
Section 38.2—Is Post-Surgery Codeine a Risk
for Children?... 434

Section 38.1

What You Need to Know about Pain Control after Surgery

"What You Need to Know About Pain Control after Surgery," © 2013 The Cleveland Clinic Foundation, 9500 Euclid Avenue, Cleveland, OH 44195. All rights reserved. Reprinted with permission. Additional information is available from the Cleveland Clinic Health Information Center, 216-444-3771, toll-free 800-223-2273 extension 43771, or at http://my.clevelandclinic.org/health.

Pain control following surgery is a major priority for both you and your doctors. While you should expect to have some pain after your surgery, your doctor will make every effort to safely minimize your pain.

We provide the following information to help you understand your options for pain treatment, to describe how you can help your doctors and nurses control your pain, and to empower you to take an active role in making choices about pain treatment.

Be sure to tell your doctor about all medications (prescribed and over-the-counter), vitamins and herbal supplements you are taking. This may affect which drugs are prescribed for your pain control.

Why Is Pain Control So Important?

In addition to keeping you comfortable, pain control can help you recover faster and may reduce your risk of developing certain complications after surgery, such as pneumonia and blood clots. If your pain is well controlled, you will be better able to complete important tasks such as walking and deep breathing exercises.

What Kinds of Pain Will I Feel after Surgery?

You may be surprised at where you experience pain after surgery. Often times the incision itself is not the only area of discomfort. You may or may not feel the following:

- **Muscle pain:** You may feel muscle pain in the neck, shoulders, back, or chest from lying on the operating table.

- **Throat pain:** Your throat may feel sore or scratchy.

- **Movement pain:** Sitting up, walking, and coughing are all important activities after surgery, but they may cause increased pain at or around the incision site.

What Can I Do to Help Keep My Pain under Control?

Important! Your doctors and nurses want and need to know about pain that is not adequately controlled. If you are having pain, please tell someone! Don't worry about being a "bother."

You can help the doctors and nurses "measure" your pain. While you are recovering, your doctors and nurses will frequently ask you to rate your pain on a scale of 0 to 10, with "0" being "no pain" and "10" being "the worst pain you can imagine." Reporting your pain as a number helps the doctors and nurses know how well your treatment is working and whether to make any changes. Keep in mind that your comfort level (that is, ability to breathe deeply or cough) is more important than absolute numbers (that is, pain score).

Are You in Pain? Please Tell Us

- 0: I'm not in pain and I do not feel uncomfortable

- 1–2: I'm not pain-free, but would be okay if no pain medication or treatment was available.

- 3–4: I'm a bit uncomfortable. It's not awful, but if Tylenol, aspirin, or ibuprofen were available, I would take it.

- 5–6: I can only concentrate on an activity for a short period of time due to my pain. I need more than Tylenol. I could wait an hour or so if I had to but I need some relief.

- 7–8: My pain is dominating my thoughts. I don't feel like doing anything unto I get some relief. Please get me something strong as soon as possible! I don't think I can wait! I need some relief.

- 9–10: I barely feel like talking. I don't want to do anything. I can't enjoy any activity at all—maybe not even eating. All I can think about is getting rid of this pain! Please give me something strong—even sooner than right now!

Who Is Going to Help Manage My Pain?

You and your surgeon will decide what type of pain control would be most acceptable for you after surgery. Your surgeon may choose to consult the Acute Pain Management Service to help manage your pain following surgery. Doctors on this service are specifically trained in the types of pain control options described in this chapter.

You are the one who ultimately decides which pain control option is most acceptable. The manager of your post-surgical pain—your surgeon or the Acute Pain Management Service doctor—will review your medical and surgical history, check the results from your laboratory tests and physical exam, then advise you about which pain management option may be best suited to safely minimize your discomfort.

After surgery, you will be assessed frequently to ensure that you are comfortable and safe. When necessary, adjustments or changes to your pain management regimen will be made.

Types of Pain-Control Treatments

You may receive more than one type of pain treatment, depending on your needs and the type of surgery you are having. All of these treatments are relatively safe, but like any therapy, they are not completely free of risk. Dangerous side effects are rare. Nausea, vomiting, itching, and drowsiness can occur. These side effects are usually easily treated in most cases.

Intravenous Patient-Controlled Analgesia (PCA)

Patient-controlled analgesia (PCA) is a computerized pump that safely permits you to push a button and deliver small amounts of pain medicine into your intravenous (IV) line, usually in your arm. No needles are injected into your muscle. PCA provides stable pain relief in most situations. Many patients like the sense of control they have over their pain management.

The PCA pump is programmed to give a certain amount of medication when you press the button. It will only allow you to have so much medication, no matter how often you press the button, so there is little worry that you will give yourself too much.

One way that you may get too much medication from the PCA pump is if a family member presses the PCA button for you. This removes the patient control aspect of the therapy, which is a major safety feature. Do not allow family members or friends to push your PCA pump button for you. You need to be awake enough to know that you need pain medication.

Patient-Controlled Epidural Analgesia

Many people are familiar with epidural anesthesia because it is frequently used to control pain during childbirth. Patient-controlled epidural analgesia uses a PCA pump to deliver pain-control medicine into an epidural catheter (a very thin plastic tube) that is placed into your back.

Placing the epidural catheter (to which the PCA pump is attached) usually causes no more discomfort than having an IV started. A sedating medication, given through your IV, will help you relax. The skin of your back will be cleaned with a sterile solution and numbed with a local anesthetic. Next, a thin needle will be carefully inserted into an area called the "epidural space." A thin catheter will be inserted through this needle into the epidural space, and the needle will then be removed. During and after your surgery, pain medications will be infused through this epidural catheter with the goal of providing you with excellent pain control when you awaken. If additional pain medication is required, you can press the PCA button.

Epidural analgesia is usually more effective in relieving pain than intravenous medication. Patients who receive epidural analgesia typically have less pain when they take deep breaths, cough, and walk, and they may recover more quickly. For patients with medical problems such as heart or lung disease, epidural analgesia may reduce the risk of serious complications such as heart attack and pneumonia.

Epidural analgesia is safe, but like any procedure or therapy, not risk free. Sometimes the epidural does not adequately control pain. In this situation, you will be given alternative treatments or be offered replacement of the epidural. Nausea, vomiting, itching, and drowsiness can occur. Occasionally, numbness and weakness of the legs can occur, which disappears after the medication is reduced or stopped. Headaches can occur, but this is rare. Severe complications, such as nerve damage and infection, are extremely rare.

Nerve Blocks

You may be offered a nerve block to control your pain after surgery. Whereas an epidural controls pain over a broad area of your body, a nerve block is used when pain from surgery affects a smaller region of your body, such as an arm or leg. Sometimes a catheter similar to an epidural catheter is placed for prolonged pain control. There are several potential advantages of a nerve block. It may allow for a significant reduction in the amount of opioid (narcotic) medication, which may result in fewer side effects, such as nausea, vomiting, itching, and drowsiness.

In some cases, a nerve block can be used as the main anesthetic for your surgery. In this case, you will be given medications during your surgery to keep you sleepy, relaxed, and comfortable. This type of anesthesia provides the added benefit of pain relief both during and after your surgery. It may reduce your risk of nausea and vomiting after surgery. You, your anesthesiologist, and your surgeon will decide before surgery if a nerve block is a suitable pain management or anesthetic option for you.

Pain Medications Taken by Mouth

At some point during your recovery from surgery, your doctor will order pain medications to be taken by mouth (oral pain medications). These may be ordered to come at a specified time, or you may need to ask your nurse to bring them to you. Make sure you know if you need to ask for the medication! Most oral pain medications can be taken every four hours.

Important! Do not wait until your pain is severe before you ask for pain medications. Also, if the pain medication has not significantly helped within 30 minutes, notify your nurse. Extra pain medication is available for you to take. You do not have to wait four hours to receive more medication.

What are some of the risks and benefits associated with pain medication?

Opioids (narcotics) after surgery: Medications such as morphine, fentanyl, hydromorphone

- *Benefits:* Strong pain relievers. Many options are available if one is causing significant side effects.

- *Risks:* May cause nausea, vomiting, itching, drowsiness, and/or constipation. The risk of becoming addicted is extremely rare.

Opioids (narcotics) at home: (Percocet, Vicodin, Darvocet, Tylenol [(#3, #4) with codeine])

- *Benefits:* Effective for moderate to severe pain. Many options available.

- *Risks:* Nausea, vomiting, itching, drowsiness, and/or constipation. Stomach upset can be lessened if the drug is taken with food. You should not drive or operate machinery while taking these medications. Note: These medications often contain acetaminophen (Tylenol). Make sure that other medications that you are taking do not contain acetaminophen, because too much of it may damage your liver.

Non-opioid (nonnarcotic) analgesics: (Tylenol, FeverAll)

- *Benefits:* Effective for mild to moderate pain. They have very few side effects and are safe for most patients. They often decrease the requirement for stronger medications, which may reduce the incidence of side effects.

- *Risks:* Liver damage may result if more than the recommended daily dose is used. Patients with pre-existing liver disease or those who drink significant quantities of alcohol may be at increased risk.

Nonsteroidal anti-inflammatory drugs (NSAIDs): Ibuprofen (Advil), naproxen sodium (Aleve), celecoxib (Celebrex)

- *Benefits:* These drugs reduce swelling and inflammation and relieve mild to moderate pain. Ibuprofen and naproxen sodium are available without a prescription, but you should ask your doctor about taking them. They may reduce the amount of opioid analgesic you need, possibly reducing side effects such as nausea, vomiting, and drowsiness. If taken alone, there are no restrictions on driving or operating machinery.

- *Risks:* The most common side effects of NSAIDs are stomach upset and dizziness. You should not take these drugs without your doctor's approval if you have kidney problems, a history of stomach ulcers, heart failure or are on "blood thinner" medications such as Coumadin (warfarin), Lovenox injections, or Plavix.

Are There Ways I Can Relieve Pain without Medication?

Yes, there are other ways to relieve pain and it is important to keep an open mind about these techniques. When used along with medication, these techniques can dramatically reduce pain.

Relaxation tapes or guided imagery is a proven form of focused relaxation that coaches you in creating calm, peaceful images in your mind—a "mental escape." For the best results, practice using the tape or CD before your surgery, and then use it twice daily during your recovery. You can get relaxation tapes at a bookstore, or rent CDs from your library. Finally, you can bring a battery-operated listening device to the hospital to play prior to surgery and during your hospital stay.

Listening to soft music and changing your position in bed are additional methods to relieve or lessen pain.

At home, heat or cold therapy may be an option that your surgeon may choose to help reduce swelling and control your pain. Specific instructions for the use of these therapies will be discussed with you by your surgical team.

If you have an abdominal or chest incision, you will want to splint the area with a pillow when you are coughing or breathing deeply to decrease motion near your incision. You will be given a pillow in the hospital. Continue to use it at home as well.

Lastly, make sure you are comfortable with your treatment plan. Talk to your doctor and nurses about your concerns and needs. This will help avoid miscommunication, stress, anxiety, and disappointment, which may make pain worse. Keep asking questions until you have satisfactory answers. You are the one who will benefit.

How Can I Control Pain at Home?

You may be given prescriptions for pain medication to take at home. These may or may not be the same pain medications you took in the hospital. Talk with your doctor about which pain medications will be prescribed at discharge.

Note: Make sure your doctor knows about pain medications that have caused you problems in the past. This will prevent possible delays in your discharge from the hospital.

Preparation for Your Discharge

Your doctors may have already given you your prescription for pain medication prior to your surgery date. If this is the case, it is best to be prepared and have your medication filled and ready for you when you come home from the hospital. You may want to have your pain pills with you on your ride home if you are traveling a long distance. Check with your insurance company regarding your prescription plan and coverage for your medication. Occasionally, a pain medication prescribed by your doctor is not covered by your insurance company.

If you do not receive your prescription for pain medication until after the surgery, make sure a family member takes your prescription and gets it filled. It is important that you are prepared in case you have pain.

Make sure you wear comfortable clothes, and keep your coughing and deep breathing pillow with you.

You may want to have your relaxation music available for your travels.

If you are traveling by plane, make sure you have your pain pills in your carry-on luggage in case the airline misplaces your checked luggage.

While at Home

Remember to take your pain medication before activity and at bedtime. Your doctor may advise you to take your pain medication at regular intervals (such as every four to six hours).

Be sure to get enough rest. If you are having trouble sleeping, talk to your doctor.

Use pillows to support you when you sleep and when you do your coughing and deep breathing exercises.

Try using the alternative methods discussed earlier. Heating pads or cold therapy, guided imagery tapes, listening to soft music, changing your position in bed, and massage can help relieve your pain.

Note: If you need to have stitches or staples removed and you are still taking pain medications, be sure to have a friend or family member drive you to your appointment. Commonly, you should not drive or operate equipment if you are taking opioid (narcotic)-containing pain medications. Check the label of your prescription for any warnings or ask your doctor, nurse, or pharmacist.

Frequently Asked Questions

I am nervous about getting "hooked" on pain pills. How do I avoid this?

The risk of becoming addicted to pain medication after surgery is very small. The bigger risk is a possible prolonged recovery if you avoid your pain medications, and cannot effectively do your required activities. If you are concerned about addiction, or have a history of substance abuse (alcohol or any drug), talk with your doctors. They will monitor you closely during your recovery. If issues arise following surgery, they will consult the appropriate specialists. [Ed. Note: Additional information about opioid medications can be found in Chapter 47—Opioid Pain Relievers.]

I am a small person who is easily affected by medicine. I am nervous that a "normal" dose of pain medication will be too much for me. What should I do?

During recovery, your healthcare team will observe how you respond to pain medication and make changes as needed. Be sure to communicate with your doctors any concerns you have prior to surgery. The relatively small doses of pain medication given after surgery are highly unlikely to have an exaggerated effect based on your body size.

I don't have a high tolerance for pain. I am afraid that the pain will be too much for me to handle. What can I do?

Concern about pain from surgery is very normal. The most important thing you can do is to talk with your surgeon and anesthesiologist about your particular situation. Setting pain control goals with your doctors before surgery will help them better tailor your pain treatment plan. Treating pain early is easier than treating it after it has set in. If you have had prior experiences with surgery and pain control, let your doctor know what worked or what did not work. Remember, there are usually many options available to you for pain control after surgery.

I normally take Tylenol if I get a headache. Can I still take Tylenol for a headache if I am on other pain medication?

As discussed earlier, before taking any other medication, be sure to talk to your doctor. Some of the medications prescribed for use at home contain acetaminophen (Tylenol) and if too much is taken, you may become ill. In order to avoid getting too much of any medication, discuss this issue with your doctor BEFORE you leave the hospital.

Play an Active Role in Your Pain Control

Ask Your Doctors and Nurses About

- Pain and pain control treatments and what you can expect from them. You have a right to the best level of pain relief that can be safely provided.
- Your schedule for pain medicines in the hospital.
- How you can participate in a pain-control plan.

Inform Your Doctors and Nurses About

- Any surgical pain you have had in the past.
- How you relieved your pain before you came to the hospital.
- Pain you have had recently or currently.
- Pain medications you have taken in the past and cannot tolerate.
- Pain medications you have been taking prior to surgery.
- Any pain that is not controlled with your current pain medications.

You Should

- Help the doctors and nurses "measure" your pain and expect staff to ask about pain relief often and to respond quickly when you do report pain.
- Ask for pain medicines as soon as pain begins.
- Tell us how well your pain is relieved and your pain relief expectations.
- Use other comfort measures for pain control—listening to relaxation or soft music, repositioning in bed, etc.

Your doctors are committed to providing you with the safest and most effective pain management strategy that is most acceptable to you.

Resources

Cleveland Clinic staff, Cleveland, Ohio

Correll DJ. Chapter 49. Perioperative Pain Management. In: Lawry GV, McKean SC, Matloff J, Ross JJ, Dressler DD, Brotman DJ, Ginsberg JS, eds. *Principles and Practice of Hospital Medicine.* New York: McGraw-Hill; 2012. http://www.accessmedicine.com/content.aspx?aID=56194340&searchStr=pain+management#56194340

D'Arcy Y. *Compact Clinical Guide to Acute Pain Management.* Philadelphia, PA: Springer Publishing; 2011

Managing Pain with Medications after Orthopaedic Surgery. American Academy of Orthopaedic Surgeons. http://orthoinfo.aaos.org/topic.cfm?topic=A00650

Pain Relief after Surgery. *Am Fam Physician*. 2001 May 15;63(10): 1985-1986. http://www.aafp.org/afp/2001/0515/p1985.html

Barrows K. Chapter e5. Complementary & Alternative Medicine. In: Papadakis MA, McPhee SJ, Rabow MW, eds. *CURRENT Medical Diagnosis & Treatment* 2013. New York: McGraw-Hill; 2013. http://www.accessmedicine.com/content.aspx?aID=22146

Section 38.2

Is Post-Surgery Codeine a Risk for Children?

"Is Post-Surgery Codeine a Risk for Kids?" Consumer Update, U.S. Food and Drug Administration (www.fda.gov), August 15, 2012.

Children are often prescribed codeine for pain relief after surgery to remove their tonsils or adenoids to treat sleep apnea, a condition in which breathing problems make it hard for them to sleep soundly.

However, some children may be at risk of developing serious side effects, or even dying, after being given codeine in amounts that are within the recommended dose range.

The Food and Drug Administration (FDA) has reviewed recent reports in medical literature of three deaths and one life-threatening case in children who took codeine for pain relief after surgery to remove their tonsils or adenoids to treat sleep apnea. The agency is warning the public that this danger exists for some children whose livers convert codeine to morphine in higher than normal amounts.

FDA wants parents and caregivers to be aware of the warning signs that could indicate their child is having trouble breathing because of this higher morphine level.

The agency is trying to determine if there have been other cases of accidental overdose or death in children taking codeine, and if there have been incidents like this when children have taken codeine after other kinds of surgical procedures, says Bob Rappaport, M.D., director of the Division of Anesthesia, Analgesia and Addiction Products (DAAAP) in FDA's Center for Drug Evaluation and Research.

The Problem

Codeine is an opioid pain reliever—a narcotic medication—used to treat mild to moderate pain. It is also used to reduce coughing, usually in combination with other medications. Codeine is available by prescription either alone or in combination with acetaminophen or aspirin, and in some cough and cold medications.

Codeine is converted to morphine in the liver by an enzyme. Some people have genetic variations that make this enzyme over-active, causing codeine to be converted to morphine faster and more completely than in other people. These "ultra-rapid metabolizers" are more likely to have higher than normal amounts of morphine in their blood after taking codeine. High levels of morphine can result in breathing difficulty, which may be fatal.

From one to seven in every 100 people are "ultra-rapid metabolizers," but they are more common among some ethnic groups. Twenty-nine percent of North African and Ethiopian populations are "ultra-rapid metabolizers," with about 6 percent of African American, Caucasian, and Greek populations also affected.

The only way to know if someone is an ultra-rapid metabolizer is to do a genetic test. There are FDA-cleared tests to check for ultra-rapid metabolism.

The cases occurred in children who showed evidence of being ultra-rapid metabolizers. The children ranged in age from two to five years old. All of the children received doses of codeine that were within the typical dose range, meaning that they were not given extra amounts of the medication.

In these cases, the signs of morphine overdose developed within one to two days after the children started taking codeine.

Signs of Trouble

FDA warns that when prescribed to treat pain after surgery, codeine should not be given on a schedule, but only when the child needs relief from pain. Children should never receive more than six doses in a day.

Parents and caregivers should watch their children closely after surgery, and after they have returned home, for signs of a morphine overdose.

There are a number of symptoms to watch for, says Rappaport. If your child shows these signs, stop giving the codeine and seek medical attention immediately by taking your child to the emergency room or calling 911:

- Unusual sleepiness, such as being difficult to wake up

- Disorientation or confusion

- Labored or noisy breathing, such as breathing shallowly with a "sighing" pattern of breathing or deep breaths separated by abnormally long pauses

- Blueness on the lips or around the mouth

"The most important thing is that caregivers should tell the 911 operator or emergency department staff that their child has been taking codeine and is having breathing problems," Rappaport says.

Talk to your child's health care professional if you have any questions or concerns about codeine. Health care professionals are being advised by FDA to prescribe the lowest effective dose for the shortest period of time when prescribing drugs that contain codeine.

If your child experiences any side effects from codeine, report them to the FDA MedWatch program (http://www.fda.gov/Safety/MedWatch/default.htm).

Chapter 39

Urological Pain

Chapter Contents

Section 39.1—Interstitial Cystitis (Painful Bladder
        Syndrome)... 438
Section 39.2—Kidney Stones.. 444

Section 39.1

Interstitial Cystitis
(Painful Bladder Syndrome)

Excerpted from "Interstitial Cystitis/Painful Bladder Syndrome,"
National Kidney and Urologic Diseases Information Clearinghouse,
a service of the National Institute of Diabetes and Digestive and
Kidney Diseases (www.niddk.nih.gov), June 29, 2012.

What is IC/PBS?

Interstitial cystitis (IC) is a condition that results in recurring discomfort or pain in the bladder and the surrounding pelvic region. The symptoms vary from case to case and even in the same individual. People may experience mild discomfort, pressure, tenderness, or intense pain in the bladder and pelvic area. Symptoms may include an urgent need to urinate, a frequent need to urinate, or a combination of these symptoms. Pain may change in intensity as the bladder fills with urine or as it empties. Women's symptoms often get worse during menstruation. They may sometimes experience pain during vaginal intercourse.

Because IC varies so much in symptoms and severity, most researchers believe it is not one, but several diseases. In recent years, scientists have started to use the terms bladder pain syndrome (BPS) or painful bladder syndrome (PBS) to describe cases with painful urinary symptoms that may not meet the strictest definition of IC. The term IC/PBS includes all cases of urinary pain that can't be attributed to other causes, such as infection or urinary stones. The term interstitial cystitis, or IC, is used alone when describing cases that meet all of the IC criteria established by the National Institute of Diabetes and Digestive and Kidney Diseases (NIDDK).

In IC/PBS, the bladder wall may be irritated and become scarred or stiff. Glomerulations— pinpoint bleeding—often appear on the bladder wall. Hunner's ulcers—patches of broken skin found on the bladder wall—are present in 10 percent of people with IC.

Some people with IC/PBS find that their bladder cannot hold much urine, which increases the frequency of urination. Frequency, however, is not always specifically related to bladder size; many people with severe frequency have normal bladder capacity when measured under anesthesia or during urologic testing. People with severe cases of IC/ PBS may urinate as many as 60 times a day, including frequent night-time urination, also called nocturia.

What are the treatments for IC/PBS?

Scientists have not yet found a cure for IC/PBS, nor can they predict who will respond best to which treatment. Symptoms may disappear with a change in diet or treatments or without explanation. Even when symptoms disappear, they may return after days, weeks, months, or years. Scientists do not know why.

Because the causes of IC/PBS are unknown, current treatments are aimed at relieving symptoms. Many people are helped for variable periods by one or a combination of treatments. As researchers learn more about IC/PBS, the list of potential treatments will change, so patients should discuss their options with a doctor.

Bladder distention: Many people with IC/PBS have noted an improvement in symptoms after a bladder distention has been done to diagnose the condition. In many cases, the procedure is used as both a diagnostic test and initial therapy. Researchers are not sure why distention helps, but some believe it may increase capacity and interfere with pain signals transmitted by nerves in the bladder. Symptoms may temporarily worsen 4–48 hours after distention, but should return to predistention levels or improve within two to four weeks.

Bladder instillation: During a bladder instillation, also called a bladder wash or bath, the bladder is filled with a solution that is held for varying periods of time, averaging 10 to 15 minutes, before being emptied.

The only drug approved by the U.S. Food and Drug Administration (FDA) for bladder instillation is dimethyl sulfoxide (Rimso-50), also called DMSO. DMSO treatment involves guiding a narrow tube called a catheter up the urethra into the bladder. A measured amount of DMSO is passed through the catheter into the bladder, where it is retained for about 15 minutes before being expelled. Treatments are given every week or two for 6–8 weeks and repeated as needed. Most people who respond to DMSO notice improvement three or four weeks after the first 6–8-week cycle of treatments. Highly motivated patients who are willing to catheterize themselves may, after consultation with their doctor, be able to have DMSO treatments at home. Self-administration is less expensive and more convenient than going to the doctor's office.

Doctors think DMSO works in several ways. Because it passes into the bladder wall, it may reach tissue more effectively to reduce inflammation and block pain. It may also prevent muscle contractions that cause pain, frequency, and urgency.

A bothersome but relatively insignificant side effect of DMSO treatments is a garlic-like taste and odor on the breath and skin that may last up to seven hours after treatment. Long-term treatment has caused cataracts in animal studies, but this side effect has not appeared in humans. Blood tests, including a complete blood count and kidney and liver function tests, should be done about every six months.

Oral drugs: Pentosan polysulfate sodium (Elmiron), the first oral drug developed for IC, was approved by the FDA in 1996. In clinical trials, the drug improved symptoms in 30 percent of patients treated. Doctors do not know exactly how the drug works, but one theory is that it may repair defects that might have developed in the lining of the bladder.

The FDA-recommended oral dosage of Elmiron is 100 milligrams (mg), three times a day. Patients may not feel relief from IC pain for the first four months. A decrease in urinary frequency may take up to six months. Patients are urged to continue with therapy for at least six months to give the drug an adequate chance to relieve symptoms. If six months of Elmiron therapy provides no benefit, it is reasonable to stop the drug.

Elmiron's side effects are limited primarily to minor gastrointestinal discomfort. A small minority of patients experienced some hair loss, but hair grew back when they stopped taking the drug. Researchers have found no negative interactions between Elmiron and other medications.

Elmiron may affect liver function, which should therefore be monitored by the doctor.

Because Elmiron has not been tested in pregnant women, the manufacturer recommends it not be used during pregnancy, except in the most severe cases. Because Elmiron has mild blood-thinning effects, it should be discontinued prior to planned surgery.

Other oral medications include aspirin and ibuprofen, which may be used as a first line of defense against mild discomfort. Doctors may recommend other drugs to relieve pain.

Some people have experienced improvement in their urinary symptoms by taking tricyclic antidepressants or antihistamines. A tricyclic antidepressant called amitriptyline (Elavil) may help reduce pain, increase bladder capacity, and decrease frequency and nocturia. Some people may not be able to take it because it makes them too tired during the day. In people with severe pain, narcotic analgesics such as acetaminophen (Tylenol) with codeine or longer-acting narcotics may be necessary.

All drugs—even those sold over the counter—have side effects. A person should always consult a doctor before using any drug for an extended amount of time.

Electrical nerve stimulation: Mild electrical pulses can be used to stimulate the nerves to the bladder—either through the skin or with an implanted device. The method of delivering impulses through the skin is called transcutaneous electrical nerve stimulation (TENS). With TENS, mild electric pulses enter the body for minutes to hours, two or more times a day either through wires placed on the lower back or just above the pubic area—between the navel and the pubic hair—or through special devices inserted into the vagina in women or into the rectum in men. Although scientists do not know exactly how TENS relieves pelvic pain, it has been suggested that the electrical pulses may increase blood flow to the bladder, strengthen pelvic muscles that help control the bladder, or trigger the release of substances that block pain.

TENS is relatively inexpensive and allows people with IC/PBS to take an active part in treatment. Within some guidelines, the patient decides when, how long, and at what intensity TENS will be used. It has been most helpful in relieving pain and decreasing frequency in people with Hunner's ulcers. Smokers do not respond as well as nonsmokers. If TENS is going to help, improvement is usually apparent in three to four months.

A person may consider having a device implanted that delivers regular impulses to the bladder. A wire is placed next to the tailbone and attached to a permanent stimulator under the skin. The FDA has approved this device, marketed as the Inter-Stim system, to treat urge incontinence, urgency-frequency syndrome, and urinary retention in people for whom other treatments have not worked.

Diet: No scientific evidence links diet to IC/PBS, but many patients find that alcohol, tomatoes, spices, chocolate, caffeinated and citrus beverages, and high-acid foods may contribute to bladder irritation and inflammation. Some people also note that their symptoms worsen after eating or drinking products containing artificial sweeteners. Eliminating various items from the diet and reintroducing them one at a time may determine which, if any, affect a person's symptoms. However, maintaining a varied, well-balanced diet is important.

Smoking: Many people feel smoking makes their symptoms worse. How the by-products of tobacco that are excreted in the urine affect IC/PBS is unknown. Smoking, however, is a major cause of bladder cancer. One of the best things smokers can do for their bladder and their overall health is to quit.

Exercise: Many patients feel that gentle stretching exercises help relieve IC/PBS symptoms.

Bladder training: People who have found adequate relief from pain may be able to reduce frequency by using bladder training techniques. Methods vary, but basically patients decide to void—empty their bladder—at designated times and use relaxation techniques and distractions to keep to the schedule. Gradually, they try to lengthen the time between scheduled voids. A diary in which to record voiding times is helpful in keeping track of progress.

Physical therapy: New evidence indicates that certain types of physical therapy, when administered by an experienced physical therapist, may improve IC/PBS symptoms. Patients should discuss this option with their health care provider.

Surgery: Surgery should be considered only if all available treatments have failed and the pain is disabling. Many approaches and techniques are used, each of which has advantages and complications that should be discussed with a surgeon. A doctor may recommend consulting another surgeon for a second opinion before taking this step. Most surgeons are reluctant to operate because some people still have symptoms after surgery.

People considering surgery should discuss the potential risks and benefits, side effects, and long- and short-term complications with a surgeon, their family, and people who have already had the procedure. Surgery requires anesthesia, hospitalization, and weeks or months of recovery. As the complexity of the procedure increases, so do the chances for complications and failure.

People should check with their doctor to locate a surgeon experienced in performing specific procedures.

Two procedures—fulguration and resection of ulcers—can be done with instruments inserted through the urethra. Fulguration involves burning Hunner's ulcers with electricity or a laser. When the area heals, the dead tissue and the ulcer fall off, leaving new, healthy tissue behind. Resection involves cutting around and removing the ulcers. Both treatments are done under anesthesia and use special instruments inserted into the bladder through a cystoscope. Laser surgery in the urinary tract should be reserved for people with Hunner's ulcers and should be done only by doctors with the special training and expertise needed to perform the procedure.

Another surgical treatment is augmentation, which makes the bladder larger. In most of these procedures, scarred, ulcerated, and inflamed sections of the patient's bladder are removed, leaving only the base of the bladder and healthy tissue. A piece of the patient's colon—also called large intestine—is then removed, reshaped, and attached to what remains of the bladder. After the incisions heal, the patient may void less frequently. The effect on pain varies greatly; IC/PBS can sometimes recur on the segment of colon used to enlarge the bladder.

Even in carefully selected patients—those with small, contracted bladders—pain, frequency, and urgency may remain or return after surgery, and they may have additional problems with infections in the new bladder and difficulty absorbing nutrients from the shortened colon. Some patients become incontinent, while others cannot void at all and must insert a catheter into the urethra to empty the bladder.

Bladder removal, called a cystectomy, is another, infrequently used surgical option. Once the bladder has been removed, different methods can be used to reroute the urine. In most cases, ureters are attached to a piece of colon that opens onto the skin of the abdomen. This procedure is called a urostomy and the opening is called a stoma. Urine empties through the stoma into a bag outside the body. Some urologists are using a second technique that also requires a stoma but allows urine to be stored in a pouch inside the abdomen. At intervals throughout the day, the patient puts a catheter into the stoma and empties the pouch. Patients with either type of urostomy must be very careful to keep the area in and around the stoma clean to prevent infection. Serious potential complications may include kidney infection and small bowel obstruction.

A third method to reroute urine involves making a new bladder from a piece of the patient's colon and attaching it to the urethra. After healing, the patient may be able to empty the newly formed bladder by voiding at scheduled times or by inserting a catheter into the urethra. Only a few surgeons have the special training and expertise needed to perform this procedure.

Even after total bladder removal, some patients still experience variable IC/PBS symptoms in the form of phantom pain. Therefore, the decision to undergo a cystectomy should be made only after testing all alternative methods and seriously considering the potential outcome.

Removing the bladder is not always done in patients with severe disease. Some urologists recommend rerouting urine to a piece of bowel connected to the abdominal wall. Urine is then collected in an external bag that is emptied periodically. While this procedure may or may not improve pelvic pain, it can decrease frequency and improve quality of life for patients who experience frequent urges to urinate.

Section 39.2

Kidney Stones

Excerpted from "Kidney Stones in Adults," National Kidney and Urologic Diseases Information Clearinghouse, a service of the National institute of Diabetes and Digestive and Kidney Diseases (www.niddk.nih.gov), January 28, 2013.

What is a kidney stone?

A kidney stone is a solid piece of material that forms in a kidney when substances that are normally found in the urine become highly concentrated. A stone may stay in the kidney or travel down the urinary tract. Kidney stones vary in size. A small stone may pass on its own, causing little or no pain. A larger stone may get stuck along the urinary tract and can block the flow of urine, causing severe pain or bleeding.

Kidney stones are one of the most common disorders of the urinary tract. Each year in the United States, people make more than a million visits to health care providers and more than 300,000 people go to emergency rooms for kidney stone problems.

Urolithiasis is the medical term used to describe stones occurring in the urinary tract. Other frequently used terms are urinary tract stone disease and nephrolithiasis. Terms that describe the location of the stone in the urinary tract are sometimes used. For example, a ureteral stone—or ureterolithiasis—is a kidney stone found in the ureter.

What are the types of kidney stones?

Four major types of kidney stones can form:

- Calcium stones are the most common type of kidney stone and occur in two major forms: calcium oxalate and calcium phosphate. Calcium oxalate stones are more common. Calcium oxalate stone formation may be caused by high calcium and high oxalate excretion. Calcium phosphate stones are caused by the combination of high urine calcium and alkaline urine, meaning the urine has a high pH.

- Uric acid stones form when the urine is persistently acidic. A diet rich in purines—substances found in animal protein such as meats, fish, and shellfish—may increase uric acid in urine. If uric acid becomes concentrated in the urine, it can settle and form a stone by itself or along with calcium.

- Struvite stones result from kidney infections. Eliminating infected stones from the urinary tract and staying infection-free can prevent more struvite stones.

- Cystine stones result from a genetic disorder that causes cystine to leak through the kidneys and into the urine, forming crystals that tend to accumulate into stones.

Kidney stones vary in size and shape. Stones may be as small as a grain of sand or as large as a pearl. Some stones are even as big as golf balls. Stones may be smooth or jagged and are usually yellow or brown.

What are the symptoms of kidney stones?

People with kidney stones may have pain while urinating, see blood in the urine, or feel a sharp pain in the back or lower abdomen. The pain may last for a short or long time. People may experience nausea and vomiting with the pain. However, people who have small stones that pass easily through the urinary tract may not have symptoms at all.

How are kidney stones treated?

Treatment for kidney stones usually depends on their size and what they are made of, as well as whether they are causing pain or obstructing the urinary tract. Kidney stones may be treated by a general practitioner or by a urologist—a doctor who specializes in the urinary tract. Small stones usually pass through the urinary tract without treatment. Still, the person may need pain medication and should drink lots of fluids to help move the stone along. Pain control may consist of oral or intravenous (IV) medication, depending on the duration and severity of the pain. IV fluids may be needed if the person becomes dehydrated from vomiting or an inability to drink. A person with a larger stone, or one that blocks urine flow and causes great pain, may need more urgent treatment, such as the following:

- **Shock wave lithotripsy:** A machine called a lithotripter is used to crush the kidney stone. The procedure is performed by a urologist on an outpatient basis and anesthesia is used. In shock wave lithotripsy, the person lies on a table or, less commonly, in a tub of water above the lithotripter. The lithotripter generates shock waves that pass through the person's body to break the kidney stone into smaller pieces to pass more readily through the urinary tract.

- **Ureteroscopy:** A ureteroscope—a long, tubelike instrument with an eyepiece—is used to find and retrieve the stone with a small basket or to break the stone up with laser energy. The procedure is performed by a urologist in a hospital with anesthesia. The urologist inserts the ureteroscope into the person's urethra and slides the scope through the bladder and into the ureter. The urologist removes the stone or, if the stone is large, uses a flexible fiber attached to a laser generator to break the stone into smaller pieces that can pass out of the body in the urine. The person usually goes home the same day.

- **Percutaneous nephrolithotomy:** In this procedure, a wire-thin viewing instrument called a nephroscope is used to locate and remove the stone. The procedure is performed by a urologist in a hospital with anesthesia. During the procedure, a tube is inserted directly into the kidney through a small incision in the person's back. For large stones, an ultrasonic probe that acts as a lithotripter may be needed to deliver shock waves that break the stone into small pieces that can be removed more easily. The person may have to stay in the hospital for several days after the procedure and may have a small tube called a nephrostomy tube inserted through the skin into the kidney. The nephrostomy tube drains urine and any residual stone fragments from the kidney into a urine collection bag. The tube is usually left in the kidney for two or three days while the person remains in the hospital.

Part Four

Medical Management of Pain

Chapter 40

Working with Your Doctor and Pain Management Team

Chapter Contents

Section 40.1—What Is the Specialty of Pain
    Medicine?.. 450
Section 40.4—Pain Management Programs 451

Section 40.1

What Is the Specialty of Pain Medicine?

"What Is Pain Medicine?" Copyright © 2012 American Board of Pain Medicine (www.abpm.org). All rights reserved.

Definition of Pain Medicine

The specialty of pain medicine, or algiatry, is a discipline within the field of medicine that is concerned with the prevention of pain, and the evaluation, treatment, and rehabilitation of persons in pain. Some conditions may have pain and associated symptoms arising from a discrete cause, such as postoperative pain or pain associated with a malignancy, or may be conditions in which pain constitutes the primary problem, such as neuropathic pains or headaches.

Pain medicine specialists use a broad-based approach to treat all pain disorders, ranging from pain as a symptom of disease to pain as the primary disease. The pain physician serves as a consultant to other physicians but is often the principal treating physician (as distinguished from the primary care physician) and may provide care at various levels, such as treating the patient directly, prescribing medication, prescribing rehabilitative services, performing pain relieving procedures, counseling patients and families, directing a multidisciplinary team, coordinating care with other health care providers and providing consultative services to public and private agencies pursuant to optimal health care delivery to the patient suffering from pain. The objective of the pain physician is to provide quality care to the patient suffering from pain. The pain physician may work in a variety of settings and is competent to treat the entire range of pain encountered in delivery of quality health care.

Pain medicine specialists typically formulate comprehensive treatment plans, which consider the patients' cultural contexts, as well as the special needs of the pediatric and geriatric populations. Evaluation techniques include interpretation of historical data; review of previous laboratory, imaging, and electrodiagnostic studies; assessment of behavioral, social, occupational, and avocational issues; and interview and examination of the patient by the pain specialist.

450

Section 40.2

Pain Management Programs

"Pain Management Programs," © 2012 American Chronic Pain Association. All rights reserved. Reprinted with permission. For additional information, visit www.theacpa.org.

Interdisciplinary Pain Management Programs

What should you be looking for?

For many people, living with pain is a way of life. Living a full and active life, however, may seem impossible. It is actually possible to increase your level of functioning and quality life while reducing your sense of suffering. The key, like anything in life, is to have the right skills, support, and direction. That is a tall order in the health care arena these days. Rarely, if ever, do we find ourselves faced with the opportunity to have time to talk with our health care providers about our state of being. There are some exceptions. Fortunately for people with pain there is a means to build a relationship with a health care provider and their staff that can, if you are willing to take an active role, help you move from a patient to an active person. The road is not an easy one, but the rewards far outweigh any temporary issues.

While medicine has made remarkable advances to eradicate some diseases, cure others, and extend life, chronic pain is still one they are struggling to understand and improve. The good news is they have made advances in helping people to manage their pain. Interdisciplinary pain programs are designed to help a person with pain become part of the treatment team and take an active role in regaining control of his or her life in spite of the pain. The programs are focused on the total person, not just the pain.

What is interdisciplinary pain management?

It involves a team of health care providers working directly with the person with pain with a variety of measurement, interventions, and strategies for self-management designed to offer a complete program from assessment, treatment, communication, education, and follow up.

The treatment is never focused on just the pain, but it takes a holistic approach meaning who you are and how you feel is as much a part of shaping your treatment as your physical self.

The team is made up of:

- "Patient" (person with pain)
- Significant others (family, friends, neighbors)
- Physicians
- Physician assistants and nurse practitioners
- Nurses
- Psychologists
- Physical therapists
- Occupational therapists
- Recreational therapists
- Vocational counselors
- Pharmacists
- Nutritionists/dietitians
- Social workers
- Support staff
- Volunteers
- Others

Team members may vary from one program to the next, but the underlying goal remains the same: help you live a full life. You might have noticed that the "patient" is at the top of the list. Without your willingness to take an active role in the program, nothing that the program has to offer will be helpful since there is currently no cure. Your efforts are key to success!

Your team shares in providing you with a well-balanced approach to treatment. They all have specific roles that complement each other to provide better care. It is the team approach working directly with the "patient" that makes this type of program effective. Team members each have personal responsibilities that, when blended together, make for a treatment option that allows the patient to make progress.

Benefits of a well-functioning team: In a typical health care environment, you may have a primary care provider, a physical therapist, a counselor, and other specialists that you see. In many cases, while they communicate occasionally, they do not come face to face as a team to focus on you. It is in an interdisciplinary pain program that a team on a regular basis will review your care and discuss it with you. They will look at the goals that have been set, what you have accomplished, where you are having difficulties and evaluate what the next best steps are for YOU.

Based on your progress they will be able to determine which team members may need to alter their approach, other areas that might need added attention, and personal communication with you as part of that team.

The team needs to have the ability to work together in an environment where there is mutual respect and a collaborative atmosphere. Freedom to express new ideas and share insights is key to the team working together for the common good of those in the program.

The bottom line is that the treatment should focus on the whole person, not a body part or symptom, and to empower the person with pain as well as their family, or caregiver.

Interdisciplinary pain program: There are a number of practices and facilities that are called pain clinics. While they may address specific pain problems, they do not offer the complete package needed to help a person regain control of their lives. It is important that a program provide you with the physical, emotional, and psychological components you need. Perhaps the most important first step is to meet the team and make sure that you feel comfortable with them. If you are not comfortable with the team, it will be much more difficult to make progress. When looking for a pain program you need to keep in mind the following things:

Qualities of a Well-Functioning Interdisciplinary Pain Team

- Share the same beliefs and mission

- The program is patient and family centered

- Work together for common, agreed upon goals

- Develop treatment plans based on individual needs

- Mutual respect and open communication as a team

- Frequent communication between primary provider and team members

- Shared goal of improvement for each person in the program is ongoing and the responsibility of all team members

- Monitoring of progress toward goal achievement

- Feedback about progress and performance is provided to you, caregivers, significant others, and primary care providers

- Formal follow-up is scheduled

Adapted from: *Interdisciplinary Pain Management:* Dennis Turk, et al. Task Force Report developed for American Pain Society. 2009.

Chapter 41

Diagnosing and Evaluating Pain

Chapter Contents

Section 41.1—Getting a Diagnosis for Chronic Pain 456

Section 41.2—X-Rays 462

Section 41.3—Magnetic Resonance Imaging 464

Section 41.4—Electromyograms and Nerve
Conduction Studies 469

Section 41.1

Getting a Diagnosis for Chronic Pain

"Getting Diagnosed" is excerpted from "The Healthy Woman: Pain," Office on Women's Health (www.womenshealth.gov), November 2008. "Pain Intensity Scales" is from the National Institutes of Health Pain Consortium (http://painconsortium.nih.gov), January 17, 2007. Citations for individual pain scales are included within the text. These are reprinted with permission from the copyright holders. Editor's note added by David A. Cooke, MD, FACP, March 2013.

Getting Diagnosed

The first step in treating your pain is a diagnosis. During your first visit, your doctor will ask you questions about these concerns:

- When your pain started

- Location of your pain

- How your pain feels (for instance, does it feel like a sharp stabbing pain, a steady burning, or a dull ache?)

- What makes your pain better or worse

- How the pain affects your activities of daily living (for instance, bathing, dressing, and eating)

- All of the medicines that you have ever used to treat your pain (both those that were prescribed by a doctor and those that you bought over the counter)

- Any side effects you may have from these medicines

The doctor may also ask you questions to find out if you are depressed. Being depressed is quite common among patients with chronic pain. For some patients, though, the depression comes first. The chronic pain may be caused by or be part of the depression. In fact, many people who are depressed complain about pain problems, such as frequent headaches, back pain, or stomach pain, rather than depression. The only way your doctor can find out and treat your real problem is for you to answer your doctor's questions honestly.

Pain Intensity Scales

The following pain intensity scales are used by researchers at the National Institutes of Health (NIH) Clinical Center to measure how intensely individuals are feeling pain and to monitor the effectiveness of treatments. Some of the scales are appropriate for children and adults; others are used for infants

0–10 Numeric Rating Scale

Indications: Adults and children (older than nine years old) in all patient care settings who are able to use numbers to rate the intensity of their pain.

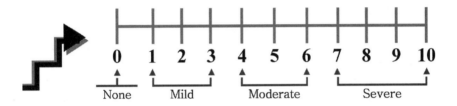

Figure 41.1. Numeric Rating Scale

Instructions

1. The patient is asked any one of the following questions:
    *   What number would you give your pain right now?
    *   What number on a 0 to 10 scale would you give your pain when it is the worst that it gets and when it is the best that it gets?
    *   At what number is the pain at an acceptable level for you?

2. When the explanation suggested in #1 above is not sufficient for the patient, it is sometimes helpful to further explain or conceptualize the Numeric Rating Scale in the following manner:
    *   0 = No pain
    *   1–3 = Mild pain (nagging, annoying, interfering little with activities of daily living [ADLs])
    *   4–6 = Moderate pain (interferes significantly with ADLs)
    *   7–10 = Severe pain (disabling; unable to perform ADLs)

3. The interdisciplinary team in collaboration with the patient/ family (if appropriate), can determine appropriate interventions in response to Numeric Pain Ratings.

Reference: McCaffery, M., & Beebe, A. (1993). *Pain: Clinical Manual for Nursing Practice*. Baltimore: V.V. Mosby Company. Reprinted with permission.

Wong–Baker FACES Pain Rating Scale

Indications: Rating scale is recommended for persons age three years and older.

Instructions: Explain to the person that each face [see Figure 41.2] is for a person who feels happy because he has no pain (hurt) or sad because he has some or a lot of pain. Face 0 is very happy because he doesn't hurt at all. Face 1 hurts just a little bit. Face 2 hurts a little more. Face 3 hurts even more. Face 4 hurts a whole lot. Face 5 hurts as much as you can imagine, although you don't have to be crying to feel this bad. Ask the person to choose the face that best describes how he is feeling.

Be specific about the pain location and at what time pain occurred (now or earlier during a procedure). The interdisciplinary team in collaboration with the patient/family (if appropriate), can determine appropriate interventions in response to FACES pain ratings.

Reference: Wong-Baker FACES Pain Rating Scale (From Hockenberry MJ, Wilson D: *Wong's essentials of pediatric nursing, ed. 8*, St. Louis, 2009, Mosby. Used with permission. Copyright Mosby, Inc.)

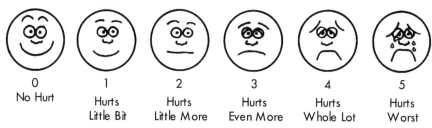

0	1	2	3	4	5
No Hurt	Hurts Little Bit	Hurts Little More	Hurts Even More	Hurts Whole Lot	Hurts Worst

Figure 41.2. Wong-Baker FACES Pain Rating Scale (From Hockenberry MJ, Wilson D: Wong's essentials of pediatric nursing, ed. 8, St. Louis, 2009, Mosby. Used with permission. Copyright Mosby, Inc.)

CRIES Pain Scale

Indications: For neonates (0–6 months)

Instructions: Each of the five (5) categories is scored from 0–2, which results in a total score between 0 and 10. The interdisciplinary team in collaboration with the patient/family (if appropriate), can determine appropriate interventions in response to CRIES Scale scores.

Crying: Characteristic cry of pain is high pitched.

0. No cry or cry that is not high-pitched

1. Cry high pitched but baby is easily consolable

2. Cry high pitched but baby is inconsolable

Requires O2 for SaO2 < 95%: Babies experiencing pain manifest decreased oxygenation. Consider other causes of hypoxemia, for example, oversedation, atelectasis, pneumothorax)

0. No oxygen required

1. < 30% oxygen required

2. > 30% oxygen required

Increased vital signs (BP and HR): Take blood pressure (BP) last as this may awaken child making other assessments difficult. Use baseline preoperative parameters from a non-stressed period. Multiply baseline heart rate (HR) by 0.2 then add to baseline HR to determine the HR that is 20% over baseline. Do the same for BP and use the mean BP.

0. Both HR and BP unchanged or less than baseline

1. HR or BP increased but increase in < 20% of baseline

2. HR or BP is increased > 20% over baseline.

Expression: The facial expression most often associated with pain is a grimace. A grimace may be characterized by brow lowering, eyes squeezed shut, deepening naso-labial furrow, or open lips and mouth.

0. No grimace present

1. Grimace alone is present

2. Grimace and non-cry vocalization grunt is present

Sleepless: Scored based upon the infant's state during the hour preceding this recorded score.

0. Child has been continuously asleep

1. Child has awakened at frequent intervals

2. Child has been awake constantly

Total Score: _____

Reference: Krechel, SW & Bildner, J. (1995). CRIES: a new neonatal postoperative pain measurement score – initial testing of validity and reliability. Paediatric Anaesthesia, 5: 53-61. Copyright © S. Krechel, M.D. and J. Bildner, RNC, MC-CNS. . Reprinted with permission.

FLACC Scale

Indications: Infants and children (2 months–7 years) unable to validate the presence of or quantify the severity of pain.

Instructions:

1. Each of the five (5) categories is scored from 0–2, which results in a total score between 0 and 10:

- (F) Faces
- (L) Legs
- (A) Activity
- (C) Cry
- (C) Consolability

2. The interdisciplinary team in collaboration with the patient/family (if appropriate), can assess the patient for distressed behaviors and determine appropriate interventions in response to FLACC Scale scores.

Face:

0. No particular expression or smile

1. Occasional grimace or frown, withdrawn, disinterested

2. Frequent to constant quivering chin, clenched jaw

Legs:

0. Normal position or relaxed

1. Uneasy, restless, tense

2. Kicking, or legs drawn up

Activity:

0. Lying quietly, normal position, moves easily

1. Squirming, shifting back and forth, tense

2. Arched, rigid, or jerking

Cry:

0. No cry (awake or asleep)

1. Moans or whimpers; occasional complaint

2. Crying steadily, screams or sobs, frequent complaints

Consolability:

0. Content, relaxed

1. Reassured by occasional touching, hugging or being talked to, distractible

2. Difficult to console or comfort

Total Score: _____

Reference: Merkel, SI, Voepel-Lewis, T., Shayevitz, JR, and Malviya, S. (1997). The FLACC: a behavioral scale for scoring postoperative pain in young children. *Pediatric Nursing*, 23(3): 293–297. © 2002 The Regents of the University of Michigan. Reprinted with permission.

Editor's Note

While various pain rating scales are frequently used in pain assessments, many experts feel that these scales are less useful in chronic pain than in acute pain. People with chronic pain frequently rate their pain at the upper end of the scale, but these ratings may not accurately reflect their ability to function. This does not necessarily mean that they are not accurately reporting how they feel; rather, chronic pain is a more complex problem, and is not simply "acute pain that doesn't go away."

For acute pain, such as after an injury or fracture, rating scales may be quite useful in guiding treatment. Chronic pain has more complex dimensions, and a focus on how the pain impacts day-to-day life is often more informative than "my pain is X out of 10."

Section 41.2

X-Rays

Printed with permission from: NASS Patient Education
Committee. *Radiographic Assessment for Back Pain.* © 2003–
2012 North American Spine Society. Available at: http://www
.knowyourback.org.

What Are Radiographic Assessments?

Radiographic assessments for low back pain involve the use of x-rays to determine the cause of the pain or discomfort. Usually, x-rays are ordered by your physician in cases in which he or she suspects congenital defects, degenerative disease, trauma, metastatic cancer, or bone deformity as a cause of lower back pain.

When Should I Get an X-Ray for Low Back Pain?

Most cases of back pain tend to get better without major medical intervention in six to eight weeks after the onset of the pain. Therefore, x-rays are usually not recommended until after back pain has been present for at least that long unless your physician suspects a problem such as spondylolisthesis or fracture may be present.

If you have had lower back pain for only six to eight weeks, have treated it with rest, mild exercise, or analgesic or antiinflammatory medications, and are seeing an improvement in your condition or are able to perform more activities, you probably do not need an x-ray.

Also, if you have had an x-ray of your back in the past two years that did not find any significant structure-related cause for your pain, your doctor may not recommended you have another x-ray unless you have had a new injury or illness.

However, there are some cases that may require x-ray assessment immediately such as when there is numbness or loss of feeling in the legs or feet, weakness, problems with urination or pain that becomes worse as time goes on.

Other Reasons for Having an X-Ray

Other factors may cause your doctor to order an x-ray assessment for low back pain prior to the six-to-eight-week point. They include:

- if you are over the age of 65, under the age of 18, or are a student athlete,

- if you have a history of osteoporosis,

- if you have a history of cancer,

- if your pain is intense while you are at rest or if it increases at night,

- if you are experiencing fever and chills along with your pain,

- if you have had a sudden and unexplained loss of weight accompanying your back pain,

- if you have experienced an injury or have been subjected to a repeated stress that may have caused a fracture in one of the bones of your spine,

- or if you have had a previous surgery or fracture in the lower back.

What Types of X-Ray Are Used?

Usually, most physicians will order anteroposterior (called AP) and/ or lateral view x-rays for low back pain. The AP view is a front-to-back image taken when you are facing the x-ray machine. Lateral views are the side-to-side images taken while you are standing sideways from the x-ray camera. Less often, the physician will request an oblique x-ray, which provides a view from an angle.

In order to get a true picture of your spine, your physician may order weight-bearing images. These are x-rays that are taken while you are standing up rather than lying down. By having the x-rays taken while you are standing, your doctor can get a better picture of the forces that affect your spine that may cause pain. Additionally, in some cases your physician may order x-rays taken while you are stretching or bending to better determine the cause of your pain. Lateral flexion and extension (bending forward and backward) x-rays may be taken to assess the degree of motion between the vertebrae.

How Effective Are X-Rays?

X-ray examination can be a useful screening tool to assess any bone abnormality of the spine. It can also complement findings from other tests such as magnetic resonance imaging (MRI) and computerized tomography (CT) scans.

Significant findings on x-rays may determine the need for additional studies and may indicate which type of test would be indicated.

As with any medical procedure, you should be fully informed on the reasons behind, and the expected results of, any test your physician prescribes for you.

Section 41.3

Magnetic Resonance Imaging

Printed with permission from: NASS Patient Education Committee. *Magnetic Resonance Imaging.* © 2002–2012 North American Spine Society. Available at: http://www.knowyourback.org.

What Is Magnetic Resonance Imaging (MRI)?

Magnetic resonance imaging (MRI) is a valuable diagnostic study that has been used by health care providers since the 1980s. MRI is a noninvasive, nonradioactive, and pain-free method of evaluating the human body. An MRI typically is ordered as part of a medical evaluation and uses strong magnets and radio waves that are evaluated using computer technology to view three-dimensional images of the body.

During MRI, radio waves are released in pulses through your body, causing movement or "excitement" in hydrogen atoms in your cells. When the radio waves stop, the hydrogen atoms relax and release energy. Different parts of the body, such as soft tissue and bones, have characteristic patterns of how they are affected by the radio waves; these patterns are displayed on a computer monitor as pictures of the anatomy of the body. A specially trained radiologist reads these images, which are presented in visual sections or slices, to help determine the cause of your pain.

MRIs are easily obtained, risk-free to most people and can usually be performed without any special preparation (such as having to drink or be injected with contrast materials or radioactive dye.) Occasionally, your doctor will order a study that requires the injection of a special drug that provides greater detail in the images.

Do I Need an MRI?

When you go to your health care provider for neck or back pain or radicular pain (pain that radiates from the neck into the arm or lower spine into the leg), it is important to determine the source of your pain. There are many possible causes.

In many cases, neck, back, and radicular pain may subside in a month or two with proper treatment. However, if the pain continues more than six or seven weeks, gets worse before that time, or if significant weakness or numbness develops, MRI is a tool that can be used by your health care provider to help pinpoint the cause and assist in choosing an appropriate treatment plan.

In some cases, neck, back, or radicular pain may indicate a serious medical condition. Therefore, it is very important that the cause is identified and addressed early.

Which Spine Problems Can Be Detected By MRI?

The usual causes of low back and radicular pain are degeneration of the spine or a disc herniation. These can also be factors in neck pain. MRI can provide information on the condition of the vertebrae, the spinal canal and the intervertebral discs (the shock-absorbing connective tissue between the vertebrae.) Scientific studies have shown that MRI is a good examination tool to provide this type of information, usually in a noninvasive manner. (Myelogram can also be an accurate test, but requires an injection.) However, keep in mind that abnormalities that show up on MRI can also be found in patients without any symptoms. Therefore, it is essential that the findings on MRI are considered together with a detailed history and physical examination.

Disc Degeneration and Herniation

MRI can determine the physical changes that occur in a disc, including the development of a herniation or bulge that can lead to neck or back pain or the development of radicular pain and tingling or numbness. Your health care provider can use the information from the MRI to determine the location and type of disc damage or herniation that may have occurred and prescribe the proper treatment.

Sometimes disc degeneration can cause pain by allowing normal everyday forces (stress and strain) to be transferred to other areas of the spine, such as to the facet joints that connect the vertebrae. MRI can reveal when these stresses have been strong enough to cause changes in the facet joints or a narrowing of the spinal canal.

Recurrent Disc Herniation

For certain tests, MRI can be used in conjunction with intravenous contrast materials to determine the cause of radiating back pain, especially following spinal surgery. MRI enhanced with gadolinium can be very effective for determining whether back pain following spine surgery is the result of a buildup of scar tissue or a reherniation of the disc—a problem that was once very difficult to verify.

Gadolinium-enhanced MRI is a technology in which the patient is injected with gadolinium, a naturally occurring metallic element that has special magnetic properties, during the procedure. This procedure usually involves two MRIs. The first is performed before the injection of gadolinium. After the initial, or baseline, MRI, the patient is injected with gadolinium. Within ten minutes of the injection, a second MRI is taken of the same area. The gadolinium will enter the scar tissue faster than the disc material or bone because scar tissue often has a greater blood supply than normal tissue. The special magnetic properties of gadolinium make scar tissue easier for the radiologist to detect, enabling him or her to tell if scar tissue or disc reherniation may be causing pain.

Spinal Stenosis

The spinal canal runs through the vertebrae from top (base of the skull) to bottom (the tailbone) and provides a passageway for the nerves running to the lower extremities. A narrowing of the spinal canal is called spinal stenosis, which can cause neck or leg pain, weakness of the arm or leg muscles and/or numbness in the arms or legs. MRI can be very effective in viewing the spinal canal from different angles, called planes, which gives your health care provider valuable structural information to confirm the diagnosis as well as aid in planning operative or nonoperative treatment.

Compression Fractures

Compression fractures are fractures of the vertebrae in which the anterior (front) part of the vertebrae compresses or wedges under the posterior (back) part. This fracture causes the vertebrae to become taller in back than in front. In some situations, it is difficult for the health care provider to determine whether a compression fracture of the vertebrae is new and if it has been caused by osteoporosis, tumor, infection or other reason. MRI can be helpful in determining the cause of these fractures, which can be very important since the recommended treatment will be different depending upon the source of the fracture.

Other Uses

MRI is also a sensitive tool for the detection of spinal infection. Studies have found MRI to be 94% accurate in the detection of osteomyelitis (infection of the bones, including those of the spine.) The results of MRI for the detection of bone infection are similar to other studies such as bone scans and gallium studies. The benefit of the MRI over those two types of studies is that you do not have to undergo the injection of radioactive isotopes.

MRI can also show evidence of infection of the intervertebral discs and other soft tissue structures of the spine and can be used to detect tumors.

How Is MRI Performed?

An MRI evaluation usually takes from 15 minutes to one hour to complete. It requires little effort from you, except to be as motionless as possible for the duration of the examination. This requirement, however, does make it difficult for those in serious pain and those who are disoriented or mentally impaired.

Technologic advances have led to many changes in the size and structure of MRI diagnostic machines. Older MRI machines consist of an elongated tube, which the patient passes through while laying on his or her back on a sliding platform. With this type of machine, there are limitations for people who are very overweight (over 350 lbs.), very young or with claustrophobia.

Newer, "open" MRI machines have more space between the magnets to allow the patient to lay flat on a table without passing through a narrow tube and provide the patient with a less constricted environment. These machines are better suited to handle patients up to 500 lbs., young children (especially children with special needs) and people with a fear of tight spaces. However, there is some debate about the effectiveness of the open MRI. Because these types of machines use a lower strength magnetic field, the images may not be as detailed as the traditional, tube-type MRI.

After the Procedure

One of the advantages of an MRI is there is usually not much preparation needed before the test. Unless you are undergoing a test that requires the injection of a contrast (such as gadolinium), there is no need to fast or restrict fluid intake prior to an MRI.

You may want to wear loose-fitting, comfortable clothing that has no metal buttons or zippers. You will be asked about any metal-containing devices in your body and will also be asked to remove any eyeglasses, jewelry, coins from your pocket, or clothing containing metallic zippers before the procedure.

Who Should Not Get an MRI?

Since the MRI is magnetically generated, they are not indicated for use in the presence of certain medical implants. People with ferromagnetic cerebral aneurysm clips, cardiac pacemakers, metal foreign bodies in their eyes, and metal cochlear implants are not suggested to have MRI. Likewise, women who are pregnant (especially those in the first trimester), people with electrical nerve stimulators, and those with severe claustrophobia are also advised against MRI.

Titanium implants are MRI compatible. People with nontitanium implants should inform the radiologist or technician prior to the procedure; however, most joint implants are firmly attached inside bone and will not pose a serious problem. People with internal metallic surgical staples from healed surgeries should also inform the radiologist or technician prior to the procedure.

People with long bone or pelvic external fixation devices or with retained bullet fragments should consult a medical expert on the use of MRI.

Although metallic instrumentation in the spine, such as pedicle screw instrumentation for spinal fusion, is not specified as a contraindication to MRI evaluation, it can obscure the results of the evaluation and therefore sometimes are not used in this group of patients who require further diagnostic testing.

Section 41.4

Electromyograms and Nerve Conduction Studies

Printed with permission from: NASS Patient Education Committee. *Electrodiagnostic Testing.* © 2003-2012 North American Spine Society. Available at: http://www.knowyourback.org.

What Is Electrodiagnostic Testing?

The term "electrodiagnostic testing" covers a whole spectrum of specialized tests, two of which are the electromyogram and the nerve conduction study. Many problems involving nerves or muscles require electrodiagnostic testing to provide information. Although they are different tests, the electromyogram and the nerve conduction study go hand in hand to give vital information regarding your nerve and muscle function.

What is an electromyogram (EMG)?

An electromyogram (EMG) is a diagnostic study that has been used by health care providers for over 50 years. An EMG provides information about the function of the muscles and the nerves in your body. An EMG examination is typically ordered by a physician to evaluate for muscle or nerve damage as part of a medical workup.

Using a specialized computer, the examiner actually sees and hears how your muscles and nerves are working. A very small needle is inserted into various muscles in the arm, leg, neck or back, depending on your symptoms. In many cases the examination will include areas away from where you are having symptoms because nerves can be very long. There is virtually no chance to catch any diseases from having an EMG because only new, sterile needles are used. An EMG is only one part of nerve testing; the other part is called the nerve conduction study.

What is a nerve conduction study (NCS)?

Like an EMG, a NCS is typically ordered by a physician to evaluate for muscle or nerve damage as part of a medical workup. The examiner places small electrodes on your skin over muscles being tested in your arms or legs. The examiner then uses a stimulator to deliver a very small electrical current to your skin near nerves being tested, causing your nerves to fire. The electrical signals produced by nerves and muscles are picked up by the computer, and the information is interpreted by a physician specially trained in electrodiagnostic medicine. The stimulator only produces a very small shock that does not cause damage to your body. Many different motor and sensory nerves are typically evaluated.

Do I Need an EMG/NCS?

When you go to your health care provider with symptoms including radicular pain (nerve pain radiating from the neck or back), numbness, weakness or tingling in an arm or leg, it is important to find out what is causing your symptoms. There are many possible causes for the above symptoms, and many cases resolve spontaneously on their own. However, if symptoms persist, an EMG/NCS is one way to assess muscle and nerve function and is often used with other tests such as MRI or CT scan that create images of the body.

What Can EMG/NCS Detect?

The EMG/NCS examines nerves from just outside the spinal cord to the skin. Nerves have long projections called axons that carry electrical signals. Axons are surrounded by supporting cells called Schwann cells, which produce myelin. Myelin acts like an insulator for the axons and makes nerve signals travel faster.

In addition, because nerves go into muscles and give signals to muscles causing muscle contraction, the EMG/NCS also tests muscles. Abnormalities with the peripheral nervous system (all nerve tissue outside the brain and spinal cord), including the insulating myelin and muscles, can all be evaluated with EMG/NCS. While EMG/NCS can detect many different problems with nerves or muscles, some of the more common are covered below.

Cervical or Lumbar Radiculopathy

A radiculopathy is the term used for nerve pain radiating from the neck (cervical) or low back (lumbar). There are many causes for radiculopathy; one is herniated discs. The intervertebral discs are one of the weight bearing structures in the neck and back. These discs can become degenerated and can herniate, pressing on nearby nerves and causing the radiating pain. An EMG/NCS can evaluate the severity of the nerve damage due to disc herniations.

Peripheral Neuropathy

Many common medical conditions like diabetes can cause nerve damage. In such cases, the longest nerves are usually affected first; hence the name peripheral neuropathy. Whether the diabetes is controlled with diet, oral or injectable medications, there is often nerve damage. An EMG/NCS can evaluate the severity and monitor any progression of a peripheral neuropathy.

Myopathy

A myopathy is a disease that is localized to the muscle and muscle supporting structures. Myopathies are hereditary (inherited from a mother or father) or acquired (from infection or underlying medical condition). A patient will usually present with proximal muscle weakness and perhaps myalgias (muscle aches). An EMG/NCS can localize the disease process in such cases and aid diagnosis.

Focal Neuropathies

A focal neuropathy is when a single nerve suffers damage at a specific site along the its course. There are an infinite number of possible focal neuropathies in the body, but the most common example is carpal tunnel syndrome. Carpal tunnel syndrome is when the nerve to the hand is squeezed at the wrist causing numbness, tingling and pain. An EMG/NCS evaluates the severity and location of such focal neuropathies.

How Should I Prepare for an EMG/NCS?

After showering on the day of your examination, do not use any creams, moisturizers or powders on your skin. If you have any bleeding disorders, let the examining physician know prior to testing. If you take blood thinners, even any aspirin or aspirin like medications let the examining physician know. You may be asked to stop blood thinners and aspirin products prior to your examination. If you have a pacemaker or other devices that are implanted in your body to deliver medications, let the examining physician know. Any history of back or neck surgery should be discussed with the examining physician, as the examination may need to be modified. Also, any recent fevers or chills may indicate current bodily infection and should be mentioned to the examining physician.

What Can I Expect on the Day of the Test?

As mentioned earlier, the electrodiagnostic testing usually includes both electromyogram (EMG) and nerve conduction studies (NCS). The EMG section includes a small sterilized needle being inserted in the muscles to be tested. There is some discomfort with needle insertion, but most tolerate the testing without difficulty. You may notice some bruising after the needle portion of the examination. Icing sore areas can help with discomfort and limit the bruising. Any time the skin is penetrated with a needle, there is a theoretical risk of infection developing.

The NCS portion of the examination includes a small stimulus applied near nerves to make them fire. In most cases a series of shocks are necessary to get the optimal response. Any discomfort is temporary, and the stimulus is not strong enough to cause damage to the body.

When Are the Results Ready?

After EMG/NCS testing, the examining physician must analyze the data and combine all the information into a report. The electrodiagnostic examination report will be added to your medical record and a copy sent to the referring physician. The time for report generation varies from lab to lab, but generally is no more than a few days. Be sure to follow up with your health care provider.

Chapter 42

Conventional and Integrative Approaches to Pain Management

Chapter Contents

Section 42.1—Pain Treatment Plans 474

Section 42.2—Pain Management Therapies 476

Section 42.3—Rehabilitation Approaches to Pain
Management 485

473

Section 42.1

Pain Treatment Plans

Excerpted from "Frequently Asked Questions," reprinted with permission from www.StopPain.org, the website of the Department of Pain Medicine and Palliative Care at Beth Israel Medical Center, New York, New York. © Continuum Health Partners, Inc., reviewed 2013.

Can Pain Be Treated?

Yes. Pain can be treated safely and effectively. There are many types of treatments for pain, including medication and non-drug treatments. It is important to treat pain. Unrelieved pain brings unnecessary suffering. Living with pain uses up a lot of energy that can be better used to fight illness or maintain activities of daily living. Pain may cause patients to:

- feel weak because of disruptions in activity, appetite, and sleep
- give up hope
- reject treatment programs
- feel helpless, anxious, and depressed
- think about suicide
- stop enjoying normal activities, such as work, recreation, and relations with others

If you are in pain, don't give up! Working with your doctor and other professionals, you can manage your pain. Sometimes pain relief can be obtained right away. In other situations, it takes time for treatment to be tailored to fit the individual and his/her unique condition.

How Can Pain Be Treated?

Pain treatment needs to be tailored to the individual. What works for one person may not work for the next. Pain can be treated through the use of:

- **Drug therapies:** Acetaminophen and nonsteroidal anti-inflammatory drugs (NSAIDs), such as aspirin, ibuprofen, naproxen, and others; opioids (also called narcotics); so-called adjuvant analgesics, which are drugs that are used primarily to treat conditions other than pain but can relieve some painful conditions. Adjuvant drugs include antidepressants, anticonvulsants, local anesthetics, and others.

- **Rehabilitation therapies:** Physical therapy, occupational therapy, treatments such as heat, cold, ultrasound, and others.

- **Psychological therapies:** Cognitive approaches, such as relaxation training, distraction techniques, hypnosis, biofeedback, and other behavioral approaches; other types of psychotherapy.

- **Anesthetic therapies:** Nerve blocks, drug infusion into the spine, spinal cord stimulation.

- **Neurostimulatory procedures:** Transcutaneous electrical nerve stimulation (TENS), acupuncture, invasive stimulatory therapies (spinal cord and brain).

- **Surgical approaches**

- **Alternative or complementary approaches**

Treatment Plans for the Elderly

The elderly are more likely to experience pain than the general population and are often undertreated for pain due to myths about their pain sensitivity, pain tolerance, and ability to benefit from opioid drugs.

If you are an older person experiencing pain, you should take the following factors into account:

- You may experience more than one source of pain;

- You may have several medical problems and be taking a number of medications at once, and this may increase the risk of analgesic drugs;

- You run a higher-than-average risk of side effects from all drugs, including analgesics like nonsteroidal anti-inflammatory drugs. It is important to report the over-the-counter pain medications you take to your health care team;

- Having chronic medical problems and an increased risk of side effects does not mean than your pain cannot, or should not, be aggressively treated. You may be a candidate for any of the many pain-relieving therapies that exist.

Treatment Plans for Children

Pain management for children should:

- Be tailored to the child's level of development, including his/her verbal skills, ability to separate from parents, and understanding of medical procedures;

- Take advantage of the child's personality and draw on his/her emotional and physical resources wherever possible;

- Respond to issues the child's pain is causing in the family.

Section 42.2

Pain Management Therapies

Excerpted from "Pain," reprinted with permission from www .StopPain.org, the website of the Department of Pain Medicine and Palliative Care at Beth Israel Medical Center, New York, New York. © Continuum Health Partners, Inc., reviewed 2013.

Treatments that can successfully control pain include:

Pharmacological Therapies (Medication)

- Non-opioid pain relievers
- Opioids
- Adjuvant medications (drugs whose primary purpose is not for pain but rather for other conditions)
- Topical treatments (drugs are applied directly to the skin, as a patch, gel, or cream)

Because the effects of a medication can vary widely from person to person, treatment of pain needs to be tailored to fit each individual. Some patients may need to try many different kinds of treatments before they find the right balance between pain relief and side effects.

Patients should be sure their doctors are aware of all medications they are taking, even for conditions unrelated to their pain or over-the-counter drugs such as aspirin. Many medications should not be taken together because they increase or decrease each other's effects or produce new adverse reactions. Of course, the doctor should also be informed if the patient is pregnant or breast-feeding.

Non-Pharmacological Treatments

Non-pharmacological treatments (treatments that do not rely primarily on medication to achieve their effect) offer a variety of approaches to pain relief. Most are non-invasive.

Simple, relatively safe non-pharmacological approaches include:

* Physiatric approaches

* Non-invasive stimulatory approaches

* Psychological approaches

* Complementary/alternative approaches

In most cases, these techniques should be used in addition to, not instead of, other approaches to pain relief.

More invasive non-pharmacological treatments include:

* Anesthesiologic approaches

* Invasive stimulatory approaches

* Surgical approaches

Physiatric Approaches

Therapeutic Exercise

Exercising is important because it can:

* Strengthen weak muscles

* Mobilize stiff joints

* Help restore coordination and balance

* Promote a sense of well-being

* Decrease anxiety and stress

* Keep the heart healthy

• Help maintain an appropriate weight

A physical therapist, exercise physiologist, or certified athletic trainer can help patients get started safely and learn exercises designed specifically to target problem areas. Even bedridden patients can benefit from range-of-motion exercises.

Heat Therapy

Heat therapy can reduce pain, especially the pain of muscle tension or spasm. Sometimes patients with other types of pain benefit. Heat therapy acts to:

• Increase the blood flow to the skin

• Dilate blood vessels, increasing oxygen and nutrient delivery to local tissues

• Decrease joint stiffness by increasing muscle elasticity

Heat should be applied for 20 minutes. Patients can use hot packs, hot water bottles, hot and moist compresses, electric heating pads, or chemical and gel packs carefully wrapped to avoid burns. Patients can also submerge themselves or the painful part in warm water.

Heat therapy is not recommended on tissue that has received radiation treatment. Pregnant women should avoid using hot tubs or any method that subjects the developing baby to prolonged heat.

Deep heat delivered to underlying tissue by short wave diathermy, microwave diathermy, or ultrasound is also sometimes used to relieve pain. Deep heat should be used with caution by patients with active cancer and should not be applied directly over a cancer site.

Cold Therapy

Cold therapy, which constricts blood vessels near the skin, sometimes can relieve the pain of muscle tension or spasm. Other types of pain also benefit in some cases. It can also reduce swelling if applied soon after an injury.

Ice packs, towels soaked in ice water, or commercially-prepared chemical gel packs should be applied for 15 minutes. Cold sources should be sealed to prevent dripping, flexible to conform to the body, and adequately wrapped to prevent irritation or damage to the skin.

Non-Invasive Stimulatory Approaches

Transcutaneous Electrical Nerve Stimulation (TENS)

Transcutaneous electrical nerve stimulation (TENS) is a method of applying a gentle electric current to the skin to relieve pain. Studies have shown that it can be effective in certain cases of chronic pain.

A small box-shaped device, which patients can put in their pocket or hang on their belt, transmits electrical impulses through wires to electrodes taped to the skin in the painful area. Patients describe the sensation of TENS as buzzing, tingling or tapping.

The patient should experiment with the placement of the electrodes and the timing, intensity, amplitude, and frequency of the electrical current to find the most effective setting. Pain relief usually lasts beyond the period when current is applied. TENS can become less effective at relieving pain over time.

TENS is usually safe and well tolerated. However, it is not recommended on inflamed, infected, or otherwise unhealthy skin, over a pregnant uterus (except for obstetric pain relief), or in the presence of a cardiac pacemaker.

Psychoeducational Approaches

Cognitive Behavioral Techniques

Cognitive behavioral techniques are used to reduce the body's unproductive responses to stress, helping to relieve pain, or improve the ability to tolerate it. Some techniques are:

Deep breathing: In this simple technique, the patient focuses his or her attention on breathing deeply. This may shift attention away from the source of pain.

Progressive muscle relaxation: In this technique, developed in the 1930s, patients contract, then relax, muscles throughout the body, group by group. Progressive muscle relaxation can help patients learn about the tension in their body and the contrast between tense and relaxed muscles.

Imagery: In this technique, patients focus on pleasant thoughts, for example waves gently hitting a sandy beach. One variation is to think of an image that represents the pain (such as a hot, blazing concrete sidewalk), then imagine it changing into an image representing a pain-free state (a pretty, snow-covered forest).

Meditation: In this technique, practiced routinely in Asia, the individual aims to empty his or her mind of thoughts, focusing instead on the sensation of breathing and the rhythms of his or her body.

Biofeedback therapy: Biofeedback is a method in which people learn to reduce their body's unproductive responses to stress, and thus decrease their sensitivity to pain. Children are particularly quick to learn from biofeedback. In biofeedback, electrodes are placed at various points on the patient's skin to measure:

- Muscle tension. As a muscle contracts, electrical activity increases
- Temperature. The stress response is related to blood flow in the hands or feet, and blood flow determines temperature
- Heart beat
- Sweating

Patients watch the monitor and listen to the tones measuring their stress indicators. They use these as a guide in learning to release tension throughout their body.

Distraction: Distraction is a pain management technique in which patients focus their attention on something other than their pain and negative emotions. To distract themselves, patients can: sing, count, listen to music, watch TV, listen to the radio, talk to friends or family, read, or listen to stories being read.

Reframing: Reframing is a pain and stress management technique that teaches patients to monitor negative thoughts and images and replace them with positive ones.

Patients can learn to have a more positive outlook by recognizing some counterproductive thought patterns, such as:

- Blaming, in which the individual avoids taking responsibility. Thoughts such as "It's my boss's fault I have this headache" can be replaced with "I'm going to focus on what I can do to feel better."

- "Should" or "must" statements, which imply that someone has failed to live up to an arbitrary standard. Statements such as "I should have been more careful" can be counteracted with "I do not have to be perfect" or "I made the best decision I could have at the time."

- Polarized thinking, in which everything is black or white, with no shades of gray. Statements such as "I'm still in pain, so this program is useless" can be counteracted with "I wish I could be

480

free of pain, but I have made some progress. Sometimes small improvements add up."

- Catastrophizing, in which the person imagines the worst possible scenario then acts as if it will surely come true. Statements such as "This pain must mean I am going downhill" can be counteracted with "I am jumping to conclusions" or "I'll find a way to cope with whatever happens."

- Control fallacy, in which the person sees him or herself as completely controlled by others (or controlling everything). Thoughts such as "My spouse doesn't think I need to see a counselor, so I can't go" can be counteracted with "I am not a helpless victim" (or thoughts such as "My family will fall apart without me" can be counteracted with "Members of my family are not helpless").

- Emotional reasoning, in which the individual believes that what he or she feels must be true. Statements such as "I'm so frightened the pain will never stop, I know it never will" can be counteracted with "I'm scared, but that does not give me an accurate view of the situation" or "When I calm down, I will think about what this means."

- Filtering, in which people focus on one thing (such as pain) to the exclusion of any other experience or point of view. Statements such as "I can't take it" can be replaced with "I have coped before and can cope again."

- Entitlement fallacy, in which individuals believe they have the right to what they want. Statements such as "Life is so unfair" or "I have been cheated" can be counteracted with "No one promised me a rose garden. I will focus on finding ways to make things better."

Psychotherapy and Social Support

Psychotherapy and social support can help a patient cope with pain. Psychotherapy may be useful for anyone whose pain is difficult to manage, who has developed clinical depression or anxiety or who has a history of psychiatric illness.

Among the goals of psychotherapy are the following:

- Emphasize the patient's past strengths

- Support the patient's use of previously successful coping strategies

- Teach new coping skills

- Establish a bond to decrease a patient's sense of isolation

- Foster a sense of self-worth

Psychological Approaches

- Group Approaches: Peer groups, in which a patient meets with others with the same condition, can help by:
- Providing support
- Showing the patient how others have coped effectively
- Helping the patient maintain a social identity
- Providing access to information and material aid

Spiritual leaders are another potential source of support for patients.

Complementary/Alternative Approaches

Acupuncture

Acupuncture is an ancient method for relieving pain and controlling disease, used in China for thousands of years. It appears to be effective for some patients with chronic pain.

Thin gold or metal needles, gently twirled for ten to twenty minutes, can be used to stimulate acupuncture points, which relieve pain in specific parts of the body (for example, a point on the leg targets stomach pain). Patients usually feel a tingling, warm sensation, similar to that of transcutaneous electrical nerve stimulation. Acupuncture points can also be stimulated with deep massage (acupressure), electric currents (electroacupuncture), or lasers.

The risk of side effects is low. Side effects can include post-needling pain, bleeding, bruising, dizziness, fainting, and local skin reactions. Rarely, organ damage can occur with deep needling techniques. Infection because of inadequately sterilized needles is a hazard; disposable needles are recommended.

Acupuncture is not recommended for patients with serious blood clotting problems. Acupuncture should be used with caution by pregnant women.

Massage

Massage can be a useful addition to a pain management program, especially for patients who are bedridden.

Massage can:

- Stimulate blood flow

- Relax muscles that are tight or in spasm
- Promote a feeling of well-being

Muscles can be stroked, kneaded or rubbed in a circular motion. A lotion can reduce friction on the skin.

Massage is not recommended in cases of swollen tissue. It should be used in addition to, and not instead of, exercise by patients who can walk.

Anesthesiologic Approaches

For patients with pain who fail conservative therapies, simple to complex interventional therapies such as nerve blocks, epidural steroid injections, intraspinal drug administration, or trigger point injections may be helpful. These therapies are typically provided by anesthesiologists with advanced training in pain management.

Nerve Blocks and Epidural Steroid Injections

Nerve blocks can relieve pain by inhibiting the impulses that travel along specific nerves in the body. To achieve a block, the doctor usually injects a local anesthetic along the course of a nerve or nerves. Although this is called a "temporary" block, in the best outcome, pain relief lasts for a long time. In very selected cases, the doctor can inject a solution that damages the nerve and produces a more permanent block.

Sympathetic nerve blocks inhibit the nerves of the sympathetic nervous system, which are responsible for increasing heart rate, constricting blood vessels, and raising blood pressure in response to stress. Sympathetic nerve blocks can be useful in treating some pains due to nerve damage, such as some types of complex regional pain syndrome (also called reflex sympathetic dystrophy or causalgia).

Blocks of somatic nerves can be targeted to any area of the body. In some cases, nerve blocks fail to provide pain relief, or provide only a brief respite.

Epidural steroids, administered through injection, can help to interrupt the passage of painful impulses through nerves.

Spinal Infusion

Intraspinal drug administration involves the delivery of low doses of analgesic drugs, such as morphine or clonidine, through a catheter inserted directly into the spine. This approach is used often to manage cancer pain.

Trigger Point Injections

[Ed. Note: Trigger point injections are another anesthesiologic approach. According to the National Cancer Institute's dictionary (available online at www.cancer.gov/dictionary), "trigger points are places on the body where injury has occurred, but the pain has been sent along nerves and is felt in another place in the body."]

Invasive Stimulatory Approaches

Invasive Nerve Stimulation

Invasive nerve stimulation can provide pain relief for some patients who have not responded to other therapies. In this technique, electrodes are implanted in the patient's body to send a gentle electrical current to nerves in the spinal column or the brain.

Spinal cord stimulation has been used for chronic back and/or leg pain following lumbar surgery, pain due to nerve damage (complex regional pain syndrome and postherpetic neuralgia) and intractable angina. Few controlled studies of this method exist.

Deep brain stimulation may help as many as half of patients with central pain, a challenging condition that can develop as a result of damage to the central nervous system from stroke.

Disadvantages of this therapy include its high cost, risks of an invasive treatment (such as infection), and difficulty predicting before a trial which patients will benefit.

Surgical Approaches

Surgery to treat pain (rather than the underlying disease) is only appropriate in cases where more conservative approaches have failed and where trained neurosurgeons and follow-up care are available.

A surgeon can cut a nerve close to the spinal cord (rhizotomy) or bundles of nerves in the spinal cord (cordotomy) to interrupt the pathways that send pain signals to the brain. In the best possible outcome, surgery relieves pain and the need for most or all pain medication.

However, surgery carries the risk of:

- Stopping the pain only briefly

- Creating new pain from nerve damage at the site of the operation

- Limiting the patient's ability to feel pressure and temperature in the region, putting him or her at risk for injury

Section 42.3

Rehabilitation Approaches to Pain Management

Excerpted from "Rehabilitation Approaches," reprinted with permission from www.StopPain.org, the website of the Department of Pain Medicine and Palliative Care at Beth Israel Medical Center, New York, New York. © Continuum Health Partners, Inc., reviewed 2013.

Physical therapy and occupational therapy may reduce pain and help restore function. Chronic pain sufferers may benefit from a supervised exercise regimen, designed by a physical therapist trained in treating chronic pain, that includes range of motion maneuvers, strengthening techniques, and aerobic conditioning. Heat and cold and other so-called modalities (for example, vibration or ultrasound) also may help alleviate pain, although they should not be applied to areas without sensation or in patients who are unable to communicate. Sources of heat or cold include heating pads, hot-water baths, ice packs, or vapocoolant sprays like ethyl chloride or Fluori-Methane.

Physical Therapy

Physical therapy can be an important part of the treatment strategy. Physical therapy techniques are useful in teaching patients to control pain, to move in safe and structurally correct ways, to improve range of motion, and to increase flexibility, strength and endurance. "Active" and "passive" modalities can both be used, but active modalities, such as therapeutic exercise, are particularly important when the goal is to improve both comfort and function.

Exercise

Exercise can have a variety of benefits. It has been suggested that regular exercise could activate pain control systems in the brain, possibly by affecting endorphin levels, and also improve the functioning of the immune system. Although these benefits are uncertain, a very large clinical experience indicates that patients can benefit from exercise in terms of better stamina and function. Exercise may reduce the risk of secondary pain problems like muscle strains, and may also lead to improved confidence and sense of well-being.

A supervised exercise regimen may include range of motion maneuvers, strengthening techniques, and aerobic conditioning. Exercise programs are particularly useful for chronic musculoskeletal pain including back, neck and shoulder pain, rheumatoid and osteoarthritis pain and fibromyalgia.

Thermal Modalities

Thermal modalities include a variety of methods that produce heating and cooling of the tissues to manage acute and chronic musculoskeletal pain. Superficial heat, such as moist hot packs, increases skin and joint temperature and blood flow, and may decrease joint stiffness and muscle spasms. However, the use of superficial heat has not been studied extensively and there is little scientific evidence to support its use in the treatment of pain. In early injury, it may actually increase swelling at the injury site (whereas cold would reduce swelling).

Diathermy involves the use of high-frequency oscillating current and ultrasound (inaudible sound wave vibrations) to create deep heating. The deep heating may reduce the perception of pain. It is believed to promote healing and decrease inflammation. While there has not been a great deal of research on the effectiveness of diathermy and ultrasound for pain relief, it appears that there are short-term beneficial effects with the use of diathermy and significant improvement in pain relief with ultrasound, as with other heating modalities.

Cryotherapy, the use of cold for the treatment of pain, decreases skin and joint temperature and decreases blood flow to the affected area. It has short-term benefits including pain relief and reduction in swelling.

Chapter 43

Complementary and Alternative Medicine (CAM) Therapies for Pain

Chapter Contents

Section 43.1—Chronic Pain and CAM 488

Section 43.2—Acupuncture 492

Section 43.3—Dietary Supplements 496

Section 43.4—Spinal Manipulation 499

Section 43.5—Massage Therapy 501

Section 43.6—Relaxation Techniques 504

Section 43.7—Yoga 507

Section 43.1

Chronic Pain and CAM

Excerpted from "Chronic Pain and CAM: At a Glance," National Center for Complementary and Alternative Medicine, September 2011. The complete text of this document, including references, can be found online at http:// nccam.nih.gov/health/pain/chronic.htm.

Introduction

Pain is one of the most common conditions for which adults use complementary and alternative therapies. Because chronic (long-term) pain can be resistant to many medical treatments and can cause serious problems, people who suffer from chronic pain often turn to complementary and alternative medicine (CAM) for relief. This section provides basic information on chronic pain and "what the science says" about the effectiveness of CAM therapies. If you are considering a CAM therapy for chronic pain, talk with your health care provider first.

About Chronic Pain

Millions of Americans suffer from pain that is chronic, severe, and not easily managed. Pain from arthritis, back problems, other musculoskeletal conditions, and headache costs U.S. businesses more than $61 billion a year in lost worker productivity.

Chronic pain is often defined as any pain lasting more than 12 weeks. Whereas acute pain is a normal sensation, chronic pain is very different. Chronic pain persists—often for months or even longer. (In a national survey, 26 percent of adults—an estimated 76.5 million Americans—reported experiencing pain that lasted more than 24 hours; of those reporting pain, 42 percent said it lasted more than a year.) Chronic pain may arise from an initial injury such as a back sprain, or there may be an ongoing cause such as a disease, or there may be no evident cause. Other health problems—such as fatigue, sleep disturbance, mood changes, and mobility limitations—may also be associated with chronic pain.

Common chronic pain conditions include low-back pain, headache, arthritis pain, pain from nerve damage (for example, diabetic neuropathy), cancer pain, and other conditions, such as fibromyalgia, in which pain is a prominent factor.

A person may have two or more co-existing chronic pain conditions. Such conditions can include chronic fatigue syndrome, endometriosis, fibromyalgia, interstitial cystitis (painful bladder syndrome), irritable bowel syndrome, temporomandibular joint dysfunction, and vulvodynia (chronic vulvar pain). It is not known whether these disorders share a common cause.

People who suffer from chronic pain take various prescription and nonprescription medications; often, these do not provide adequate relief and have unwanted side effects. Other approaches to pain management, such as cognitive behavioral therapy (which emphasizes the role of thought patterns), physical therapy, exercise, and various CAM therapies, are also widely used.

About Scientific Evidence on CAM Therapies

Scientific evidence on CAM therapies includes results from laboratory research (for example, animal studies) as well as clinical trials (studies in people). It encompasses both "positive" findings (evidence that a therapy may work) and "negative" findings (evidence that it probably does not work or that it may be unsafe). Scientific journals publish study results, as well as review articles that evaluate the evidence as it accumulates; fact sheets from the National Center for Complementary and Alternative Medicine (NCCAM) base information about CAM research primarily on the most rigorous review articles, known as systematic reviews and meta-analyses. Authors of such reviews often conclude that more research and/or better designed studies are needed.

A comprehensive description of scientific research on all the CAM therapies that people use for chronic pain is beyond the scope of this text. The rest of this section highlights the research status of some of the therapies used for common kinds of pain.

Low-back pain: Reviews of research on acupuncture, massage, and spinal manipulation for chronic low-back pain have found evidence that these therapies may be beneficial. Clinical practice guidelines issued by the American College of Physicians/American Pain Society in 2007 recommend these therapies and five other nonpharmacologic (nondrug) approaches for patients with back pain who do not improve with medication, education, and self-care (the other recommended approaches are cognitive-behavioral therapy, exercise therapy, progressive relaxation, intensive interdisciplinary rehabilitation, and yoga). Reviews of research on other CAM therapies that people sometimes use for chronic low-back pain, such as various herbal remedies and prolotherapy injections, generally have found limited or no evidence to support their use for this purpose, or the evidence is mixed.

Arthritis: Among CAM approaches that have been studied for pain relief in osteoarthritis are acupuncture, glucosamine/chondroitin, herbal remedies, mineral baths (balneotherapy), and tai chi. Many of these approaches have also been studied for rheumatoid arthritis. Overall, although some studies of CAM practices for arthritis have had promising results, the evidence generally is limited or mixed. A systematic review article on acupuncture for osteoarthritis concluded that acupuncture may lead to small improvements in pain and function. However, in a large clinical study, known as GAIT (Glucosamine/chondroitin Arthritis Intervention Trial), the popular dietary supplements glucosamine and chondroitin sulfate alone or in combination did not significantly relieve knee osteoarthritis pain among all participants, although the combination did help a subgroup who had moderate-to-severe pain. Reviews have found evidence that gamma linolenic acid (GLA, from evening primrose and certain other plant oils) may relieve rheumatoid arthritis pain, although further research is needed. Reviews have also noted evidence that dietary supplements known as ASUs (avocado-soybean unsaponifiables) and devil's claw may provide relief from osteoarthritis pain.

Headache: Reviews of research on acupuncture for reducing the frequency and intensity of migraine and tension-type headaches conclude that patients may benefit from acupuncture therapy. One review found evidence that spinal manipulation may help patients suffering from chronic tension-type or cervicogenic (neck-related) headaches. Some research suggests that the herb feverfew may prevent migraine attacks, but results from clinical trials are mixed, and additional research is needed.

Neck pain: Reviews of research on manual therapies (primarily manipulation or mobilization) and acupuncture for chronic neck pain have found mixed evidence regarding potential benefits and have emphasized the need for additional research. One review noted that clinical guidelines often endorse the use of manual therapies for neck pain, although there is no overall consensus on the status of these therapies.

Other types of pain: Various CAM approaches have also been studied for other types of chronic pain, such as facial pain, including from temporomandibular joint (jaw) disorder; nerve pain associated with diabetes and other conditions; cancer pain; and pain experienced by people with fibromyalgia. For example, a small study found that people with fibromyalgia may benefit from practicing tai chi. In general, research reviews have found some promising evidence of effectiveness for some CAM therapies but often emphasize that additional research is needed before treatment recommendations can be made.

Other CAM approaches: People suffering from various types of chronic pain sometimes turn to other CAM practices, such as hypnotherapy, meditation, or qi gong. Again, reviews of the research on these therapies have found some evidence of effectiveness but note the need for further studies. Although static magnets are widely marketed for pain control, a review of the related research concludes that the evidence does not support this practice.

If You Are Considering CAM for Chronic Pain

- Do not use a CAM therapy as a replacement for conventional care or to postpone seeing a doctor about chronic pain or any other medical problem.

- Learn about the therapy you are considering, especially the scientific evidence on its safety and whether it works.

- Talk with the health care providers you see for chronic pain. Tell them about the therapy you are considering and ask any questions you may have. They may know about the therapy and be able to advise you on its safety, use, and likely effectiveness.

- If you are considering a practitioner-provided CAM therapy such as chiropractic manipulation, massage, or acupuncture, ask a trusted source (such as your doctor or a nearby hospital) to recommend a practitioner. Find out about the training and experience of any practitioner you are considering. Ask whether the practitioner has experience working with your pain condition.

- If you are considering dietary supplements, keep in mind that they can act in the same way as medications. They can cause medical problems if not used correctly, and some may interact with prescription or nonprescription medications or other dietary supplements you take. Your health care provider can advise you. If you are pregnant or nursing a child, or if you are considering giving a child a dietary supplement, it is especially important to consult your health care provider.

• Tell all your health care providers about any complementary and alternative practices you use. Give them a full picture of what you do to manage your health. This will help ensure coordinated and safe care.

Section 43.2

Acupuncture

Excerpted from "Acupuncture for Pain," National Center for Complementary and Alternative Medicine, August 2010. The complete text of this document, including references, can be found online at http://nccam.nih.gov/health/acupuncture/acupuncture-for-pain.htm.

Use of Acupuncture for Pain

Acupuncture, among the oldest healing practices in the world, is part of traditional Chinese medicine. Acupuncture practitioners stimulate specific points on the body—most often by inserting thin needles through the skin. In traditional Chinese medicine theory, this regulates the flow of qi (vital energy) along pathways known as meridians.

According to the 2007 National Health Interview Survey, which included a comprehensive survey of complementary and alternative medicine (CAM) use by Americans, 1.4 percent of respondents (an estimated 3.1 million Americans) said they had used acupuncture in the past year. A special analysis of acupuncture data from an earlier National Health Interview Survey (NHIS) found that pain or musculoskeletal complaints accounted for seven of the top ten conditions for which people use acupuncture. Back pain was the most common, followed by joint pain, neck pain, severe headache/migraine, and recurring pain.

What the Science Says about Acupuncture for Pain

Acupuncture has been studied for a wide range of pain conditions, such as postoperative dental pain, carpal tunnel syndrome, fibromyalgia, headache, low-back pain, menstrual cramps, myofascial pain, osteoarthritis, and tennis elbow.

Overall, it can be very difficult to compare acupuncture research results from study to study and to draw conclusions from the cumulative body of evidence. This is because studies may use different acupuncture techniques (for example, electrical vs. manual), controls (comparison groups), and outcome measures.

One particularly complex factor in acupuncture research is choosing the controls for a clinical trial. The choice depends in part on whether the researchers want to study a particular aspect of acupuncture (for example, effects on the brain) or to determine whether acupuncture is useful compared with other forms of care. Examples of control groups include study participants who receive no acupuncture, simulated acupuncture (procedures that mimic acupuncture, sometimes also referred to as "placebo" or "sham"), or other treatments (in addition to or in place of acupuncture or simulated acupuncture).

An emerging theme in acupuncture research is the role of the placebo. For example, a 2009 systematic review of research on the pain-relieving effects of acupuncture compared with placebo (simulated) or no acupuncture was inconclusive. The reviewers found a small difference between acupuncture and placebo and a moderate difference between placebo and no acupuncture; the effect of placebo acupuncture varied considerably, and the effect of acupuncture appeared unrelated to the specific kind of placebo procedure used. All of the study participants received standard care, typically consisting of analgesic drugs and physical therapy.

The following sections summarize research on acupuncture for a variety of pain conditions, including those reported by NHIS respondents who had used acupuncture. In general, acupuncture appears to be a promising alternative for some of these pain conditions; however, further research is needed.

About Scientific Evidence on CAM Therapies

Carpal tunnel syndrome: Although a 1997 National Institutes of Health (NIH) consensus statement on acupuncture concluded that acupuncture was promising for carpal tunnel syndrome, additional research confirming acupuncture's efficacy for this condition is scant.

Fibromyalgia: Evidence on acupuncture for fibromyalgia is mixed. Some reviews of the scientific literature have found the evidence promising. However, another review that focused on the few rigorous randomized controlled trials on acupuncture as an adjunct therapy for fibromyalgia did not find a benefit. Additionally, a 2003 assessment by the Agency for Healthcare Research and Quality concluded that the evidence was insufficient and the beneficial effects of acupuncture for fibromyalgia could not be determined.

Headache/migraine: Study results on acupuncture for headache are conflicting. Some literature reviews found evidence to support the use of acupuncture for headache, but others noted that most of the studies were of poor quality. A 2008 review of randomized trials on acupuncture highlighted a few well-designed trials whose findings indicate that acupuncture reduces migraine symptoms and is as effective as headache medications. In addition, a 2009 review found that acupuncture may help relieve tension headaches. However, two large trials that looked at acupuncture for migraines found no difference between actual and simulated acupuncture, both of which were equal to conventional care or superior to no treatment.

Low-back pain: According to clinical practice guidelines issued by the American Pain Society and the American College of Physicians in 2007, acupuncture is one of several CAM therapies physicians should consider when patients with chronic low-back pain do not respond to conventional treatment. In early, small studies, combining actual acupuncture with conventional treatment was more effective than conventional treatment alone for relieving chronic low-back pain; but actual acupuncture was not more effective than simulated acupuncture or conventional treatment. However, a large, rigorously designed clinical trial reported in May 2009 found that actual acupuncture and simulated acupuncture were equally effective—and both were more effective than conventional treatment—for relieving chronic low-back pain. There is insufficient evidence to draw definite conclusions about the effectiveness of acupuncture for acute low-back pain.

Menstrual cramps: Two literature reviews have suggested that acupuncture may help with pain from menstrual cramps, but the research is limited.

Myofascial pain: The evidence for acupuncture and myofascial pain (in which pain occurs in sensitive areas, known as trigger points, in the muscles) is mixed. Some literature reviews have found the evidence promising, but another review indicated that "needling therapies" for myofascial trigger point pain were not more effective than placebo.

Neck pain: Studies of acupuncture for chronic neck pain have found that acupuncture provided better pain relief than some simulated treatments. However, the studies varied in terms of design and most had small sample sizes.

494

Osteoarthritis/knee pain: Acupuncture appears to be effective for osteoarthritis, particularly in the area of knee pain. Recent literature reviews have found that acupuncture provides pain relief and improves function for people with osteoarthritis of the knee. However, authors of a 2007 systematic literature review suggested that although some large, high-quality trials have shown that acupuncture may be effective for osteoarthritis of the knee, differences in the design, size, and protocol of the studies make it hard to draw any definite conclusions from the body of research. These authors concluded that it is too soon to recommend acupuncture as a routine part of care for patients with osteoarthritis.

Postoperative dental pain: Although recent data on acupuncture for postoperative dental pain are scant, literature reviews based on earlier evidence have identified acupuncture as a promising treatment for dental pain—especially pain following tooth extraction. For example, a 1999 study of 39 dental surgery patients found that acupuncture was superior to placebo (simulated acupuncture) in preventing postoperative pain. However, a 2005 study of 200 dental surgery patients found no significant analgesic effect for acupuncture compared to simulated acupuncture, although patients who believed they received acupuncture reported significantly less pain than those who believed they received a placebo.

Tennis elbow: Study results on the use of acupuncture for tennis elbow (lateral epicondyle) pain are mixed. An early review of clinical trials reported that data on acupuncture for lateral epicondyle pain were insufficient and of poor quality; however, recent reviews have found the evidence promising, noting strong evidence that acupuncture provides short-term pain relief for lateral epicondyle pain.

Other research: Acupuncture has also been studied for a variety of other pain conditions, including arm and shoulder pain, pregnancy-related pelvic and back pain, and temporomandibular joint (jaw) dysfunction. Although some studies have produced some positive results, more evidence is needed to determine the efficacy of acupuncture for any of these conditions.

There is evidence that people's attitudes about acupuncture can affect outcomes. In a 2007 study, researchers analyzed data from four clinical trials of acupuncture for various types of chronic pain. Participants had been asked whether they expected acupuncture to help their pain. In all four trials, those with positive expectations reported significantly greater pain relief.

In addition to studying acupuncture's efficacy, researchers are looking at potential biomechanisms—that is, how acupuncture might work to relieve pain. There are several theories about these biomechanisms (for example, acupuncture activates opioid systems in the brain that respond to pain); additional research is still needed to test the theories. Researchers are using neuroimaging techniques such as functional magnetic resonance imaging (fMRI) to look at the effects of acupuncture on various regions of the brain.

Side Effects and Risks

Acupuncture is generally considered safe when performed by an experienced practitioner using sterile needles. Relatively few complications from acupuncture have been reported. Serious adverse events related to acupuncture are rare, but include infections and punctured organs. Additionally, there are fewer adverse effects associated with acupuncture than with many standard drug treatments (such as anti-inflammatory medication and steroid injections) used to manage painful musculoskeletal conditions like fibromyalgia, myofascial pain, osteoarthritis, and tennis elbow.

Section 43.3

Dietary Supplements

Excerpted from "Using Dietary Supplements Wisely," National Center for Complementary and Alternative Medicine, March 2010. The complete text of this document, including references, can be found online at http://nccam.nih.gov/health/supplements/wiseuse.htm.

About Dietary Supplements

Dietary supplements were defined in a law passed by Congress in 1994 called the Dietary Supplement Health and Education Act (DSHEA). According to DSHEA, a dietary supplement is a product that is intended to supplement the diet; contains one or more dietary ingredients (including vitamins, minerals, herbs or other botanicals, amino acids, and certain other substances) or their constituents; is intended to be taken by mouth, in forms such as tablet, capsule, powder, softgel, Gelcaps, or liquid; and is labeled as being a dietary supplement.

Herbal supplements are one type of dietary supplement. An herb is a plant or plant part (such as leaves, flowers, or seeds) that is used for its flavor, scent, and/or therapeutic properties. *Botanical* is often used as a synonym for herb. An herbal supplement may contain a single herb or mixtures of herbs.

Research has shown that some uses of dietary supplements are effective in preventing or treating diseases. For example, scientists have found that folic acid (a vitamin) prevents certain birth defects, and a regimen of vitamins and zinc can slow the progression of the age-related eye disease macular degeneration. Also, calcium and vitamin D supplements can be helpful in preventing and treating bone loss and osteoporosis (thinning of bone tissue).

Research has also produced some promising results suggesting that other dietary supplements may be helpful for other health conditions (for example, omega-3 fatty acids for coronary disease), but in most cases, additional research is needed before firm conclusions can be drawn.

The federal government regulates dietary supplements through the U.S. Food and Drug Administration (FDA). The regulations for dietary supplements are not the same as those for prescription or over-the-counter drugs. In general, the regulations for dietary supplements are less strict. A manufacturer does not have to prove the safety and effectiveness of a dietary supplement before it is marketed. A manufacturer is permitted to say that a dietary supplement addresses a nutrient deficiency, supports health, or is linked to a particular body function (for example, immunity), if there is research to support the claim. Such a claim must be followed by the words "This statement has not been evaluated by the U.S. Food and Drug Administration (FDA). This product is not intended to diagnose, treat, cure, or prevent any disease."

Safety Considerations of Dietary Supplements

If you are thinking about or are using a dietary supplement, here are some points to keep in mind.

Tell your health care providers about any complementary and alternative practices you use, including dietary supplements. Give them a full picture of what you do to manage your health. This will help ensure coordinated and safe care. It is especially important to talk to your health care provider if you are thinking about replacing your regular medication with one or more dietary supplements or if you are taking any medications (whether prescription or over-the-counter), as some dietary supplements have been found to interact with medications. If you are planning to have surgery, talk to your doctor before taking any dietary supplements because certain dietary supplements may increase the risk of bleeding or affect the response to anesthesia. Also, be sure to talk to your doctor if you are pregnant or nursing a baby, or are considering giving a child a dietary supplement. Most dietary supplements have not been tested in pregnant women, nursing mothers, or children.

If you are taking a dietary supplement, read the label instructions. Talk to your health care provider if you have any questions, particularly about the best dosage for you to take. If you experience any side effects that concern you, stop taking the dietary supplement, and contact your health care provider. You can also report your experience to the FDA's MedWatch program. Consumer safety reports on dietary supplements are an important source of information for the FDA.

Keep in mind that although many dietary supplements (and some prescription drugs) come from natural sources, "natural" does not always mean "safe." For example, the herbs comfrey and kava can cause serious harm to the liver. Also, a manufacturer's use of the term "standardized" (or "verified" or "certified") does not necessarily guarantee product quality or consistency.

Be aware that an herbal supplement may contain dozens of compounds and that its active ingredients may not be known. Researchers are studying many of these products in an effort to identify active ingredients and understand their effects in the body. Also consider the possibility that what's on the label may not be what's in the bottle. Analyses of dietary supplements sometimes find differences between labeled and actual ingredients.

Section 43.4

Spinal Manipulation

Excerpted from "Spinal Manipulation for Low-Back Pain," National Center for Complementary and Alternative Medicine, April 2012. The complete text of this document, including references, can be found online at http://nccam.nih.gov/health/pain/spinemanipulation.htm.

About Spinal Manipulation

Spinal manipulation—sometimes called spinal manipulative therapy—is practiced by health care professionals such as chiropractors, osteopathic physicians, naturopathic physicians, physical therapists, and some medical doctors. Practitioners perform spinal manipulation by using their hands or a device to apply a controlled force to a joint of the spine. The amount of force applied depends on the form of manipulation used. The goal of the treatment is to relieve pain and improve physical functioning.

Reviews have concluded that spinal manipulation for low-back pain is relatively safe when performed by a trained and licensed practitioner. The most common side effects are generally minor and include feeling tired or temporary soreness.

Reports indicate that cauda equina syndrome (CES), a significant narrowing of the lower part of the spinal canal in which nerves become pinched and may cause pain, weakness, loss of feeling in one or both legs, and bowel or bladder problems, may be an extremely rare complication of spinal manipulation. However, it is unclear if there is actually an association between spinal manipulation and CES, since CES usually occurs without spinal manipulation. In people whose pain is caused by a herniated disc, manipulation of the low back appears to have a very low chance of worsening the herniation.

What the Science Says about Spinal Manipulation for Low-Back Pain

Overall, studies have shown that spinal manipulation is one of several options—including exercise, massage, and physical therapy—that can provide mild-to-moderate relief from low-back pain. Spinal manipulation also appears to work as well as conventional treatments such as applying heat, using a firm mattress, and taking pain-relieving medications.

In 2007 guidelines, the American College of Physicians and the American Pain Society included spinal manipulation as one of several treatment options for practitioners to consider when low-back pain does not improve with self-care. More recently, a 2010 Agency for Healthcare Research and Quality (AHRQ) report noted that complementary health therapies, including spinal manipulation, offer additional options to conventional treatments, which often have limited benefit in managing back and neck pain. The AHRQ analysis also found that spinal manipulation was more effective than placebo and as effective as medication in reducing low-back pain intensity. However, the researchers noted inconsistent results when they compared spinal manipulation with massage or physical therapy to reduce low-back pain intensity or disability.

Researchers are also exploring how spinal manipulation affects the body. In an study funded by the National Center for Complementary and Alternative Medicine (NCCAM) of a small group of people with low-back pain, spinal manipulation affected pain perception in specific ways that other therapies (stationary bicycle and low-back extension exercises) did not.

Managing Low-Back Pain

A review of evidence-based clinical guidelines for managing low-back pain resulted in several recommendations for primary care physicians and pointed to potential benefits of nondrug therapies including spinal manipulation, as well as exercise, massage, and physical therapy:

Acute low-back pain: Routine imaging (x-rays or MRIs) generally is not necessary for patients who have had nonspecific low-back pain for a short time. These patients often improve on their own and usually should remain active, learn about back pain and self-care options, and consider nondrug therapies, including spinal manipulation, if pain persists longer than four weeks.

Chronic low-back pain: Long-term use of opioid drugs usually does not improve functioning for patients with chronic low-back pain. However, these patients may benefit from nondrug therapies, including spinal manipulation. Psychological and social factors also may play a role in chronic low-back pain. Most patients will not become pain free; a realistic outlook focuses on improving function in addition to reducing pain.

Section 43.5

Massage Therapy

Excerpted from "Massage Therapy: An Introduction," National Center for Complementary and Alternative Medicine, August 2010. The complete text of this document, including references, can be found online at http://nccam.nih.gov/health/massage/massageintroduction.htm.

History of Massage

Massage therapy dates back thousands of years. References to massage appear in writings from ancient China, Japan, India, Arabic nations, Egypt, Greece (Hippocrates defined medicine as "the art of rubbing"), and Rome.

Massage became widely used in Europe during the Renaissance. In the 1850s, two American physicians who had studied in Sweden introduced massage therapy in the United States, where it became popular and was promoted for a variety of health purposes. With scientific and technological advances in medical treatment during the 1930s and 1940s, massage fell out of favor in the United States. Interest in massage revived in the 1970s, especially among athletes.

People use massage for a variety of health-related purposes, including to relieve pain, rehabilitate sports injuries, reduce stress, increase relaxation, address anxiety and depression, and aid general wellness.

The term "massage therapy" encompasses many different techniques. In general, therapists press, rub, and otherwise manipulate the muscles and other soft tissues of the body. They most often use their hands and fingers, but may use their forearms, elbows, or feet.

In Swedish massage, the therapist uses long strokes, kneading, deep circular movements, vibration, and tapping. Sports massage is similar to Swedish massage, adapted specifically to the needs of athletes. Among the many other examples are deep tissue massage and trigger point massage, which focuses on myofascial trigger points—muscle "knots" that are painful when pressed and can cause symptoms elsewhere in the body.

The Practice of Massage Therapy

Massage therapists work in a variety of settings, including private offices, hospitals, nursing homes, studios, and sport and fitness facilities. Some also travel to patients' homes or workplaces. They usually try to provide a calm, soothing environment.

Therapists usually ask new patients about symptoms, medical history, and desired results. They may also perform an evaluation through touch, to locate painful or tense areas and determine how much pressure to apply.

Typically, the patient lies on a table, either in loose-fitting clothing or undressed (covered with a sheet, except for the area being massaged). The therapist may use oil or lotion to reduce friction on the skin. Sometimes, people receive massage therapy while sitting in a chair. A massage session may be fairly brief, but may also last an hour or even longer.

Research Status

Although scientific research on massage therapy—whether it works and, if so, how—is limited, there is evidence that massage may benefit some patients. Conclusions generally cannot yet be drawn about its effectiveness for specific health conditions.

According to one analysis, however, research supports the general conclusion that massage therapy is effective. The studies included in the analysis suggest that a single session of massage therapy can reduce "state anxiety" (a reaction to a particular situation), blood pressure, and heart rate, and multiple sessions can reduce "trait anxiety" (general anxiety-proneness), depression, and pain.

There are numerous theories about how massage therapy may affect the body. For example, the "gate control theory" suggests that massage may provide stimulation that helps to block pain signals sent to the brain. Other theories suggest that massage might stimulate the release of certain chemicals in the body, such as serotonin or endorphins, or cause beneficial mechanical changes in the body. However, additional studies are needed to test the various theories.

Safety

Massage therapy appears to have few serious risks—if it is performed by a properly trained therapist and if appropriate cautions are followed. The number of serious injuries reported is very small. Side effects of massage therapy may include temporary pain or discomfort, bruising, swelling, and a sensitivity or allergy to massage oils.

Cautions about massage therapy include the following:

- Vigorous massage should be avoided by people with bleeding disorders or low blood platelet counts, and by people taking blood-thinning medications such as warfarin.

- Massage should not be done in any area of the body with blood clots, fractures, open or healing wounds, skin infections, or weakened bones (such as from osteoporosis or cancer), or where there has been a recent surgery.

- Although massage therapy appears to be generally safe for cancer patients, they should consult their oncologist before having a massage that involves deep or intense pressure. Any direct pressure over a tumor usually is discouraged. Cancer patients should discuss any concerns about massage therapy with their oncologist.

- Pregnant women should consult their health care provider before using massage therapy.

If You Are Thinking about Using Massage Therapy

- Do not use massage therapy to replace your regular medical care or as a reason to postpone seeing a health care provider about a medical problem.

- If you have a medical condition and are unsure whether massage therapy would be appropriate for you, discuss your concerns with your health care provider. Your health care provider may also be able to help you select a massage therapist. You might also look for published research articles on massage therapy for your condition.

- Before deciding to begin massage therapy, ask about the therapist's training, experience, and credentials. Also ask about the number of treatments that might be needed, the cost, and insurance coverage.

- If a massage therapist suggests using other CAM practices (for example, herbs or other supplements, or a special diet), discuss it first with your regular health care provider.

- Tell all your health care providers about any complementary and alternative practices you use. Give them a full picture of what you do to manage your health. This will ensure coordinated and safe care.

Section 43.6

Relaxation Techniques

Excerpted from "Relaxation Techniques for Health: An Introduction," National Center for Complementary and Alternative Medicine, August 2011. The complete text of this document, including references, can be found online at http://nccam.nih.gov/health/stress/relaxation.htm.

About Relaxation Techniques

Relaxation is more than a state of mind; it physically changes the way your body functions. When your body is relaxed breathing slows, blood pressure and oxygen consumption decrease, and some people report an increased sense of well-being. This is called the "relaxation response." Being able to produce the relaxation response using relaxation techniques may counteract the effects of long-term stress, which may contribute to or worsen a range of health problems including depression, digestive disorders, headaches, high blood pressure, and insomnia.

Relaxation techniques often combine breathing and focused attention on pleasing thoughts and images to calm the mind and the body. Most methods require only brief instruction from a book or experienced practitioner before they can be done without assistance. These techniques may be most effective when practiced regularly and combined with good nutrition, regular exercise, and a strong social support system.

Relaxation response techniques include the following:

- **Autogenic training:** When using this method, you focus on the physical sensation of your own breathing or heartbeat and picture your body as warm, heavy, and/or relaxed.

- **Biofeedback:** Biofeedback-assisted relaxation uses electronic devices to teach you how to consciously produce the relaxation response. Biofeedback is sometimes used to relieve conditions that are caused or worsened by stress.

- **Deep breathing or breathing exercises:** To relax using this method, you consciously slow your breathing and focus on taking regular and deep breaths.

- **Guided imagery:** For this technique, you focus on pleasant images to replace negative or stressful feelings and relax. Guided imagery may be directed by you or a practitioner through storytelling or descriptions designed to suggest mental images (also called visualization).

- **Progressive relaxation** (also called Jacobson's progressive relaxation or progressive muscle relaxation): For this relaxation method, you focus on tightening and relaxing each muscle group. Progressive relaxation is often combined with guided imagery and breathing exercises.

- **Self-hypnosis:** In self-hypnosis you produce the relaxation response with a phrase or nonverbal cue (called a "suggestion"). Self-hypnosis may be used to relieve pain (tension headaches, labor, or minor surgery) as well as to treat anxiety and irritable bowel syndrome.

Mind and body practices, such as meditation and yoga are also sometimes considered relaxation techniques.

How Relaxation Techniques May Work

To understand how consciously producing the relaxation response may affect your health, it is helpful to understand how your body responds to the opposite of relaxation—stress.

When you're under stress, your body releases hormones that produce the "fight-or-flight response:" Heart rate and breathing rate go up and blood vessels narrow (restricting the flow of blood). This response allows energy to flow to parts of your body that need to take action, for example the muscles and the heart. However useful this response may be in the short term, there is evidence that when your body remains in a stress state for a long time, emotional or physical damage can occur. Long-term or chronic stress (lasting months or years) may reduce your body's ability to fight off illness and lead to or worsen certain health conditions. Chronic stress may lead to high blood pressure, headaches, stomach ache, and other symptoms. Stress may worsen certain conditions, such as asthma. Stress also has been linked to depression, anxiety, and other mental illnesses.

In contrast to the stress response, the relaxation response slows the heart rate, lowers blood pressure, and decreases oxygen consumption and levels of stress hormones. Because relaxation is the opposite of stress, the theory is that voluntarily creating the relaxation response through regular use of relaxation techniques could counteract the negative effects of stress.

Relaxation Techniques and Pain-Related Concerns

In the past 30 years, there has been considerable interest in the relaxation response and how inducing this state may benefit health. Research has focused primarily on illness and conditions in which stress may play a role either as the cause of the condition or as a factor that can make the condition worse.

- **Pain:** Some studies have shown that relaxation techniques may help reduce abdominal and surgery pain.

- **Headache:** There is some evidence that biofeedback and other relaxation techniques may be helpful for relieving tension or migraine headaches. In some cases, these mind and body techniques were more effective than medications for reducing the frequency, intensity, and severity of headaches.

- **Fibromyalgia:** Although some preliminary studies report that using relaxation or guided imagery techniques may sometimes improve pain and reduce fatigue from fibromyalgia, more research is needed.

- **Irritable bowel syndrome:** Some studies have indicated that relaxation techniques may prevent or relieve symptoms of irritable bowel syndrome (IBS) in some participants. One review of the research found some evidence that self-hypnosis may be useful in the treatment of IBS.

- **Temporomandibular disorder** (pain and loss of motion in the jaw joints): A review of the literature found that relaxation techniques and biofeedback were more effective than placebo in decreasing pain and increasing jaw function.

Many of the studies of relaxation therapy and health have followed a small number of patients for weeks or months. Longer studies involving more participants may reveal more about the cumulative effects of using relaxation techniques regularly.

Side Effects and Risks

Relaxation techniques are generally considered safe for healthy people. There have been rare reports that certain relaxation techniques might cause or worsen symptoms in people with epilepsy or certain psychiatric conditions, or with a history of abuse or trauma. People with heart disease should talk to their doctor before doing progressive muscle relaxation.

Relaxation techniques are often used as part of a treatment plan and not as the sole treatment for potentially serious health conditions.

Section 43.7

Yoga

Excerpted from "Yoga for Health," National Center for Complementary and Alternative Medicine, May 2012. The complete text of this document, including references, can be found online at http://nccam.nih.gov/health/yoga/introduction.htm.

About Yoga

Yoga in its full form combines physical postures, breathing exercises, meditation, and a distinct philosophy. There are numerous styles of yoga. Hatha yoga, commonly practiced in the United States and Europe, emphasizes postures, breathing exercises, and meditation. Hatha yoga styles include Ananda, Anusara, Ashtanga, Bikram, Iyengar, Kripalu, Kundalini, Viniyoga, and others.

Yoga is generally low-impact and safe for healthy people when practiced appropriately under the guidance of a well-trained instructor.

Overall, those who practice yoga have a low rate of side effects, and the risk of serious injury from yoga is quite low. However, certain types of stroke as well as pain from nerve damage are among the rare possible side effects of practicing yoga.

Women who are pregnant and people with certain medical conditions, such as high blood pressure, glaucoma (a condition in which fluid pressure within the eye slowly increases and can damage the eye's optic nerve), and sciatica (pain, weakness, numbing, or tingling that can extend from the lower back to the calf, foot, or even the toes), should modify or avoid some yoga poses.

Many people who practice yoga do so to maintain their health and well-being, improve physical fitness, relieve stress, and enhance quality of life. In addition, yoga is also used to address specific health conditions, such as back pain, neck pain, arthritis, and anxiety.

What the Science Says about Yoga

Current research suggests that a carefully adapted set of yoga poses may reduce low-back pain and improve function. Other studies also suggest that practicing yoga (as well as other forms of regular exercise) might improve quality of life; reduce stress; lower heart rate and blood pressure; help relieve anxiety, depression, and insomnia; and improve overall physical fitness, strength, and flexibility. But some research suggests yoga may not improve asthma, and studies looking at yoga and arthritis have had mixed results.

Training, Licensing, and Certification

There are many training programs for yoga teachers throughout the country. These programs range from a few days to more than two years. Standards for teacher training and certification differ depending on the style of yoga.

There are organizations that register yoga teachers and training programs that have complied with a certain curriculum and educational standards. For example, one nonprofit group (the Yoga Alliance) requires at least 200 hours of training, with a specified number of hours in areas including techniques, teaching methodology, anatomy, physiology, and philosophy. Most yoga therapist training programs involve 500 hours or more. The International Association of Yoga Therapists is developing standards for yoga therapy training.

Everyone's body is different, and yoga postures should be modified based on individual abilities. Carefully selecting an instructor who is experienced with and attentive to your needs is an important step toward helping you practice yoga safely. Ask about the physical demands of the type of yoga in which you are interested and inform your yoga instructor about any medical issues you have.

Tell all your health care providers about any complementary health practices you use. Give them a full picture of what you do to manage your health. This will help ensure coordinated and safe care.

Chapter 44

Over-the-Counter Pain Relievers

A Guide to Safe Use of Pain Medicine

If you've ever been treated for severe pain from surgery, an injury, or an illness, you know just how vital pain relief medications can be.

Pain relief treatments come in many forms and potencies, are available by prescription or over-the-counter (OTC), and treat all sorts of physical pain—including that brought on by chronic conditions, sudden trauma, and cancer.

Pain relief medicines (also known as *analgesics* and *painkillers*) are regulated by the U.S. Food and Drug Administration (FDA). Some analgesics act on the body's peripheral and central nervous systems to block or decrease sensitivity to pain. Others act by inhibiting the formation of certain chemicals in the body. Among the factors health care professionals consider in recommending or prescribing them are the cause and severity of the pain.

OTC Pain Medications

These relieve the minor aches and pains associated with conditions such as headaches, fever, colds, flu, arthritis, toothaches, and menstrual cramps.

This chapter includes excerpts from "A Guide to Safe Use of Pain Medicine," U.S. Food and Drug Administration (FDA; www.fda.gov), updated August 9, 2012; and excerpts from "The Best Way to Take Your Over-the-Counter Pain Reliever? Seriously," FDA, April 27, 2012.

There are basically two types of OTC pain relievers: acetaminophen and non-steroidal anti-inflammatory drugs (NSAIDs).

Acetaminophen is an active ingredient found in more than 600 OTC and prescription medicines, including pain relievers, cough suppressants, and cold medications.

NSAIDs are common medications used to relieve fever and minor aches and pains. They include aspirin, naproxen, and ibuprofen, as well as many medicines taken for colds, sinus pressure, and allergies. They act by inhibiting an enzyme that helps make a specific chemical.

Use as Directed

Pain medications are safe and effective when used as directed. However, misuse of these products can be extremely harmful and even deadly.

Consumers who take pain relief medications must follow their health care professional's instructions carefully. If a measuring tool is provided with your medicine, use it as directed. Do not change the dose of your pain relief medication without talking to your doctor first. Also, pain medications should never be shared with anyone else. Only your health care professional can decide if a prescription pain medication is safe for someone.

Here are other key points to remember with acetaminophen:

- Taking a higher dose than recommended will not provide more relief and can be dangerous.

- Too much can lead to liver damage and death. Risk for liver damage may be increased in people who drink three or more alcoholic beverages a day while using acetaminophen-containing medicines.

- Be cautious when giving acetaminophen to children. Infant drop medications can be significantly stronger than regular children's medications. Read and follow the directions on the label every time you use a medicine. Be sure that your infant is getting the infants' pain formula and your older child is getting the children's pain formula.

Here are other key points to remember with NSAIDs:

- Too much can cause stomach bleeding. This risk increases in people who are over 60 years of age, are taking prescription blood thinners, are taking steroids, have a history of stomach bleeding or ulcers, and/or have other bleeding problems.

- Use of NSAIDs can also cause kidney damage. This risk may increase in people who are over 60 years of age, are taking a diuretic (a drug that increases the excretion of urine), have high blood pressure, heart disease, or pre-existing kidney disease.

Know the Active Ingredients

A specific area of concern with OTC pain medicines is when products sold for different uses have the same active ingredient. A cold and cough remedy may have the same active ingredient as a headache remedy or a prescription pain reliever.

To minimize the risks of an accidental overdose, consumers should avoid taking multiple medications with the same active ingredient at the same time. All OTC medicines must have all of their active ingredients listed on the package. For prescription drugs, the active ingredients are listed on the container label.

Talk with your pharmacist or another health care professional if you have questions about using OTC medicines, and especially before using them in combination with dietary supplements or other OTC or prescription medicines.

The Best Way to Take Your Over-the-Counter Pain Reliever

Over-the-counter (OTC) pain relievers/fever reducers can cause serious problems when used by people with certain conditions or taking specific medicines. They can also cause problems in people who take too much, or use them for a longer period of time than the product's Drug Facts label recommends. That is why it is important to follow label directions carefully. If you have questions, talk to a pharmacist or health care professional.

There are two categories of over-the-counter pain relievers/fever reducers: acetaminophen and nonsteroidal anti-inflammatory drugs (NSAIDs). Acetaminophen is used to relieve headaches, muscle aches and fever. It is also found in many other medicines, such as cough syrup and cold and sinus medicines. OTC NSAIDs are used to help relieve pain and reduce fever. NSAIDs include aspirin, naproxen, ketoprofen and ibuprofen, and are also found in many medicines taken for colds, sinus pressure and allergies.

These products, when used occasionally and taken as directed, are safe and effective. Read the labels of all your over-the-counter medicines so you are aware of the correct recommended dosage. If a measuring tool is provided with your medicine, use it as directed.

511

Using too much acetaminophen can cause serious liver damage, which may not be noticed for several days. NSAIDs, for some people with certain medical problems, can lead to the development of stomach bleeding and kidney disease.

There are many OTC medicines that contain the same active ingredient. If you take several medicines that happen to contain the same active ingredient, for example a pain reliever along with a cough-cold-fever medicine, you might be taking two times the normal dose and not know it. So read the label and avoid taking multiple medicines that contain the same active ingredient or talk to your pharmacist or health care professional.

Before using any medicine, remember to think SAFER:

- **S**peak up

- **A**sk questions

- **F**ind the facts

- **E**valuate your choices

- **R**ead the label

Chapter 45

Topical Pain Relievers

Creams, gels, sprays, liquids, patches, or rubs applied on the skin over a painful muscle or joint are called topical pain relievers or topical analgesics. Many are available without a prescription.

Topical agents should be distinguished from transdermal medications, which are also applied directly to the skin. Whereas topical agents work locally and must be applied directly over the painful area, transdermal drugs have effects throughout the body and work when applied away from the area of pain (currently available transdermal drugs include fentanyl, buprenorphine, and clonidine). Transdermal medication in a patch is absorbed through the skin by the bloodstream over a period of time (in general, you should never cut a transdermal patch into smaller pieces, but topical lidocaine patches may be cut into smaller sizes with scissors as noted on the packaging).

Some of the OTC topical agents contain salicylates, a family of drugs that reduce inflammation and pain. They come from the bark of the willow tree and are the pain relieving substances found in aspirin. Small amounts relieve mild pain. Larger amounts may reduce both pain and inflammation. Salicylates decrease the ability of the nerve endings in the skin to sense pain.

Counterirritants, another group of topical agents, are specifically approved for the topical treatment of minor aches and pains of muscles

Excerpted from "ACPA Resource Guide to Chronic Pain Medication and Treatment," © 2012 American Chronic Pain Association. All rights reserved. Reprinted with permission. For additional information, visit www.theacpa.org.

and joints (simple backache, arthritis pain, strains, bruises, and sprains). They stimulate nerve endings in the skin to cause feelings of cold, warmth, or itching. This produces a paradoxical pain-relieving effect by producing less severe pain to counter a more intense one. Some topical pain relievers are methyl salicylate, menthol, camphor, eucalyptus oil, turpentine oil, histamine dihydrochloride, and methyl nicotinate.

Counterirritants come in various forms such as balms, creams, gels, and patches under several brands such as BenGay, Icy Hot, Salonpas, and Thera-Gesic for ease of application. The balms, creams, and gels can be applied to the painful area(s) three to four times a day (usually for up to one week). When using the BenGay patch product, one patch can be applied for up to 8 to 12 hours; if pain is still present, a second patch may be applied for up to 8 to 12 hours (maximum: two patches in 24 hours for no longer than three days of consecutive use). The Salonpas Pain Relief Patch (10% methyl salicylate and 3% menthol) is currently the only U.S. Food and Drug Administration (FDA)-approved OTC topical analgesic patch and can be applied up to three to four times/day for seven days; the patch may remain in place for up to eight hours. It is approved for temporary relief of mild to moderate aches and pains of muscles and joints associated with strains, sprains, simple backache, arthritis, and bruises.

Even though these products are sold without a prescription, they still carry some risk of adverse effects (mostly skin irritation). Topical products containing NSAIDs (methyl salicylate) carry less risk of side effects versus the oral NSAIDs (that is, ibuprofen), but they still apply. Also, these products should not be applied on wounds, damaged skin, or the face. Lastly, after application, be sure to wash your hands thoroughly to avoid getting these products in sensitive areas such as your eyes. When removing and discarding used patches, fold the used patches so that the adhesive side sticks to itself. Safely discard used patches where children and pets cannot get to them.

Topical agents have also gained popularity for use in certain neuropathic pain conditions such as diabetic neuropathy, postherpetic neuralgia (PHN), or neuroma pain. They are also prescribed in (complex regional pain syndrome) CRPS states.

Aspirin in chloroform or ethyl ether, capsaicin (Zostrix, Zostrix-HP), EMLA (eutectic mixture of local anesthetics) cream, and local anesthetics such as the lidocaine patch 5% (Lidoderm) are topical treatments for neuropathic pain. Of these, the topical lidocaine patch 5% is the only FDA-approved treatment for neuropathic pain, and it requires a prescription. There are additional topical agent combinations which can be compounded at your local pharmacy. These compounded mixtures are prepared uniquely for each individual but have not passed rigorous scientific study. Any benefit from such compounded creams is anecdotal.

Capsaicin is the active ingredient in hot peppers which produces a characteristic heat sensation when applied to the skin (dermal drug delivery). Several studies have suggested that capsaicin (cap-SAY-sin) can be an effective analgesic in at least some types of neuropathic pain and arthritic conditions (osteoarthritis and rheumatoid arthritis). An adequate trial of capsaicin usually requires four applications daily, around the clock, for at least three to four weeks. Some individuals may experience a burning sensation, which usually lessens within 72 hours with repeated use. Gloves should be worn during application, and hands should be washed with soap and water after application to avoid contact with the eyes or mucous membranes.

In late 2009, the FDA approved Qutenza (capsaicin) 8% patch for the management of neuropathic pain attributed to PHN that may occur after an episode of herpes zoster (shingles). The Qutenza patch releases a synthetic form of capsaicin through a dermal delivery system at a much stronger dosage than capsaicin cremes available over the counter. Only physicians or health care professionals under the close supervision of a physician are to administer Qutenza. Qutenza is applied for 60 minutes and may be repeated every three months or as warranted by the return of pain (not more frequently than every three months). Before patch application, a physician must identify and mark the painful area, including areas of hypersensitivity and allodynia. A topical anesthetic is applied before Qutenza application. In clinical trials, the most common adverse reactions were application site redness, pain, itching, and papules. The majority of these reactions were transient and self-limited. Among patients treated with Qutenza, 1% discontinued treatment prematurely due to an adverse event. Serious adverse reactions included application-site pain and increased blood pressure. Information can be found at http://www.qutenza.com/_docs/qutenza_full_PI_.pdf.

Topical anesthetics, such as EMLA (Eutectic Mixture of Local Anesthetic) cream and L.M.X.4, are used primarily prior to painful procedures such as venipuncture (blood drawing), lumbar puncture (spinal tap), and wart removal. EMLA cream may be effective in the treatment of postherpetic neuralgia, ischemic (decreased blood supply) neuropathy, and a variety of other neuropathic conditions.

EMLA cream is a combination of the local anesthetics lidocaine and prilocaine. This combination results in a relatively constant release of dissolvable local anesthetics that can diffuse through the skin and soft tissue. A thick layer of EMLA cream is applied to intact skin and covered with an occlusive dressing. The minimal application time to obtain reliable superficial pain relief is one hour. However, the cream may be left on the skin for up to two hours, depending on the degree of the procedure performed. Analgesia can be expected to increase for up to three hours under occlusive dressing and persist for one to two hours after removal of the cream. Side effects to EMLA cream include skin blanching, redness, and swelling. In younger individuals or in cases in which too much has been applied, negative effects can occur to hemoglobin (red blood cells). Therefore, EMLA cream should be avoided in individuals less than one month old and in patients with a predisposition to methemoglobinemia (a problem with the red cell). EMLA cream should also not be applied to broken skin or mucous membranes (for example, mouth).

L.M.X.4 contains 4% lidocaine and is available without a prescription. It has a shorter application time (30 minutes) and a shorter duration of action (30 minutes) than EMLA. It has not been shown to be effective for chronic pain most likely because of its short duration.

Lidoderm 5% (lidocaine) patches can be cut to fit over the area of pain. The 5% lidocaine patch is the only topical anesthetic agent to receive FDA approval for the treatment of a neuropathic pain condition, specifically PHN. It measures 10 cm x 14 cm and has a clear plastic backing that must be removed before application of the patch to the skin. The manufacturer states that up to three patches can be applied simultaneously to intact skin for up to 12 hours in any 24-hour period; however, research has shown that four patches worn continuously for 24 hours then replaced with new patches is safe.

Side effects of topical local anesthetics are usually minimal and include localized skin irritation and swelling that generally disappear within two to three hours after the local anesthetic is removed from the skin. As a rule, blood concentrations of topical local anesthetics are well below toxic levels.

Potential hazards still exist, however. In 2007, the FDA issued a public health advisory to notify consumers and health care professionals of potential life-threatening side effects associated with the use of topical anesthetics, particularly before cosmetic procedures. At risk are consumers, especially those without the supervision of a health care professional. They may apply large amounts of anesthetics or cover large areas of the skin, leave these products on for long periods of time, or use materials, wraps, or dressings to cover the skin after anesthetic application. Application to areas of skin irritation, rash, or broken skin may also increase the risk of systemic absorption. The FDA recommends that if topical anesthetics are needed prior to medical or cosmetic procedures, consumers ask their healthcare provider for instructions on the safe use of these products, use only FDA-approved products, and use products with the lowest amount of anesthetic while applying the least amount possible to relieve pain.

Compounded Medications

Compounded medications are not commercially available; rather, they are prescribed by a health care professional and prepared by a pharmacist to meet an individual's unique needs. These compounded medications do not go through the same FDA approval process that is required for commercially available prescription drugs. Therefore, trials may or may not be conducted to determine safety and efficacy. Such studies are not a legal requirement for compounding medications.

The most common compounded medications are topical gels. They typically contain ingredients such as lidocaine, amitriptyline, gabapentin, or ketoprofen. Most of them use PLO (Pluronic Lecithin Organogel) as a vehicle to help deliver the active ingredients through the skin. The benefit to this type of delivery system is that medication is localized to the area of pain. Studies show less systemic absorption for ingredients like lidocaine and amitriptyline when used in PLO gels. Lidocaine 5% in PLO gel has been shown in studies to be effective in relieving pain with a minimal enough amount of systemic absorption to alleviate fears of approaching toxic levels. Studies regarding the efficacy of amitriptyline in PLO gels have been more ambiguous; more research needs to be conducted to determine its role in compounded topical pain medications.

Chapter 46

Non-Opioid
Analgesic Pain Relievers

Aspirin, NSAIDs and acetaminophen are the most widely used medications for most pain conditions. But these drugs are not without risk. Unlike opioids, these medications have an analgesic "ceiling effect." This means that after a certain dose, additional quantities do not provide added pain relief.

NSAIDs can cause gastric distress with ulceration and bleeding, while acetaminophen can cause liver toxicity, particularly when taken in excess. Fortunately, non-opioids do not produce physical or psychological dependence. There is some evidence suggesting that long-term use of common analgesics, such as aspirin, acetaminophen, or NSAIDs, appears to increase the risk for hypertension.

Aspirin and acetaminophen are available OTC while NSAIDs are available both by prescription and some by non-prescription OTC purchase.

These non-opioid analgesic pain relievers are effective for pain and fever. Aspirin and the NSAIDs are also indicated for pain that involves inflammation, whereas acetaminophen does not have anti-inflammatory activity.

Some of these medications are more effective than others in some individuals, which indicates that it makes sense to try several different ones to determine which medication works best for you.

Excerpted from "ACPA Resource Guide to Chronic Pain Medication and Treatment," © 2012 American Chronic Pain Association. All rights reserved. Reprinted with permission. For additional information, visit www.theacpa.org.

The cyclooxygenase-2 (COX-2) inhibitors are NSAIDs that have a lower risk of gastrointestinal (GI) side effects with short term use. Currently available in the United States is celecoxib (Celebrex), which is more expensive than some other NSAIDs and does not provide any better pain relief. Although celecoxib is associated with a lower risk for developing a stomach ulcer when taken for less than six months, serious stomach ulceration can still occur without warning with this drug. As with other NSAIDs, patients should be monitored during long-term use. There is no evidence that some COX-2 selective NSAIDs such as meloxicam (Mobic), etodolac (Lodine, Lodine XL), and nabumetone (Relafen) have fewer GI side effects. NSAIDs additionally are associated with potential kidney effects and heart (cardiovascular) complications, especially when taken for prolonged periods. Remember also that when acetaminophen (Tylenol) is used in combination with NSAIDs, there is an increased risk of developing kidney problems. This effect is usually only seen with long-term use.

While the increased risk of cardiovascular events, such as stroke and myocardial infarction, associated with COX-2 inhibitors has been well established, data are emerging that demonstrate similar risk increases associated with NSAIDs that are not selective for COX-2. Currently, it appears that doses of celecoxib 200 mg or less per day do not seem to increase the risk of cardiovascular events any more than the risk associated with traditional NSAIDs. You are advised to discuss the risk-benefit ratio of NSAIDs with your health care professional. The risk of experiencing adverse events or side effects with NSAIDs increases with the duration of use and the dose. Therefore, it is often recommended that you use these medications for the shortest period and at the lowest dose required to achieve therapeutic improvement. Individuals taking aspirin for its ability to protect the heart should consult with their health care professional prior to utilizing NSAIDs on a long-term basis. The regular use of NSAIDs inhibits aspirin's ability to protect the heart.

In order to improve the side effect profile of NSAIDs, topical NSAIDs have been developed and approved by the FDA. Diclofenac Gel (Voltaren 1% Gel) has been approved for the treatment of chronic pain associated with osteoarthritis in joints close to the skin surface (for example, hands, knees, and ankles). By applying the drug topically to the joint, one is able to receive the pain relieving benefits of the medication while at the same time having lower levels of the drug in the body. Therefore, the risk of experiencing systemic side effects from the medication is theoretically reduced. However, in December 2009, the FDA issued a warning about the potential for liver damage during treatment with all diclofenac products, including the gel. The smallest effective amount should be applied for the shortest time possible to minimize the potential for an adverse liver-related event. After applying the gel, the area should not be covered for at least 10 minutes, and showering and bathing should be avoided for a least one hour after application. Skin irritation (for example, rash, dry skin) may occur with topical diclofenac administration.

In 2007, a topical NSAID patch containing diclofenac (Flector) was approved by the FDA for the treatment of acute pain due to minor strains, sprains, and contusions. The Flector patch has not been approved for the treatment of chronic pain from osteoarthritis. In 2009, the FDA issued an advisory that transdermal and topical patches that contain metal, which includes Flector, need to be removed prior to MRI procedures.

Intravenous (IV) formulations of the NSAIDs ibuprofen (Caldolor) and ketorolac (Toradol) are given most often in the inpatient setting to manage moderate to severe pain; ketorolac may also be given intramuscularly (IM). In November 2010, IV acetaminophen (Ofirmev) was FDA approved for the management of mild to moderate pain, severe pain with adjunctive opioid analgesics, and reduction of fever. Similar to the IV NSAIDs, IV acetaminophen is administered in an inpatient setting and helps reduce the amount of opioid medication needed to manage pain. The side effect profile for IV acetaminophen is the same as other acetaminophen dosage forms; headache, agitation, nausea, vomiting, and constipation. Injection site reactions such as redness and swelling may occur with any of the IV non-opioids.

Gastrointestinal (GI) Protective Medications

As has been mentioned earlier, the NSAID medications can increase your risk of ulcers and other problems with your stomach and digestion. Often people are prescribed an additional medication to help protect their GI system, sometimes called cytoprotective medications, which are medications that protect cells from noxious chemicals or other harmful stimuli.

There are four commonly used cytoprotective classes of drugs:

1. Misoprostol (Cytotec)—(often combined with diclofenac and distributed as Arthrotec)

2. Sucralfate (Carafate)

3. Histamine type 2 (H2) receptor blockers: famotidine (Pepcid), nizatidine (Axid), ranitidine (Zantac), cimetidine (Tagamet), etc.

4. Proton pump inhibitors (PPIs): esomeprazole (Nexium), lansoprazole (Prevacid), omeprazole (Prilosec), pantoprazole (Protonix), rabeprazole (AcipHex).

Taking cytoprotective agents along with your NSAID pain medication is recommended for individuals who will benefit from an NSAID but also have a high GI risk factor profile. Individuals considered being at elevated risk includes those with a history of prior GI bleed, the elderly, diabetics, and cigarette smokers. Long-term NSAID treatment increases the risk among those most susceptible, although any patient can potentially develop an adverse effect at any time.

PPIs have been shown to reduce the risk of GI ulcers. A study published in 2006 raised concerns because the chronic use of PPIs might have a significant impact on the rate of hip fractures. The authors think that acid-suppressive therapy may increase the risk of hip fractures by decreasing calcium absorption. Thus, as with all medications, PPIs must be used with caution, and the disadvantages must be weighed against the benefits.

Misoprostol (Cytotec) mimics naturally occurring prostaglandins in the body. Prostaglandins play many roles, which include regulating blood pressure, the amount of stomach acid secretion, body temperature, and platelet aggregation; controlling inflammation; and affecting the action of certain hormones. Misoprostol inhibits gastric acid secretion via direct interaction on stomach cells called parietal cells. Misoprostol also exhibits mucosal protective effects which enables it to be a positive treatment for stomach ulcers. Prostaglandins increase the contraction ability in the uterus, so females should not take misoprostol if pregnant or planning to become pregnant.

Sucralfate (Carafate) works via interactions with hydrochloric acid found in the stomach. The combination forms a glue-like substance which acts as an acid buffer, protecting the stomach.

Treatment with antacids, such as TUMS and H2 blockers offer little if any protection against duodenal and gastric ulcers. Many of the studies on H2 blockers show that they have no value in the protection of the gastric mucosa.

Non-Opioid Analgesic Drugs and Their Uses

The following information summarizes the uses and cautions that apply to many of the non-opioid analgesic medications now on the market.

Medications (generic) and brand names (brand names are the trademarked property of the medication's manufacturer):

Aspirin (Bayer; Bufferin)

- **May be useful for:** Headache, muscle ache, fever, menstrual cramps, arthritis pain and inflammation. May reduce the risk of heart attack and stroke.

- **Pros:** Anti-inflammatory; inexpensive.

- **Cons:** May irritate stomach. Inhibits platelets and can cause prolonged bleeding. Can precipitate asthma in aspirin-sensitive patients.

- **Comments:** May cause Reye syndrome in children and teen-agers and should not be used during viral syndromes; may be harmful for women in late pregnancy, people with kidney or liver disease, asthma, high blood pressure, or bleeding disorders.

Salicylate Salts: choline salicylate (Arthropan); choline magnesium trisalicylate (Trilisate)

- **May be useful for:** Pain, osteoarthritis and rheumatoid arthritis.

- **Pros:** Fewer GI side effects than other NSAIDs.

- **Cons:** May irritate stomach.

- **Comments:** Do not affect bleeding time or platelet aggregation.

Acetaminophen (FeverAll; Tylenol)

- **May be useful for:** Headache, muscle ache, backache, fever, and arthritis pain (especially osteoarthritis).

- **Pros:** More gentle to the stomach than NSAIDs; safer for children. Does not promote bleeding (or protect against heart attack, stroke).

- **Cons:** Does not reduce inflammation; may be less effective than aspirin for soft tissue pain.

- **Comments:** May be harmful for people with kidney or liver disease or those who drink alcohol heavily. May increase bleeding time in individuals receiving anticoagulation therapy.

Ibuprofen (Advil; Motrin)

- **May be useful for:** Headache, muscle ache, fever, sprains, menstrual cramps, backache, and arthritis pain.

- **Pros:** Stronger and generally longer lasting than aspirin.
- **Cons:** May irritate stomach.
- **Comments:** May be harmful for people with kidney or liver disease, asthma, bleeding disorders, or those who drink alcohol heavily.

Ketoprofen (Orudis; Oruvail)

- **May be useful for:** Headache, muscle ache, fever, menstrual cramps, cold or flu aches.
- **Pros:** Helps reduce inflammation. More gentle to the stomach than aspirin.
- **Cons:** Less gentle to the stomach than naproxen sodium, ibuprofen, acetaminophen.
- **Comments:** May be harmful for people with kidney or liver disease or those who drink alcohol heavily. Not recommended for children without a health care professional's supervision.

Naproxen Sodium (Aleve [OTC]; Anaprox; Naprelan; Naprosyn)

- **May be useful for:** Headache, muscle ache, fever, menstrual cramps, backache, arthritis pain and inflammation.
- **Pros:** Stronger and generally longer lasting than aspirin for menstrual cramps, toothache, and inflammation.
- **Cons:** May irritate stomach; tends to be higher in cost.
- **Comments:** Not recommended for children without a health care professional's supervision.

Meloxicam (Mobic)

- **May be useful for:** Arthritis pain.
- **Pros:** Associated with less risk of ulcers than other NSAIDs.
- **Cons:** Still a risk for stomach irritation. Tends to cost more.
- **Comments:** Generally well-tolerated but still need to be concerned about GI side effects.

COX-2 Inhibitors (Celebrex)

- **May be useful for:** Muscle aches, joint pain, arthritis, pain and inflammation.

- **Pros:** Helps reduce inflammation; less stomach irritation than other NSAIDs.

- **Cons:** Still a risk for stomach irritation. Tends to cost more.

- **Comments:** Generally well-tolerated but still need to be concerned about GI side effects. No effect on bleeding time. These agents are available by prescription only. Use caution with sulfa allergies and celecoxib.

Other NSAIDs Include the Following

- Diclofenac (Cataflam, Voltaren, others)

- Diflunisal (Dolobid)

- Etodolac (Lodine, Lodine XL)

- Fenoprofen (Nalfon)

- Flurbiprofen (Ansaid)

- Indomethacin (Indocin, Indocin SR)

- Mefenamic acid (Ponstel)

- Nabumetone (Relafen)

- Oxaprozin (Daypro)

- Piroxicam (Feldene)

- Sulindac (Clinoril)

- Tolmetin (Tolectin)

- Ketorolac (Toradol, others)—NSAID injectable formulation (intramuscular and intravenous)

- Ibuprofen (Caldolor)—NSAID available intravenous for acute pain and fever

Chapter 47

Opioid Pain Relievers

Chapter Contents

Section 47.1—Commonly Prescribed Opioid Medications 528

Section 47.2—Opioid Use for Chronic, Non-Terminal
Pain Is Controversial 541

Section 47.1

Commonly Prescribed Opioid Medications

Excerpted from "ACPA Resource Guide to Chronic Pain Medication and Treatment," © 2012 American Chronic Pain Association. All rights reserved. Reprinted with permission. For additional information, visit www.theacpa.org.

The Opioid Dilemma

Considerable controversy exists about the use of opioids for the treatment of chronic pain of non-cancer origin. Many health care professionals think that chronic pain is inadequately treated and that opioids can play an important role in the treatment of all types of chronic pain, including non-cancer pain. Others caution against the widespread use of opioids, noting problems with tolerance, loss of benefit with time, and escalating usage with decreasing function in some individuals.

The use of opioids (or for that matter any treatment) makes sense when the benefits outweigh the risks and negative side effects. Benefit is suggested when there is a significant increase in the person's level of functioning, a reduction or elimination of pain complaints, a more positive and hopeful attitude, and when side effects are minimal or controllable.

Opioids are not harmless drugs. The dilemma with the long-term use of opioids is that while opioid treatment may be prescribed to reduce pain and improve function, the treatment may actually result at times in just the opposite.

It is well known that in the opioid naïve (someone new to opioid use) patient, the use of opioids may heighten the risk of accidental death from respiratory depression.

It is well known that prolonged use of opioids may result in problems including tolerance, hyperalgesia (increased pain sensitivity), hormonal effects (decreased testosterone levels, decreased libido and sex drive, irregular menses), depression, impaired sleep patterns, and suppression of the immune system. The long-term use of opioids may also impair functional improvement in an individual's recovery from surgery or with long-standing musculoskeletal disorders.

Research shows that chronic use of large quantities of opioids may interfere with the body's natural pain relievers, the endorphins. Since physical activity is thought to promote release of endorphins, it is also possible that opioids could inhibit the body's own mechanism of reducing pain by causing a person to be less active. Additionally, long-term opioid use may cause depression in some patients, which may impede their ability to recover.

Fifty-one percent of all patients taking oral opioids experience at least one adverse event/effect. Approximately 20% of all patients taking oral opioids discontinue their use because of an adverse event or an associated side effect.

In an article published by the U.S. Department of Health and Human Services, Centers for Disease Control and Prevention, National Center for Health Statistics, titled "Increase in Fatal Poisonings Involving Opioid Analgesics in the United States, 1999–2006," opioid poisoning was noted to be the second leading cause of injury death overall and the leading cause of injury death for people aged 35–54 years, surpassing both firearm- related and motor vehicle-related deaths in this age group. The number of poisoning deaths and the percentage of these deaths involving opioid analgesics increased each year from 1999 through 2006.

Due to the seriousness of this problem, the U.S. Food and Drug Administration (FDA) is now requiring that special safety procedures called REMS (Risk Evaluation and Mitigation Strategies) be put into place to protect people. One of the components of REMS requires that patients who receive opioids must be given an informational brochure called a "Medication Guide" for the specific drug they receive each time they get a new prescription. The "Medication Guide" is designed to inform patients about the serious risks associated with the drug. It should be read each time a new prescription is received, even if the specific opioid being used has not changed, since there may be important new information added. The FDA is also working in cooperation with other governmental agencies, state professional licensing boards, and societies of healthcare professionals to increase prescribers' knowledge about appropriate prescribing and safe use of opioids. There is renewed emphasis on home storage and safe disposal of unused medication to help patients protect their families and the continued availability of opioids to patients.

What Are Opioids?

Opioid Agonists

Opioids are morphine-like substances and have been available for centuries to relieve pain. The term opioid is derived from opium, which is an extract from the poppy plant. There are naturally occurring (opiate), synthetic (opioid), and semisynthetic forms.

Most opioids are agonists, a drug that binds to a receptor of a cell and triggers a response by the cell. An agonist produces an action. It is the opposite of an antagonist, which acts against and blocks an action.

Examples of opioid agonists include morphine, hydromorphone, fentanyl, and oxycodone. There are a number of opioid receptors in the body that mediate analgesia. In 1975, it was discovered that the body generates its own (internal or endogenous) opioids (called endorphins, enkephalins, and dynorphins).

There are numerous opioids available by prescription (see information below). The potency, speed of onset, and duration are unique to each drug. All of the opioids have similar clinical effects that vary in degree from one drug to another.

There are both short- and long-acting opioid formulations. Some opioids are used around-the-clock in scheduled doses, while others are used as needed for intermittent or breakthrough pain.

Opioid Mixed Agonists/Antagonists

There are a number of opioid analgesics (pain relievers) that are partial agonists and mixed agonists/antagonists. The mixed agonists/antagonists are characterized as having an analgesic "ceiling" effect in which the analgesic benefit plateaus, and no further benefit is obtained by increasing the dose.

Given their antagonist nature, these medications can reverse the effects (analgesia and side effects) of full agonist opioids, such as morphine, fentanyl, hydromorphone, and oxycodone, and therefore should be used with caution in those taking a full agonist opioid. A partial agonist/antagonist is occasionally initiated in a person already taking an agonist opioid. The doses should be adjusted gradually to avoid symptoms of opioid withdrawal. In most cases, these two types of agents should not be used together.

Symptoms of withdrawal include sweating, gooseflesh or goose bumps (a temporary local change in the skin when it becomes rougher due to erection of little muscles, as from cold, fear, or excitement), runny nose, abdominal cramping, diarrhea, nervousness, agitation, hallucinations, and a fast heartbeat. Tell your health care professional or pharmacist if you have these or other side effects.

Opioid Delivery

Opioids are available orally (by mouth), intravenously, by intramuscular injection, via nasal spray, transdermally (through the skin), oral transmucosally (absorbed under the tongue and the inside of the cheek), buccally (absorbed via the inside of the cheek), via suppository, epidurally, and intrathecally.

Short-Acting and Long-Acting Opioid Agonists

Short-acting oral opioids, also called immediate-release (IR) opioids, often contain an opioid as the only active ingredient (for example, morphine, hydromorphone, oxycodone, and oxymorphone), while others contain a combination of an opioid and a non-opioid such as acetaminophen or ibuprofen.

Examples of short-acting opioid combination products include:

- oxycodone with acetaminophen (Percocet)

- oxycodone with aspirin (Percodan)

- oxycodone with ibuprofen (Combunox)

- hydrocodone with acetaminophen (Lorcet, Lortab, Vicodin, Norco)

- hydrocodone with ibuprofen (Vicoprofen)

- tramadol hydrochloride with acetaminophen (Ultracet)

Short-acting oral opioids, true to their description, exert a rapid-onset but short-lived therapeutic effect. These agents typically start working 15–30 minutes after administration, with peak analgesic effect within one to two hours. Sustained pain relief is maintained for only about four hours. They are a potent option for treating acute pain (for example, from a serious athletic injury or after a root canal) and are usually prescribed for pain that is anticipated to last only a few days.

Because of their short half-life and rapid clearance from the body, short-acting opioids must be taken every three to four hours. Therefore, these drugs are not ideal for long-term therapy of chronic pain.

Short-acting opioids may be effective, however, as an initial "trial" therapy in patients with moderate or severe chronic pain who have not previously received opioid treatment. In this case, short-acting agents are used to establish an individual patient's response and tolerance to opioid therapy and lay the groundwork for long-term dosing of long-acting opioid therapy.

In addition to their importance in managing acute pain and initiating therapy for chronic pain, short-acting agents can be used with a long-acting agent during long-term therapy as "rescue medication." Rescue medication may be necessary for addressing breakthrough pain that occurs despite ongoing, long-term analgesic treatment.

Long-acting (sometimes called slow-release) medications are the opioid treatment of choice for patients with continuous moderate to severe chronic pain. They have a more lasting therapeutic effect than short-acting agents. Long-acting formulations are described as having sustained, extended, or controlled release of drug and are abbreviated as SR, ER, or CR, respectively.

Examples of long-acting opioids include:

- morphine (oral sustained release, e.g., MS Contin, Avinza, Kadian)

- oxycodone (oral controlled release, e.g., OxyContin)

- oxymorphone (oral extended release Opana ER)

- hydromorphone (oral extended release Exalgo)

- methadone (oral) (e.g., Dolophine, Methadose)

- fentanyl transdermal system (Duragesic)

The prolonged effects of these agents are due to their long half-lives or slow delivery into the body via controlled-release opioid preparations. Because of the slower release of active drug, long-acting opioids can provide prolonged, steady pain relief for 8–12 hours. Long-acting drug preparations are given at regularly scheduled times, such as every 12 hours.

Slow-release tablets should be swallowed whole and are not to be broken, chewed, dissolved, or crushed. Taking broken, chewed, dissolved, or crushed slow-release pills can lead to rapid release and absorption of a potentially fatal dose of the drug.

Examples of Medical Opioid Agonists*

Codeine (with acetaminophen—Tylenol with codeine No. 2, No. 3, No. 4): Codeine is metabolized by the liver to morphine. Some individuals do not have the enzyme required to convert codeine to morphine, and therefore the medication is ineffective. Even though they do not receive benefit, they are still at risk for the associated side effects. Codeine often is associated with higher levels of nausea and vomiting and constipation compared to other opioids.

Dihydrocodeine bitartrate, aspirin, caffeine (Synalgos-DC): This combination drug of dihydrocodeine, aspirin and caffeine is rarely prescribed in chronic pain states.

Fentanyl (Actiq lozenge, Fentora and ONSOLIS buccal tablets, Duragesic transdermal patch): There have been reports of death and other serious side effects from overdoses while on fentanyl transdermal patches. Furthermore, patients that have not been on opioids (opioid naïve) should not be initially started on the fentanyl transdermal patch because of the inherent inaccuracies in dosing which can lead to an overdose. Exposure to heat (hot bath, heating pad, hot sun, etc.) can increase the speed of fentanyl release. The directions for using the fentanyl skin patch must be followed exactly to prevent death or other serious side effects from overdose.

Oral transmucosal fentanyl is available in three formulations (Actiq, Fentora, and ONSOLIS) for the treatment of breakthrough pain in cancer patients receiving opioid treatment and who have become tolerant to it. The FDA warns that serious adverse events, including deaths, can occur in patients treated with oral fentanyl. The deaths that have occurred were due to respiratory depression as a result of improper patient selection, improper dosing, and/or improper product substitution.

Actiq (oral transmucosal fentanyl lozenge on a plastic stick) is absorbed by swabbing the drug-containing lozenge over and under the tongue and between the cheeks and gums. It is contraindicated for acute postoperative pain and migraine headache.

Fentora is an effervescent tablet that is administered by placing the tablet between the upper molar and cheek. Similar to Actiq, Fentora is contraindicated for migraine and acute postoperative pain.

ONSOLIS (a fentanyl buccal soluble film) is administered by placing the nickel-sized film on the inside of the cheek. It is indicated only for the management of breakthrough pain in patients with cancer, 18 years of age and older, who are already receiving and who are tolerant to opioid therapy for their underlying persistent cancer pain.

Hydrocodone (with acetaminophen—Anexsia, Lorcet, Lortab, Norco, Vicodin, Hycet, Xodol, Co-Gesic, Zydone; with ibuprofen—Reprexain, Vicoprofen; with aspirin—Azdone, Lortab ASA, Panasal): Hydrocodone is a short-acting opioid available only in combination with other ingredients, and different combination products are prescribed for different uses. Some hydrocodone products are used to relieve moderate to severe pain. Other hydrocodone products are used to relieve cough.

Hydromorphone (Dilaudid, Dilaudid-5, EXALGO):* EXALGO tablets are an extended-release oral formulation.

Levorphanol (Levo-Dromoran): Levorphanol has the same properties as morphine with respect to the potential for habituation, tolerance, physical dependence and withdrawal syndrome. It is four to eight times as potent as morphine and has a longer half-life.

Meperidine (Demerol): Due to its low potency, short duration of action, and unique toxicity (that is, seizures, delirium, and other neuropsychological effects) relative to other available opioid analgesics, meperidine has fallen out of favor and is not recommended or typically used in chronic pain states.

Methadone (Dolophine, Methadose): Although methadone possesses analgesic properties, it must be used carefully and with a great deal of caution. It has a long half-life and can accumulate in the body which can lead to an overdose. It interacts with a large number of other medications, including OTC drugs. It is strongly recommended that the individual on methadone not use any OTC or herbal medications without clearing them with the prescribing health care professional. The addition of other commonly used pain medications (for example, antidepressants, anticonvulsants, and nonsteroidal anti-inflammatory drugs [NSAIDs]) can increase the likelihood of methadone negatively influencing the heart's ability to conduct electrical signals properly. Prior to starting methadone, patients should undergo an electrocardiogram to check for any pre-existing heart abnormalities that may contraindicate its use. Methadone can also be associated with the development of central sleep apnea. Benzodiazepines should be utilized with extreme caution by individuals on methadone secondary to the synergistic negative respiratory and cardiac effects.

Morphine (Avinza, Duramorph, Kadian, MS Contin, Oramorph SR, Roxanol):* Morphine is considered to be the prototypical opioid and is available in many formulations.

Oxycodone (OxyContin, OxyIR, Roxicodone):

- Combunox (containing ibuprofen, oxycodone)
- Endocet (containing acetaminophen, oxycodone)
- Endodan (containing aspirin, oxycodone)
- Lynox (containing acetaminophen, oxycodone)
- Magnacet (containing acetaminophen, oxycodone)

- Narvox (containing acetaminophen, oxycodone)
- Percocet (containing acetaminophen, oxycodone)
- Percodan (containing aspirin, oxycodone)
- Perloxx (containing acetaminophen, oxycodone)
- Primlev (containing acetaminophen, oxycodone)
- Roxicet (containing acetaminophen, oxycodone)
- Roxiprin (containing aspirin, oxycodone)
- Taxadone (containing acetaminophen, oxycodone)
- Tylox (containing acetaminophen, oxycodone)
- Xolox (containing acetaminophen, oxycodone)

Recently, the manufacturer of OxyContin reformulated its product. The previous OxyContin product contained an immediate-release component (38%) as well as an extended-release component (62%). The reformulated OxyContin is 100% extended-release. The reformulated OxyContin is harder to crush or chew and therefore serves as a better deterrent for abuse. The previous OxyContin had an imprint of "OC" on the tablet, whereas the reformulated OxyContin has an imprint of "OP." There is currently no generic for the reformulated OxyContin, which is the only form available in the United States. With the older formulation, many patients experienced euphoria, which was essentially due to the initial high levels of the oxycodone in the blood. Often times the euphoria feeling has been equated with better pain control, although research has not shown this to be the case. The new tablet formulation takes longer to reach peak levels, which can be incorrectly associated with inadequate pain control.

Oxymorphone (Numorphan, Opana and Opana ER):* Opana ER is an extended-release oral formulation of oxymorphone.

Tapentadol (Nucynta, Nucynta ER):* Tapentadol is an opioid with both opioid and nonopioid activity. The drug binds to opioid receptors and also inhibits the reuptake of the neurotransmitter norepinephrine. The dual mechanism of action inhibits the transmission of pain signals in both the ascending and descending pathways. In pre-clinical studies, this drug has a lower affinity than morphine for the opioid receptor. The short-acting formulation is approved for acute pain treatment, and the extended-release formulation is approved for continuous moderate to severe chronic pain. Tapentadol may have an improved GI side effect profile in comparison with other opioids.

535

Tramadol (Ultram, Ultram ER)* and Tramadol combined with acetaminophen (Ultracet) considered a "weak" opioid: Tramadol is a weak opioid analgesic that acts on the central nervous system in two ways. It binds modestly to opioid receptors and thus produces some analgesia by the same mechanism as opioids. It also affects certain neurotransmitters in the brain to decrease the perception of pain. While a weak opioid, tramadol is not completely free of this risk and may trigger addiction even in those without a history of drug abuse or previous addiction. Tramadol reduces the respiratory rate to a lesser extent than opioids in overdoses and does not cause the sort of GI irritation produced by NSAIDs. Tramadol reduces the threshold for seizures, which may occur in overdose. Seizures may also be provoked in those with a history of seizure disorders, head trauma, etc., or in those taking other drugs that reduce the seizure threshold. Since tramadol is a centrally acting synthetic analgesic, not an NSAID, it has no anti-inflammatory activity. Also unlike NSAIDs, tramadol does not have the potential to compromise the efficacy of certain antihypertensive agents (diuretics and ACE-inhibitors). Tramadol should be used cautiously, if at all, in patients with underlying liver and kidney disease.

*__Slow-release__ (for example, extended-release, controlled-release, and sustained-release) oral opioid formulations should be swallowed whole and are not to be broken, chewed, dissolved, or crushed. Taking broken, chewed, dissolved, or crushed slow-release pills can lead to rapid release and absorption of a potentially fatal dose of the drug.

Examples of Medical Opioid Mixed Agonists/ Antagonists

Buprenorphine (Buprenex, Butrans Transdermal, Subutex)—also used for the treatment of opioid dependence: In addition to its use for the treatment of chronic pain, buprenorphine is used to help alleviate unpleasant withdrawal symptoms associated with opioid detoxification. Buprenorphine exhibits a ceiling effect, which means increasing the dose of buprenorphine beyond a certain point results in no additional pain control. Doses greater than 32 mg/day are ineffective. The ceiling effect demonstrated with buprenorphine offers advantages when compared to other medications used to manage addiction because there is a lower abuse potential, lower level of both physical dependence and withdrawal, and there is a decreased incidence of dose related side effects.

Buprenorphine/naloxone (Suboxone)—also used for the treatment of opioid dependence: Buprenorphine/naloxone (Suboxone) is a combination drug. Naloxone is a pure opioid antagonist, meaning it blocks the effects that opioid drugs have on the receptors. When given sublingually, naloxone has no significant effects on buprenorphine. However if Suboxone is crushed or injected, naloxone will block the effects of buprenorphine. This characteristic discourages misuse. If Suboxone is swallowed instead of dissolved under the tongue, the patient may experiences no effect due to the poor bioavailability and first pass metabolism. Naloxone inhibits respiratory depression, hypotension, sedation, and analgesia.

Butorphanol (Stadol): Available in injection or nasal spray formulations but not typically used for chronic pain treatment.

Nalbuphine (Nubain): Administered subcutaneously, intramuscularly or intravenously but not used for chronic pain treatment.

Pentazocine (Talwin; with acetaminophen—Talacen; with aspirin—Talwin Compound): Side effects are similar to those of morphine, but pentazocine may be more likely to cause hallucinations and other psychosis-like effects. Not used for chronic pain treatment.

Pentazocine/naloxone (Talwin NX): Talwin NX is a combination of pentazocine and naltrexone, an opioid antagonist. This oral formulation was developed to prevent tampering and reduce abuse. The goal of this drug design is to reduce the possible misuse of this medication when it is tampered with by crushing, chewing, or injecting. If the drug is taken as directed, the naloxone will not release and will pass through the body with no effect.

Alert: Propoxyphene (Darvon, Darvocet)—Discontinued for Sale in the USA

In December 2010, propoxyphene, the active ingredient found in Darvocet and Darvon, a mild opioid analgesic structurally related to methadone, was discontinued for sale in the United States by the manufacturer. Propoxyphene is an opioid pain reliever that was used for many years for treatment of mild to moderate pain. Even when used at therapeutic doses, propoxyphene can lead to heart problems better known as arrhythmias, although the risk of this goes away when the medication is discontinued. Furthermore, propoxyphene has not been shown to alleviate pain any better than acetaminophen. If you have been previously prescribed propoxyphene, contact your health care professional as soon as possible to be switched to another medication to adequately manage pain. Do not abruptly stop taking this medication. It is best to titrate down to avoid withdrawal symptoms such as anxiety, diarrhea, nausea, and shaking. The health care professional may recommend switching to an NSAID, tramadol, tapentadol, or opioid therapy to best accommodate you. Propoxyphene tablets must be properly disposed. Unused propoxyphene should be disposed of in the following manner set forth by the Federal Drug Disposal Guidelines. Before throwing propoxyphene in the trash, take it out of the original container and mix it with coffee grounds or cat litter. By doing so, the drug becomes unattractive for any interested party, including children and pets. Finally, place the unused medication (with the coffee grounds or cat litter) in a zip lock bag or empty can and place it into the garbage bag.

General Opioid Adverse Side Effects

Common opioid side effects, particularly with higher doses, include nausea, vomiting, constipation, thought and memory impairment, and drowsiness. The majority of these side effects can usually be treated with dose adjustments, wane over time (with the exception of constipation), or can be offset by other alternate medications. Psychostimulants can be useful in selected patients to treat mild sedation.

Approximately 40% of individuals taking opioid therapy for non-cancer pain experience constipation (less than three bowel movements per week) secondary to opioid treatment. Most individuals taking opioid medications will not develop tolerance to the side effect/adverse effect of constipation. Therefore, an effective preventive bowel regimen including diet changes and a stimulant laxative plus a stool softener will have to be maintained throughout the course of opioid treatment. Even individuals that utilize appropriate laxative therapy often still experience constipation that may impede the appropriate use of opioid pain medication and thus result in higher levels of pain, so attention to and prevention of this side effect is essential.

Non-pharmacological interventions that can be taken to assist with constipation include: 1) increasing dietary fiber intake, 2) increasing fluid intake, 3) increasing physical activity, and 4) encouraging daily bowel movements at the same time, often after a meal. Pharmacological treatments that can be utilized include stool softeners and stimulant laxatives. In cases that do not respond, other forms of laxative treatment can be considered. Bulk forming laxatives, such as psyllium, are often not useful and can actually worsen opioid-induced constipation by producing colon obstruction. New approaches to treating opioid induced constipation are being developed. Currently, these new medications have only been FDA approved for the postoperative period and the treatment of opioid-induced constipation in patients with advanced illness.

Mild sedation and impaired judgment or coordination also should be anticipated. Until tolerance or a baseline is reached, the patient and family need to be warned against driving and the potential for falls.

Mild nausea is also common with opioid therapy. It can be treated with medications, but if it does not resolve within a few days, a trial of an alternate opioid may be appropriate.

A side effect of long-term opioid use is a decrease in certain hormones, particularly sex hormones. This reduction may cause you to lose your "sex drive," sometimes called libido. This tends to be associated with using these medications regularly for many years.

A serious side effect, particularly in opioid-naïve individuals (those who have not been taking opioids regularly), is respiratory depression (slowed rate of breathing or loss of urge to breathe). Tolerance to respiratory depression occurs with regular opioid use.

A genuine allergy to opioids is very rare. If an allergy does occur, opioids from another class should be chosen. For example, morphine, hydromorphone, oxycodone, and oxymorphone belong to the same class of opioid. Fentanyl and meperidine belong to a different class.

Summary of Possible Opioid Side Effects

- Central nervous system

  - A sense of emotional well-being and euphoria

  - Drowsiness, sedation, and sleep disturbance

  - Hallucinations

  - Potential for diminished psychomotor performance

  - Dysphoria and agitation

  - Dizziness and seizures

  - Aberrant behavior

  - Hyperalgesia

- Respiratory system

  - Respiratory depression is rare but the most serious adverse effect and may result from toxicity

539

- Diminution of pain or pain relief by other modalities may exacerbate respiratory depression
- Ocular system
  - Constriction of the pupil of the eye
- Gastrointestinal system
  - Constipation, nausea and vomiting
  - Delayed gastric emptying
- Genitourinary
  - Urinary retention
- Endocrine
  - Hormonal and sexual dysfunction
- Cardiovascular
  - Decreased blood pressure
  - Slowed heart rate
  - Peripheral edema (swelling)
- Musculoskeletal system
  - Muscle rigidity and contractions
  - Osteoporosis
- Skin system
  - Itching is common and not an allergic reaction
- Immune system
  - There is data suggesting that long term administration of opioids suppresses the immune system. Research is being conducted to determine its clinical significance.
- Pregnancy and breast feeding
  - All opioids cross the placenta
  - No teratogenic effects have been observed
  - Neonatal central nervous system depression can occur if opioids are used during labor; attention to peak times is essential
  - Use with caution in breast feeding; appropriate timing of opioid dose administration is important for safe opioid use during breast feeding

- Analgesic tolerance

  - Decreased duration of analgesia and then decreased effectiveness

- Withdrawal syndrome

  - Withdrawal symptoms may occur with abrupt opioid cessation and can include runny nose, shivering, "gooseflesh," diarrhea, and dilation of the pupil of the cye

Section 47.2

Opioid Use for Chronic, Non-Terminal Pain Is Controversial

"Opiate Use for Chronic Non-Terminal Pain Is Controversial," by David A. Cooke, MD, FACP, © 2013 Omnigraphics. Dr. Cooke is a pain management specialist with the University of Michigan Health Care System.

Treatment of chronic pain that is not due to cancer or other terminal conditions with opiates remains controversial. Although some have advocated liberal use to avoid under-treatment of pain, many experts and government agencies are urging greater caution.

Despite their widespread use for chronic pain, there are actually no published studies of opiate use for more than a year at a time; most studies lasted 12 weeks or less. Long-term toxicity from opiate use is being increasingly recognized, and complications include increased pain, worsening psychiatric disease, hormonal abnormalities, and immunosuppression. Additionally, while estimates vary, the risk of opiate addiction and abuse for patients with chronic pain appears to be much higher than previously believed.

Deaths related to prescription opiate use have skyrocketed in recent years; the Centers for Disease Control and Prevention (CDC) has declared that opiate-related deaths have reached "epidemic" levels. In most parts of the United States, deaths related to prescription opiates now exceed deaths from automobile accidents. Emergency department visits and hospitalizations for complications of prescription opiate use vastly outnumber visits related to heroin use.

There is also recognition among those who treat patients with chronic pain that many patients treated with opiates do not see significant improvements in their function. It is quite common to see patients report constant 10/10 pain and remain homebound, despite taking extremely high doses of opiates. It is difficult to see how they can be said to be benefitting from treatment. Study data suggests that only one third of patients with chronic pain see meaningful improvements with opiate therapy.

Given the increasingly clear toxicities and risk of death, there is an emerging consensus that long-term opiate use should be limited to cases where they result in substantial and meaningful improvements in functionality and quality of life.

If opiates allow people with chronic pain to work full or part-time, participate in volunteer activities, be more active with their families, or perform more self-care, there is meaningful benefit, and continued treatment may be appropriate. If the medication produces subjective pain relief, but does not result in significant changes in any of these domains, opiates should probably be stopped.

As with all medications, opiates should be initially prescribed on a trial basis. If they do not provide significant benefits, they should be stopped. Patients who remain on opiates need to be reassessed regularly. If benefits are lost over time, the opiates should be tapered and stopped. Some patients with chronic pain on heavy doses of opiates see dramatic improvements in their level of function after being weaned off their medications.

The goal of pain management is improvement in function and quality of life. Opiates can sometimes provide these benefits, but also carry very serious risks. For individual patients, the benefits of long-term opiate therapy must clearly outweigh risks.

Chapter 48

Other Medications Used for Pain Management

Antidepressants

One of the most important classes of drugs used to treat chronic pain is the antidepressant group. It is important to note that a response to drugs that were originally developed for psychiatric illness does not mean that the pain is psychiatric in origin. Antidepressant drugs have been used for many years to relieve pain.

There has long been a known association between depression and chronic pain. Not surprisingly, the chemicals (neurotransmitters such as serotonin and norepinephrine) in your brain and nervous system that play a key role in depression are also involved in chronic pain.

- They do not work for pain only by relieving depression. In fact, they work as well for non-depressed people with pain as for those with depression.

- They do not work equally well for all types of pain. For example, they tend to be helpful for fibromyalgia, headache, and pain due to nerve ("neuritic") damage (for example, diabetic neuropathy), but generally are less helpful for most acute musculoskeletal sports-type injuries.

Excerpted from "ACPA Resource Guide to Chronic Pain Medication and Treatment," © 2012 American Chronic Pain Association. All rights reserved. Reprinted with permission. For additional information, visit www.theacpa.org.

- How well they work has little to do with how effective they are as antidepressants. Some very effective antidepressants have virtually no ability to reduce pain.

How Antidepressants May Help

While most people know that pain signals go up the spinal cord to reach the brain, they may not be aware that there are signals coming down the spinal cord that can increase or reduce pain transmission. By increasing levels of chemicals (norepinephrine and serotonin) at nerve endings, antidepressants appear to strengthen the system that inhibits pain transmission.

The antidepressants that increase norepinephrine seem to have better pain relieving capabilities than those that increase scrotonin. This helps to explain why the selective serotonin reuptake inhibitors (SSRIs) work well for depression but do not have the same ability to control pain.

Some antidepressants may be useful in chronic pain because they effectively reduce anxiety and improve sleep without the risks of habit-forming medications. Some people with chronic pain are depressed, and treating the depression may also help reduce the perception of pain. Many people with chronic pain find that antidepressants, along with learning other pain management skills, can help them regain control of their lives and keep their pain under control.

Antidepressants Commonly Used for Chronic Pain

There are three main classes of antidepressant medications used in the management of chronic pain.

Tricyclic antidepressants (TCAs): The first class is the tricyclic antidepressants (TCAs) and includes the antidepressants amitriptyline (Elavil), doxepin (Sinequan), imipramine (Tofranil), desipramine (Norpramin), nortriptyline (Aventyl, Pamelor), protriptyline (Vivactil), trimipramine (Surmontil), and clomipramine (Anafranil). Also included are maprotiline (Ludiomil) and mirtazapine (Remeron), which are tetracyclic antidepressants.

The TCAs have been used to treat depression for a long time. TCAs and related drugs can be roughly divided into those with additional sedative and relaxing properties and those that are less so. Agitated and anxious patients tend to respond best to antidepressants with sedative properties whereas withdrawn individuals and those with less energy will often obtain the most benefit from less sedating antidepressants. These antidepressants have been proven to have pain-relieving effects, typically at lower doses than required to treat depression.

The different tricyclic drugs have varied side effects which may sometimes be used to the patient's advantage. For the overweight patient with lethargy and tiredness, the clinician may choose a TCA with more noradrenergic selectivity (for example, desipramine), which may be activating and can cause some anorexia. Desipramine is considered to have the lowest side effects profile of the TCAs. For others with poor sleep hygiene, the sedating properties of certain TCAs, such as amitriptyline or doxcpin, may be helpful.

Common side effects caused by the tricyclic antidepressants include dry mouth, blurred vision, constipation, difficulty urinating, worsening of glaucoma, impaired thinking, and tiredness. These antidepressants can also lower blood pressure and may cause palpitations (pounding heart). They may increase appetite and be associated with weight gain. Go to the following web site for further information about TCA toxicity: http://www.emedicine.com/emerg/topic616.htm.

Mirtazapine (Remeron) can cause sedation, increased appetite, weight gain, increased cholesterol, dizziness, dry mouth, and constipation.

Selective serotonin reuptake inhibitors SSRIs): The second main class of drugs, the selective serotonin reuptake inhibitors (SSRIs), includes fluoxetine (Prozac), sertraline (Zoloft), paroxetine (Paxil), fluvoxamine (Luvox), citalopram (Celexa), and escitalopram (Lexapro).

The SSRIs have fewer side effects and are less sedating than the tricyclic antidepressants. They are effective for headache prevention but less effective for other types of pain.

SSRIs have been disappointing for neuropathic pain. Most studies of the serotonin-selective type (non-tricyclic) antidepressants have shown little or no pain relief.

Some of the side effects that can be caused by SSRIs include dry mouth, stomach distress with nausea and vomiting, diarrhea, sweating, poor appetite, dizziness, tremors, drowsiness, anxiety, nervousness, insomnia, headache, increased blood pressure, increased heart rate, increased cholesterol levels, and sexual problems.

SSRIs should be used with caution in patients with epilepsy, history of mania, cardiac disease, diabetes, angle-closure glaucoma, concomitant use of drugs that increase risk of bleeding, history of bleeding disorders (especially GI bleeding), disorders of the liver and kidneys, pregnancy and breast-feeding. SSRIs, particularly paroxetine, may also impair performance of skilled tasks (for example, driving) by causing drowsiness. Use within 14 days of an MAO inhibitor should be avoided.

Abrupt withdrawal of SSRIs should be avoided (associated with headache, nausea, burning or tingling sensation in the extremities, dizziness, and anxiety).

While trazodone (Desyrel), venlafaxine (Effexor), bupropion (Wellbutrin, Zyban) and duloxetine (Cymbalta) are often placed into this class of drugs, trazodone is a serotonin-2 receptor antagonist, and venlafaxine, bupropion and duloxetine are mixed norepinephrine and serotonin inhibitors (SNRIs).

Selective serotonin and norepinephrine reuptake inhibitors (SNRIs): The third class includes a number of drugs that are mixed norepinephrine and serotonin inhibitors or SNRIs.

Duloxetine, venlafaxine, milnacipran (Savella) and bupropion are the SNRIs that are most commonly encountered in association with pain management.

Duloxetine has been approved for management of painful diabetic peripheral neuropathy, fibromyalgia, anxiety disorder, depression, and in 2010 for chronic musculoskeletal pain including osteoarthritis and chronic low back pain.

Milnacipran has been approved for the management of fibromyalgia. Milnacipran more potently inhibits the reuptake of norepinephrine than duloxetine and venlafaxine.

These medications have no cholinergic inhibition and, thus, they are associated with fewer side effects.

Venlafaxine has been shown to have therapeutic benefit in the treatment of neuropathic pain. Venlafaxine is available in an extended-release formulation which has a better tolerability profile than the immediate-release formulation. Blood pressure should be monitored in these patients because venlafaxine can increase systolic blood pressure.

Although marketed for different indications, Wellbutrin and Zyban contain the same active ingredient and therefore should not be taken concurrently without close health care professional supervision.

Side effects of SNRIs can include nausea, vomiting, dizziness, sleepiness, trouble sleeping, abnormal dreams, constipation, sweating, dry mouth, yawning, tremor, gas, anxiety, agitation, abnormal vision such as blurred vision or double vision, headache, and sexual dysfunction.

Other antidepressants: Trazodone is a serotonin-2 receptor antagonist. Some of the most common side effects of trazodone are sedation, dry mouth, and nausea. Although trazodone was developed for the treatment of depression, it is more frequently used today to alleviate insomnia.

The monoamine oxidase inhibitors (MAOIs) are generally not used to treat chronic pain. Those such as phenelzine (Nardil), tranylcypromine (Parnate), isocarboxazid (Marplan), and selegiline (Eldepryl) commonly cause weakness, dizziness, headaches, and tremor. While selegiline is used to treat Parkinson disease, the other MAOIs are antidepressants. They also have many drug-drug and drug-food interactions.

Antidepressants have significant implications for drug-drug interactions when used in conjunction with many other medications.

Anticonvulsant (Antiepileptic) Drugs

Anticonvulsant medications have been found to be widely effective in various neuropathic pain conditions.

Several drugs that were developed for the prevention of epileptic seizures (convulsions) have been found to help certain pain conditions. For example, carbamazepine (Carbatrol, Tegretol) is approved by the U.S. Food and Drug Administration (FDA) for relieving the pain of trigeminal neuralgia. Gabapentin (Neurontin) is approved for the management of postherpetic neuralgia (PHN; pain that lasts one to three months after shingles has healed). Pregabalin (Lyrica) is approved for PHN, painful diabetic neuropathic pain, and more recently, fibromyalgia. Nevertheless, most use of anticonvulsants for pain is "off label." Although these medications are not habit forming, abrupt discontinuation can be hazardous. They should be stopped only after discussing how to do so with a health care professional. Common side effects are drowsiness, peripheral edema (lower extremity swelling), and unsteady gait or poor balance. These symptoms tend to diminish over time.

Gabapentin (Neurontin) is widely utilized and has proven to be effective in many people for nerve injury or neuropathic pain. Decreased mental alertness or awareness is possible at higher doses (for example, 3600 mg/day) but this is variable and is person specific. Generic gabapentin is now available. A similar but newer drug, pregabalin (Lyrica), has been found effective in postherpetic neuralgia, fibromyalgia, and diabetic neuropathy. Its primary advantage over gabapentin is thought to be pregabalin's longer duration of action, allowing a twice daily dosing and improved absorption; however, there is no evidence that this translates to an increased clinical effect. Pregabalin is not associated with significant drug interactions and can be used over a wide dose range (150–600 mg/day). Its side effect profile is similar to gabapentin, and it is generally well tolerated. Side effects are mostly mild to moderate and transient, with dizziness and somnolence being the most common. Other adverse effects include dry mouth, peripheral edema, blurred vision, weight gain, and concentration or attention difficulties. Often gabapentin and pregabalin require a period of time before their effectiveness in treating a patient's pain is seen because the medications need to be titrated to the appropriate dose. Recently, the FDA has issued a warning on the use of anticonvulsants and the risks of suicidal thoughts and suicide. Patients utilizing anticonvulsants for pain control should be monitored for any signs and symptoms of suicidal thoughts.

Anticonvulsants Possibly Useful in Chronic Pain

Only gabapentin and pregabalin are approved by the FDA and for which there is solid evidence of efficacy in general neuropathic pain.

- **Gabapentin (Neurontin):** Has proven to be effective in some people for nerve injury or neuropathic pain. Seems safer, easier to use. Some mental fuzziness possible at higher doses.

- **Pregabalin (Lyrica):** Found effective in postherpetic neuralgia and diabetic neuropathy. Some advantage over gabapentin. It is generally well tolerated.

- **Carbamazepine (Tegretol):** Interacts with some other drugs, can affect the liver and white blood cells. Used for trigeminal neuralgia.

- **Valproic acid (Depakote):** Used in headache or nerve pain. May affect platelets as an adverse effect.

- **Phenytoin (Dilantin):** Stronger evidence supports the use of the above agents over phenytoin. The risk of adverse effects and drug interactions also precludes its regular use.

- **Clonazepam (Klonopin):** A benzodiazepine (Valium, Xanax family).

- **Lamotrigine (Lamictal):** May be useful for pain refractory to carbamazepine. Used in trigeminal neuralgia, central pain. May cause dizziness, constipation, nausea, decreased mental awareness, etc.

- **Tiagabine (Gabitril):** Used in combination with other anticonvulsant agents in the management of partial seizures. Possibly useful in treating neuropathic pain. Most common side effects include nonspecific dizziness, drowsiness, and difficulty with concentration. Has been associated with new onset seizures and status epilepticus in patients without epilepsy.

- **Lacosamide (Vimpat):** Lacosamide is being studied as an anticonvulsant with potential for reducing diabetic neuropathic pain.

- **Topiramate (Topamax):** Generally well tolerated but sometimes causes confusion, dizziness, fatigue, and problems with coordination and concentration. Possibly useful in treating neuropathic and sympathetically maintained pain. It is also being used as a preventive migraine treatment. Side effects include strange sensations and loss of appetite. May cause secondary angle closure glaucoma and, if left untreated, may lead to permanent vision loss. It may also cause dose-related weight loss, and cause or predispose to kidney stones.

- **Levetiracetam (Keppra):** Indicated for use as adjunctive therapy in the treatment of partial seizures in adults. It is possibly effective in neuropathic pain.

- **Oxcarbazepine (Trileptal):** Indicated for the treatment of partial seizures. Possibly useful in treating neuropathic pain. Probably useful for trigeminal neuralgia.

- **Zonisamide (Zonegran):** Indicated for use as adjunctive therapy for treatment of partial seizures (or focal seizures) in adults with epilepsy. Possibly useful in treating neuropathic pain.

Sodium Channel Blocking and Oral Anti-Arrhythmic Agents

Intravenous lidocaine has strong sodium channel blocking properties and has demonstrated efficacy in several uncontrolled studies on neuropathic pain. Some pain centers used intravenous lidocaine both as a diagnostic tool to assess responsiveness to a subsequent oral sodium channel blocker (for example, mexiletine, oxcarbazepine, and carbamazepine) as well as a therapeutic tool when delivered in an inpatient setting.

Those anti-arrhythmics with local anesthetic properties are occasionally used in refractory or difficult to treat pain. They are approved for the prevention of disturbances in heart rhythm but, just as they interrupt premature firing of heart fibers, they also diminish premature firing of damaged nerves. This leads to less firing of the nerve, and hence less capability of the nerve to trigger pain.

Due to safety concerns, the only anti-arrhythmics that are used for chronic pain are mexiletine (Mexitil) and flecainide (Tambocor). They reduce pain in diabetic neuropathy, post stroke pain, complex regional pain syndrome (CRPS) or reflex sympathetic dystrophy (RSD), and traumatic nerve injury.

Mexiletine is chemically similar to lidocaine, an anesthetic frequently used by dentists. Common side effects of mexiletine include dizziness, anxiety, unsteadiness when walking, heartburn, nausea, and vomiting. Consult a health care professional if you are pregnant, have a history of heart attack, are a smoker, or take any of the following medications: amiodarone, fluvoxamine, dofetilide (Tikosyn), bupropion, or sodium bicarbonate. It should be taken three times daily with food to lessen stomach irritation. Infrequent adverse reactions include sore throat, fever, mouth sores, blurred vision, confusion, constipation, diarrhea, headache, and numbness or tingling in the hands and feet. Serious symptoms occur with overdose including seizures, convulsions, chest pain, shortness of breath, irregular or fast heartbeat, and cardiac arrest.

Flecainide (Tambocor) was approved to treat arrhythmias and can slow a fast heart rate. It has also been effective for treating certain painful conditions related to neuropathic pain. Although cardiac side effects with flecainide may be infrequent, they can be catastrophic. Therefore, an ECG is recommended before treatment is started, and this drug should probably not be used for pain management in patients with a history of CVD or heart failure because it may cause your heart rate to slow. Inform your health care professional if you have kidney or liver problems, because this may lead to monitoring of drug levels or a dosage reduction. Flecainide interacts with amiodarone, several anti-psychotic and anti-arrhythmic medications, and ranolazine (Ranexa). Common side effects, which usually occur within the first two to four weeks of therapy, are nausea or vomiting, constipation, headache, dizziness, visual disturbances, edema, and tremor.

Sedatives, Anti-Anxiety Medications, and Tranquilizers

Proper sleep hygiene is critical to the individual with chronic pain and often is hard to obtain. Various medications may provide short-term benefit. While sleeping pills, so-called minor tranquilizers, and anti-anxiety agents are commonly prescribed in chronic pain, pain specialists rarely, if ever, recommend them for long-term use. They can be habit-forming, and they may impair function and memory more than opioid pain relievers. There is also concern that they may increase pain and depression over the long-term.

Zolpidem tartrate (Ambien) is a non-benzodiazepine and is used for the short-term treatment of insomnia (difficulty falling asleep, staying asleep, or early awakening). Side effects that are more common may include allergy, daytime drowsiness, dizziness, drugged feeling, headache, indigestion, and nausea. Some people using Ambien, especially those taking serotonin-boosting antidepressants, have experienced unusual changes in their thinking and/or behavior. Ambien and other sleep medicines can cause a special type of memory loss. Older adults, in particular, should be aware that they may be more apt to fall. Ambien should be used with caution in people who have liver problems. If it is taken for more than a week or two, it should not be stopped abruptly. It should not be used in people who use alcohol. It can increase the drug's side effects. If you have breathing problems, they may become worse when you use Ambien.

Another sleep aid, eszopiclone (Lunesta), reportedly has fewer side effects and can be taken for longer periods of time. Initial testing suggests fewer side effects than other sleep medications, but individuals taking eszopiclone or any other sedative drug may develop dependence on the drug for sleep. They may also experience withdrawal symptoms when the drug is discontinued. The most common side effects of eszopiclone are dizziness and loss of coordination.

Ramelteon (Rozerem) is a melatonin receptor agonist with high affinity for MT-1 and MT-2 receptors. These receptors are believed to regulate the body's circadian rhythm. It is indicated for the treatment of insomnia characterized by difficulty with sleep onset. According to the manufacturer, the most common adverse effects are somnolence, dizziness, and fatigue. The recommended dose is 8 mg nightly, taken within 30 minutes of going to bed. Ramelteon has been shown to be safe and effective to use for up to one year. Ramelteon should not be taken with fluvoxamine (Luvox) or given to patients with severe liver disease.

Many pain specialists believe that anxiety and insomnia in those with chronic pain are best treated with antidepressants when possible.

Non-medication approaches to proper sleep hygiene are best but are not the focus of the "ACPA Resource Guide to Chronic Pain Medication and Treatment" [from which this information is excerpted].

Benzodiazepines

Most people experience anxiety at one time or another in their lives. Anxiety can present as nervousness or sweaty palms, irritability, uneasiness, feelings of apprehension, tight muscles, and difficulty sleeping. Anxiety is often mild, but if it becomes severe, counseling or medications may be needed. The most widely prescribed drugs for anxiety are benzodiazepines, like diazepam (Valium), lorazepam (Ativan), clonazepam (Klonopin), flurazepam (Dalmane), triazolam (Halcion), temazepam (Restoril), and alprazolam (Xanax). They are also used as muscle relaxants and for insomnia (difficulty sleeping). Their use as sleep aids is limited as they do not work well when used continuously each night to produce sleep.

One of these benzodiazepines, diazepam (Valium), is recognized for causing depression and physical dependence when used for long periods.

Most benzodiazepines are not recommended for chronic pain, but clonazepam (Klonopin) is an anticonvulsant that appears to have some use with neuropathic pain.

Side effects are similar to those of alcohol and include sedation, slurred speech, and gait unsteadiness. Other adverse reactions include chest pain and a pounding heartbeat, psychological changes, headache, nausea, restlessness, vision problems, nightmares, and unexplained fatigue. Alcohol and tobacco should be avoided while taking these drugs.

Because of withdrawal symptoms, these drugs should be discontinued slowly under a health care professional's supervision. Withdrawal reactions may be mistaken for anxiety since many of the symptoms are similar. Left unattended, benzodiazepine withdrawal can be associated with seizures or even death.

Muscle Relaxants

Many drugs have been marketed as muscle relaxants, even though most do not seem to have any direct effect on muscle. Perhaps they should be called "brain relaxants," since they are all sedating, and this may be how they actually work. Sedation is a concern for those who drive, operate machinery, or otherwise are engaged in safety sensitive jobs. Some also have analgesic (pain reducing) properties. Cyclobenzaprine (Flexeril, Amrix–extended release) is chemically similar to the tricyclic antidepressants and may have a similar mechanism. Muscle relaxants have limited efficacy in chronic pain but may be used to treat acute flare-ups. There are no studies to support the long-term use of muscle relaxants, especially for low back pain. Also, the long-term use of muscle relaxants for low back pain does not improve functional recovery and can also hinder recovery.

Drugs Used as Muscle Relaxants in Chronic Pain

- **Carisoprodol (Soma):** Converted by the body into meprobamate, a barbiturate-like drug. It may cause physical dependence. It should be avoided in kidney or liver disease. With prolonged use, it is associated with dependence. Long-term use in chronic pain should be avoided.

- **Cyclobenzaprine (Flexeril, Amrix):** Skeletal muscle relaxant that is structurally similar to the TCAs. Side effects include dizziness, drowsiness, dry mouth, constipation, confusion, and loss of balance. Long-term use in chronic pain should be avoided.

- **Methocarbamol (Robaxin):** Skeletal muscle relaxant with sedative properties. Side effects include drowsiness and urine discoloration to brown, black, or green.

- **Metaxalone (Skelaxin):** Skeletal muscle relaxant. It should be used with caution in liver disease.

- **Chlorzoxazone (Parafon Forte DSC):** Skeletal muscle relaxant with sedative properties. It should be used with caution in liver disease.

- **Baclofen (Lioresal):** Reduces spasticity after neurological illness or injury. Withdrawal should not be abrupt and can be life-threatening (mainly with intrathecal therapy). Inhibits transmission at the spinal level and also depresses the central nervous system. The dose should be increased slowly to avoid the major side effects of sedation and muscle weakness (other adverse events are uncommon). Baclofen is known to be safer for long-term use.

- **Dantrolene (Dantrium):** A true muscle relaxant that acts directly on skeletal muscle and produces fewer central adverse effects. Can have significant liver toxicity. The dose should be increased slowly.

- **Orphenadrine (Norflex):** A skeletal muscle relaxant with analgesic properties.

- **Tizanidine (Zanaflex):** A drug indicated for spasticity associated with multiple sclerosis or spinal cord injury but being used off label for chronic pain. This drug may increase liver enzyme levels. Tizanidine interacts with blood pressure medications and causes low blood pressure.

- **Diazepam (Valium):** Other benzodiazepines also have muscle-relaxant properties. Most pain specialists avoid prescribing diazepam for muscle spasm. Toxicity of benzodiazepines is discussed at www.emedicine.com/emerg/topic58.htm.

Anti-Psychotic Medications

This class of drugs was marketed primarily because of its ability to reduce hallucinations and psychotic thinking, although some members of the class are used to treat nausea and migraine.

Common ones include chlorpromazine (Thorazine), aripiprazole (Abilify), clozapine (Clozaril), haloperidol (Haldol), olanzapine (Zyprexa, Zydis), quetiapine (Seroquel), risperidone (Risperdal), and ziprasidone (Geodon).

In general, their use in chronic pain is poorly established, and they have the potential to cause a permanent neurological condition called tardive dyskinesia. In mild cases, this consists of movements of the mouth and tongue, which is mostly a cosmetic problem; however, in more severe cases there can be severe muscle activity that interferes with ability to function and even to breathe. For these reasons, they are usually considered "last resort" drugs. Toxicity of anti-psychotics is discussed at http://www.emedicine.com/EMERG/topic338.htm.

Anti-Hypertensive Medications

Clonidine (Catapres, Catapres-TTS patch) is a centrally acting alpha-agonist that lowers blood pressure and has also been shown to have pain-relieving properties in sympathetically maintained pain conditions such as complex regional pain syndrome (CRPS) or reflex sympathetic dystrophy (RSD). It is available as tablets for oral administration, as an injectable solution for administration in an epidural or implanted pump, or as a once-weekly patch.

Side effects can include dry mouth, drowsiness, dizziness, and constipation. Transient localized skin reactions can occur with the patch.

It should not be discontinued suddenly as this can result in symptoms such as nervousness, agitation, headache, and tremor accompanied or followed by a rapid rise in blood pressure. Some individuals can develop an allergy to clonidine with a generalized rash, itching, or swelling. It should be used with caution in patients with severe heart disease, cerebrovascular disease (stroke), or chronic kidney failure. To avoid hypertensive crisis, clonidine should not be used with tricyclic antidepressants.

Botulinum Toxins

Botulinum toxins, BOTOX (onabotulinumtoxinA), Dysport (abobotulinumtoxinA), Xeomin (incobotulinumtoxinA) and Myobloc (rimabotulinumtoxinB) have been found to be effective in decreasing tone in overactive (hypertonic) muscles, which may be present in a number of chronic pain conditions. A recent review article by Dr. Bahman Jabbari summarizes that botulinum toxins have the most evidence to control pain of cervical dystonia, chronic migraine, and chronic lateral epicondylitis—tennis elbow (*Pain Med* 2011; 12:1594-1606). There appears to be pain relieving properties of botulinum toxin Type A irrespective of muscle relaxation.

Botox, Dysport, Xeomin and Myobloc are FDA approved for the treatment of the postural abnormalities and pain associated with cervical dystonia—also known as torticollis (head tilting, neck pain, and neck muscle spasms). Only one botulinum toxin (BOTOX, onabotulinumtoxinA) is approved by the FDA for the treatment of chronic migraine type headache and spasticity treatment in the upper limb in adults.

The efficacy of botulinum toxins in back, neck, and extremity muscle pain has been studied, off label, with mixed results. In some studies on myofascial pain, botulinum toxin has not been found to be more effective than traditional trigger point injections with local anesthetic or saline.

The dosage unit for botulinum toxins are unique to each product and are not interchangeable. In addition the FDA has specified new nonproprietary names for each drug to help prevent medication errors. Many physicians are using botulinum toxins off-label for other painful conditions including other types of headache, osteoarthritis of the knee and shoulder, and various muscle pain syndromes (myofascial pain) although the evidence for such use is not conclusive.

Botulinum toxins typically demonstrate efficacy within three to five days after intramuscular administration and lasts for an average of 12 weeks.

Side effects may occur after receiving botulinum (see FDA warning below). Muscle weakness is the most common side effect. Swallowing problems can develop when treating cervical muscle problems, especially with injections into the sternocleidomastoid muscle. Other adverse effects include dry mouth, pain at the injection site, swallowing problems, neck pain, headache, and flu-like symptoms. Additionally, adverse effects may include local bruising, generalized fatigue, lethargy, dizziness, and difficulty speaking or hoarseness.

FDA Warning: Distant Spread of Botulinum Toxin Effect

Postmarketing reports indicate that the effects all botulinum toxin products may spread from the area of injection to produce symptoms consistent with botulinum toxin effects. These may include asthenia, generalized muscle weakness, diplopia, ptosis, dysphagia, dysphonia, dysarthria, urinary incontinence, and breathing difficulties. These symptoms have been reported hours to weeks after injection. Swallowing and breathing difficulties can be life threatening and there have been reports of death. The risk of symptoms is probably greatest in children treated for spasticity but symptoms can also occur in adults treated for spasticity and other conditions, particularly in those patients who have an underlying condition that would predispose them to these symptoms. In unapproved uses, including spasticity in children, and in approved indications, cases of spread of effect have been reported at doses comparable to those used to treat cervical dystonia and at lower doses.

Migraine Headache Treatment

Migraine headache treatment has been revolutionized with the advent of the triptans. These include sumatriptan (Imitrex—also available by injection or nasal spray), zolmitriptan (Zomig—also available by nasal spray or as orally disintegrating tablets), naratriptan (Amerge), rizatriptan (Maxalt—also available as orally disintegrating tablets) and almotriptan (Axert). More recently introduced triptans include frovatriptan (Frova) and eletriptan (Relpax).

The key to effective treatment, however, is still a combination of avoidance of migraine triggers, stress management, and relaxation techniques, and non-medication symptom relief through the use of locally applied heat or cold, massage, hot showers, and rest in a quiet, darkened room. Some people benefit from complementary or alternative therapies such as relaxation techniques, training in self-hypnosis, biofeedback, yoga, aromatherapy, acupuncture, spinal manipulation, and homeopathic remedies.

Unfortunately, while migraine headaches can now be better controlled, it is unrealistic to expect instant, complete or permanent pain relief for what is essentially a chronic, recurring disease.

Effective migraine treatment begins with the early recognition that an attack is pending followed by immediate treatment. Migraine sufferers are encouraged to take an active role in managing their headaches by avoiding common triggers, making lifestyle changes, and taking their medication at the first sign of migraine pain.

For patients who are diagnosed with chronic migraine, a neurological disorder characterized by patients who experience headaches on 15 or more days per month with headaches lasting four hours a day or longer, BOTOX was granted approval in 2010 as a preventive treatment option. It is not known whether BOTOX is safe or effective to prevent headaches in patients with migraine who have 14 or fewer headache days each month (episodic migraine).

Patients taking certain migraine and antidepressant medications together may be at risk for a dangerous chemical imbalance.

Antidepressant medications included in this warning are Prozac, Zoloft, Paxil, Lexapro, Cymbalta, and Effexor. Migraine drugs include Amerge, Axert, Imitrex, and Zomig. Serotonin is a brain hormone that keeps our mood stable and our appetite in check, as well as serving other functions. When you take two or more drugs that affect serotonin levels, it can increase the amount of serotonin and may lead to bothersome or dangerous symptoms. This is called "serotonin syndrome."

An excellent medical review on migraine headaches can be found in the *Cleveland Clinic Journal of Medicine* in January 2003 at www .ccjm.org/pdffiles/Mannix103.pdf.

Treximet is a product that was FDA-approved in August 2008 as a combination medication for migraine treatment that contains naproxen 500 mg and sumatriptan 85 mg. Treximet works to relieve the pain of migraines in two ways; the sumatriptan portion works by increasing the amount of the hormone serotonin in the blood vessels and causing constriction of the arteries in the head, and the naproxen works to decrease inflammation and pain. Treximet has a "Black Box Warning" with cardiovascular and gastrointestinal (GI) risks. This combination may cause an increased risk of serious cardiovascular complications including heart attack and stroke. Also since this product contains naproxen (an NSAID) there is an increased risk of GI adverse reactions including bleeding, ulceration, and perforation of stomach or intestines. Caution should be used in patients with a history of kidney or liver disease.

Chapter 49

Corticosteroid Injections for Relieving Pain

Cortisone is a type of steroid that is produced naturally by a gland in your body called the adrenal gland. Cortisol is released from the adrenal gland when your body is under stress. Natural cortisone is released into the blood stream and is relatively short-acting.

Injectable cortisone is synthetically produced and has many different trade names (e.g., Celestone, Kenalog, etc.), but is a close derivative of your body's own product. The most significant differences are that synthetic cortisone is not injected into the blood stream, but into a particular area of inflammation. Also, the synthetic cortisone is designed to act more potently and for a longer period of time (days instead of minutes).

Steroids are a group of molecular compounds that all share some common structural characteristics. Not all different steroids are the same! Types of steroids include cortisone, cholesterol, and sex hormones. Cortisone is not the same type of steroid as a performance enhancing drug.

How It Helps

Cortisone is a powerful anti-inflammatory medication. Cortisone is not a pain relieving medication; it only treats the inflammation. When pain is decreased from cortisone it is because the inflammation

"What Is a Cortisone Shot?" © 2013 Jonathan Cluett, M.D. (http://orthopedics .about.com/). Used with permission of About Inc., which can be found online at www.about.com. All rights reserved.

is diminished. By injecting the cortisone into a particular area of inflammation, very high concentrations of the medication can be given while keeping potential side-effects to a minimum. Cortisone injections usually work within a few days, and the effects can last up to several weeks.

Why Use Cortisone

Many conditions where inflammation is an underlying problem are amenable to cortisone shots. These include, but are certainly not limited to:

- Shoulder bursitis

- Arthritis

- Trigger finger

- Tennis elbow

- Carpal tunnel syndrome

Painful Shot?

The shot can be slightly painful, especially when given into a joint, but in skilled hands it usually is well tolerated. Often the cortisone injection can be performed with a very small needle that causes little discomfort. However, sometimes a slightly larger needle must be used, especially if your physician is attempting to removed fluid through the needle prior to injecting the cortisone. Numbing medication, such as Lidocaine or Marcaine, is often injected with the cortisone to provide temporary relief of the affected area. Also, topical anesthetics can help numb the skin in an area being injected.

Side-Effects of Cortisone

Yes. Probably the most common side-effect is a "cortisone flare," a condition where the injected cortisone crystallizes and can cause a brief period of pain worse than before the shot. This usually lasts a day or two and is best treated by icing the injected area. Another common side-effect is whitening of the skin where the injection is given. This is only a concern in people with darker skin, and is not harmful, but patients should be aware of this.

Other side-effects of cortisone injections, although rare, can be quite serious. The most concerning is infection, especially if the injection is given into a joint. The best prevention is careful injection technique, with sterilization of the skin using iodine and/or alcohol. Also, patients with diabetes may have a transient increase in their blood sugar which they should watch for closely.

Because cortisone is a naturally occurring substance, true allergic responses to the injected substance do not occur. However, it is possible to be allergic to other aspects of the injection, most commonly the Betadine many physicians use to sterilize the skin.

How Much Cortisone?

There is no rule as to how many cortisone injections can be given. Often physicians do not want to give more than three, but there is not really a specific limit to the number of shots. However, there are some practical limitations. If a cortisone injection wears off quickly or does not help the problem, then repeating it may not be worthwhile. Also, animal studies have shown effects of weakening of tendons and softening of cartilage with cortisone injections. Repeated cortisone injections multiply these effects and increase the risk of potential problems. This is the reason many physicians limit the number of injections they offer to a patient.

Sources

Cole BJ and Schumacher HR "Injectable Corticosteroids in Modern Practice" *J. Am. Acad. Ortho. Surg.*, January/February 2005; 13:37–46.

Fadale PD and Wiggins ME "Corticosteroid Injections: Their Use and Abuse" *J. Am. Acad. Ortho. Surg.*, May 1994; 2:133–140.

Chapter 50

Invasive and Implanted Pain Interventions

Intra-Articular Steroid Injections

Invasive therapeutic interventions for osteoarthritis include steroids injections into the joint. Intra-articular steroids are effective for short-term (one to three weeks) pain relief but do not seem to improve function or to provide pain relief for longer time periods. The number of steroid injections should be limited secondary to associated side effects including fat necrosis, loss of skin pigmentation, skin atrophy, avascular necrosis of the femoral head, and in some cases acceleration of joint degeneration. Following a steroid injection, the treated joint should be rested (limit its use) for a minimum of 24 hours in order to prolong and to improve effects on function and pain control.

Viscosupplementation

Viscosupplementation may also be used for osteoarthritis (OA) of the knee. Viscosupplementation involves injecting lubricating substances (hyaluronic and hylan derivatives) into the knee joint in order to restore the lubrication of the joint and, therefore, decrease pain and improve mobility. Although viscosupplementation may be effective short term treatment for osteoarthritis of the knee, the improvements in pain and

---

Excerpted from "ACPA Resource Guide to Chronic Pain Medication and Treatment," © 2012 American Chronic Pain Association. All rights reserved. Reprinted with permission. For additional information, visit www.theacpa.org.

function are relatively small. Viscosupplementation seems to have a more prolonged pain relieving effect than intra-articular steroids.

There are currently five available products on the market; Orthovisc, Synvisc, Hyalgan, Supartz, and Euflexxa. In 2009, Synvisc-One (hylan G-F 20) was approved as a single-injection viscosupplement for the treatment of OA knee pain in the United States.

Spinal Cord Stimulation (SCS)

Neurostimulation therapy is delivered with a small device implanted under the skin, typically in the abdomen or buttock area. The neurostimulator generates mild electrical signals, which are delivered to an area near the spine. The impulses travel from the device to this spinal area over thin insulated wires called leads.

Medical researchers are still investigating how SCS exactly controls pain and are considering multiple theories. One is the gate control theory, which was the originally proposed mechanism of action of SCS. This theory states that by providing a pleasant vibratory and touch sensation via the SCS system, pain signals that reach the brain are decreased. Recently, it has been discovered that spinal cord stimulation modifies the chemical makeup of the spinal cord.

The current SCS devices are programmable via a remote control, which allows the patient to adjust the therapy within certain limits to help them receive the best pain relief each day, depending on their activity level or changes in pain during the day. It is not uncommon for patients being considered for a SCS to have a psychological evaluation as a part of the overall evaluation process. These are often done by psychologists or psychiatrists. The purpose of this evaluation is to see if there are any emotional or other difficulties in your life that may adversely affect the surgery or your recovery. During the psychological evaluation, you can expect to be asked questions about how the pain is currently affecting your sleep, mood, relationships and your work, household and recreational activities. You may also be asked to complete some paper-and-pencil tests as well. The results of this evaluation should be shared with you and with your doctor who will consider all the information to determine if you are a good candidate for a SCS.

Two stages are involved in SCS implantation. In both stages, a physician, guided by an x-ray, places a lead into the epidural space located within the bony spinal canal. The first stage is the trial phase, which provides information to predict the success of permanent implantation.

Together, the healthcare provider and the patient decide whether or not to advance to permanent implantation. In this stage, the lead is again placed and implanted underneath the skin with a power source the size of a pacemaker battery. Either a rechargeable or non-rechargeable power source is implanted. For the non-rechargeable systems, the battery cannot be recharged and needs replacement every several years with a minor surgical procedure. The rechargeable system needs recharging when the power source runs low. While it typically lasts longer (up to nine years) than a conventional system, eventually it will need to be replaced with a minor surgical procedure when it can no longer be recharged in a reasonable period of time. The SCS recipient goes home with a remote-control and battery charger (if they have a rechargeable battery). The patient is instructed to limit activity for about 12 weeks to allow for healing.

The reader should understand that this discussion of SCS systems is limited. These devices are expensive, and their use is limited to selected individuals as a treatment alternative for specific conditions, after consideration of the risks, after failure of a reasonable trial of less invasive methods, and following a successful temporary trial. A psychological evaluation is recommended prior to implantation.

When utilized, spinal cord stimulation should be part of an overall rehabilitation treatment strategy combining behavioral and physical medicine approaches to pain management. Effectively treating pain by implanting an SCS system requires a responsive, long-term relationship between the person with pain and his or her healthcare provider. A significant advantage of a SCS system is that it is a reversible and nondestructive treatment option.

Occasional re-programming will be needed to optimize coverage of the painful area.

Furthermore, it is important for the patient and healthcare provider to have realistic expectations regarding treatment, with the goal being pain reduction and control rather than complete elimination. As with most treatments for chronic pain, it is important for people with SCS to involve themselves in a multidisciplinary treatment plan if they are to get the best results. In appropriately selected individuals, SCS treatment can be an important tool in a treatment plan and significantly reduces pain and associated limitations.

In general terms, spinal cord stimulation is primarily suited to certain neuropathic and ischemic (loss of oxygenated blood flow) pain states. Currently, conditions that can respond favorably to SCS treatment include:

* Failed back surgery syndrome

* Complex regional pain syndrome (previously known as RSD and causalgia)

- Peripheral neuropathic pain

- Peripheral vascular disease

- Ischemic heart disease

SCS has been proven to be effective for many of these conditions with lasting results in terms of pain relief, pain medication reduction, and improvement in quality-of-life indices and satisfaction scores. Although SCS can also be quite effective in relieving ischemic pain due to peripheral vascular disease and even coronary artery disease, these are currently not U.S. Food and Drug Administration (FDA)-approved indications.

Potential complications that may occur include lead migration or fracture and infection. Lead migration after implantation may require revision surgery to regain appropriate coverage. An infection of any kind requires an immediate assessment by the physician. An unrecognized and untreated infection around the hardware can progress to more serious complications such as an epidural abscess or meningitis.

Implanted Intrathecal Drug Delivery Systems ("Pain Pumps")

Unlike medications that circulate through your body and in your bloodstream, intrathecal drug delivery systems release medication directly into the fluid surrounding your spinal cord, which may lead to fewer or more tolerable side effects, and in some instances is the only route possible for certain drugs.

With Intrathecal Drug Delivery Therapy

- Pain medication is delivered via a drug pump directly to the fluid around the spinal cord, in an area called the intrathecal space.

- The drug pump is connected to a thin, flexible tube called a catheter.

- Both the pump and the catheter are surgically implanted under the skin.

The reader should understand that this discussion of implanted drug delivery systems is limited.

These systems are expensive, and their use is limited to selected individuals as an end-stage treatment alternative for specific conditions, after consideration of the risks, after failure of a reasonable trial of less invasive methods, and following a successful temporary trial. It is not uncommon for patients being considered for an intrathecal pump to have a psychological evaluation as a part of the overall evaluation process. These are often done by psychologists or psychiatrists. The purpose of this evaluation is to see if there are any emotional or other difficulties in your life that may adversely affect the surgery or your recovery. During the psychological evaluation, you can expect to be asked questions about how the pain is currently affecting your sleep, mood, relationships and your work, household and recreational activities. You may also be asked to complete some paper-and-pencil tests as well. The results of this evaluation should be shared with you and with your doctor who will consider all the information to determine if you are a good candidate for an intrathecal pump.

A decision to proceed with an implanted drug delivery system should include:

- Failure of six months of other conservative treatment modalities (medication, surgical, psychological or physical);

- Intractable pain secondary to a disease state with objective documentation of pathology;

- Documentation that further surgical intervention is not indicated;

- Psychological evaluation has been obtained and evaluation states that the pain is not primarily psychological in origin and that benefit would occur with implantation despite any psychiatric comorbidity;

- No contraindications to implantation exist such as sepsis or coagulopathy; and

- If the above criteria are met, a temporary trial of spinal (epidural or intrathecal) opiates has been successful prior to permanent implantation as defined by at least a 50% to 70% reduction in pain and documentation in the medical record of improved function and associated reduction in oral pain medication use.

Opioids (for example, morphine) are the most common medications delivered by intraspinal infusion. Other medications (bupivacaine, clonidine, and baclofen) may be added to opioids, particularly in patients with nerve injury pain states (neuropathic pain). In patients with intraspinal infusions, monitoring is needed to check for the development of a mass at the tip of the catheter. Numerous case reports have recently been published demonstrating granulomas (an abnormal tissue growth) at the tip of these catheters which can compress the spinal cord or associated nerve roots. The doses of intraspinal opioids should be limited to the lowest dose possible required to achieve pain relief.

Constipation, urinary retention, nausea, vomiting, and pruritus are typical early adverse effects of intrathecal morphine and are readily managed symptomatically. Other potential adverse effects include amenorrhea, loss of libido, edema, respiratory depression, and technical issues with the intrathecal system.

Ziconotide (Prialt) is a non-opioid analgesic used for the management of severe chronic pain and is reserved for patients intolerant or refractory to other therapies. The drug is delivered intrathecally, that is, by continuous infusion through a pump directly into the fluid surrounding the spinal cord. Common side effects include dizziness, nausea, vomiting, confusional states, and nystagmus (inability to control eye movements). Rarely, adverse events such as meningitis, psychosis, convulsions, and rhabdomyolysis (muscle breakdown) have been reported. Ziconotide should be titrated slowly to the appropriate therapeutic effect.

The only drugs that have been approved by the FDA for continuous intrathecal use with implanted intrathecal delivery devices include ziconotide, morphine, and baclofen.

Epidurals, Nerve and Facet Blocks, and Radiofrequency Ablation (Rhizotomy)

An epidural steroid injection involves the injection of steroid into the epidural space in the cervical spine (neck) or lumbar spine (low back). Sometimes, a local anesthetic (numbing medicine) may be injected with the steroid. The epidural space is located in the spine just outside of the sac containing the spinal fluid. Epidural steroid injections are often provided to individuals with herniated discs, degenerative disc disease, or spinal stenosis that have associated nerve pain in their arm or leg. The steroids are injected into the epidural space in order to reduce inflammation in and surrounding the spinal nerve roots and adjacent tissues. By reducing inflammation and compression, the level of pain may be decreased. Epidurals are most useful in patients with acute nerve pain from the above conditions. Since a majority of individuals (80 to 90%) with acute low back pain and associated nerve pain will recover spontaneously within three months, these injections should be viewed as a way to facilitate earlier pain relief and return to function. These injections have not been demonstrated to provide long-term successful pain relief for patients solely suffering from chronic (long-standing) back pain or chronic nerve pain. Epidurals rarely provide long lasting benefit but may be useful in these chronic pain conditions for a flare-up. Some patients who have residual pain after the first injection may receive a second epidural steroid injection. Patients who do not receive any relief from the first injection are unlikely to benefit from a second injection. Furthermore, the number of steroid injection per year should be limited in order to avoid side effects that may occur including osteoporosis (weakening of the bones) and avascular necrosis (bone cell death often seen in the hip). Diabetic patients receiving epidural steroids should monitor their blood sugars closely following the procedure since elevations can occur.

Nerve and facet blocks use a combination of local anesthetic and steroid for diagnostic purposes to identify pain generators. These blocks can also be used therapeutically to "block" a painful condition. Unfortunately, these procedures do not provide lasting benefit and are best used as part of an overall treatment plan to relieve discomfort temporarily while engaging in an active rehabilitation program.

Radiofrequency ablation (rhizotomy) or lesioning involves inserting a probe to destroy the nerve that supplies the facet joint. The facet joint, a small joint that connects the back portion of your spine, can become arthritic and cause neck or back pain. Facet joints allow you to bend and twist your back and neck. For an individual with facet joint disease, these movements can be very painful and may limit daily activities. Patients with lumbar (low back) facet joint syndrome often complain of (1) hip and buttock pain, (2) low back stiffness and (3) pain that is made worse by prolonged sitting or standing. Patients with cervical (neck) facet joint syndrome often complain of (1) neck pain, (2) headache, and/or (3) shoulder pain. In addition, they will often have pain when they rotate or bend their neck.

In order to determine if facet joints are responsible for neck or back pain, medial branch blocks are performed. A medial branch block is a block that is performed under fluoroscopy (x-ray), and local anesthetic (numbing medicine) is injected on the nerves in the back or neck that supply the facet joint. Following the procedure, patients are asked to keep a pain diary to record any pain relief, the amount of pain relief, and for how long. Based on the response to this block, it can be determined if you are a candidate for medial branch radiofrequency ablation (rhizotomy). Patient selection is important to achieving successful results.

Following radiofrequency ablation, patients are often asked to resume physical therapy for flexibility and strengthening exercises. Radiofrequency usually blocks the signal for a prolonged period of time (six months to a year). Eventually, the nerve grows back and can allow the pain signal to be transmitted again. If this happens, the procedure can be repeated. This procedure often does not relieve all back pain, but it relieves the pain associated with facet joint arthritis.

As with any procedure, there are certain risks involved which should be discussed with a treating physician. In order to achieve optimal results, it is important that these interventions be incorporated into a multidisciplinary treatment plan.

Chapter 51

Surgical Procedures for Pain Relief

Chapter Contents

Section 51.1—Types of Back Surgery 572

Section 51.2—Minimally Invasive Spine Surgery..................... 577

Section 51.3—Nerve Blocks.. 580

Section 51.4—Joint Replacement Surgery 583

Section 51.1

Types of Back Surgery

Excerpted from "Back Pain and Sciatica,"
© 2013 A.D.A.M., Inc. Reprinted with permission.

The health care provider should give patients complete information on the expected course of their low back pain and self-care options before discussing surgery. Patients should ask their health care provider about evidence favoring surgery or other (nonsurgical) treatments in their particular case. They should also ask about the long-term outcome of the recommended treatment. Would the improvements last and, if so, for how long? Another consideration when surgery is an option is the overall safety of the recommended procedure, weighed against its potential short-term benefits and its benefits in the long run.

Patients should generally try all possible non-surgical treatments before opting for surgery. The vast majority of back pain patients will not need aggressive medical or surgical treatments.

The most common reasons for surgery for low back pain are disk herniation and spinal stenosis. In general, surgery has been found to provide better short term and possibly quicker relief for selected patients when compared to non-surgical treatment. However, over time, nonsurgical treatments are as effective.

Many approaches and procedures are available or being investigated. However, there have been few well-conducted studies to determine if any type of back pain surgery works better than others, or if a single procedure is better than no surgery at all.

It should be noted that surgery does not always improve outcome and, in some cases, can even make it worse. Surgery can be an extremely effective approach, however, for certain patients whose severe back pain does not respond to conservative measures.

Discectomy

Discectomy is the surgical removal of the diseased disk. The procedure relieves pressure on the spine. It has been performed for 40 years, and increasingly less invasive techniques developed over time.

However, few studies have been conducted to determine the procedure's real effectiveness. In appropriate candidates it provides faster relief than medical treatment, but long-term benefits (over five years) are uncertain.

Discectomy is recommended when a herniated disk causes one or more of the following:

- Leg pain or numbness that is severe or persistent, making it hard for the patient to perform daily tasks

- Weakness in the muscles of the lower leg or buttocks

- An inability to control bowel movements or urination

Most other people with low back or neck pain, numbness, or even mild weakness are often first treated without surgery. Often, many of the symptoms of low back pain caused by a herniated disc get better or disappear over time, without surgery.

Microdiscectomy

Microdiscectomy is the current standard procedure. It is performed through a small incision (1 to 1½ inch). The back muscles are lifted and moved away from the spine. After identifying and moving the nerve root, the surgeon removes the injured disk tissue under it. The procedure does not change any of the structural supports of the spine, including joints, ligaments, and muscles.

Other, less invasive procedures are available, including endoscopic discectomy, percutaneous discectomy (PAD), and laser discectomy. The long-term benefits of these procedures are unknown, however. There is no evidence that any of these less-invasive procedures are as effective as the standard microdiscectomy.

Complications and Outlook

Most people achieve pain relief and can move better after microdiscectomy. Numbness and tingling should get better or disappear. Your pain, numbness, or weakness may NOT get better or go away if the disk damaged your nerve before surgery.

Scar tissue is a potential problem, since it can cause persistent low back pain afterward. Other complications of spinal surgery can include nerve and muscle damage, infection, and the need for another operation.

Patients are usually up and walking soon after disk surgery. It may take four to six weeks for full recovery, however. Gentle exercise may be recommended at first. Starting intensive exercise four to six weeks after a first-time disk surgery appears to be very helpful for speeding up recovery. Little or no physical therapy is usually needed.

Laminectomy

Laminectomy is surgery to remove either the lamina, two small bones that make up a vertebra, or bone spurs in your back. Laminectomy opens up your spinal canal so your spinal nerves or spinal cord have more room. It is often done along with a discectomy, foraminotomy, and spinal fusion.

Laminectomy is frequently done to treat spinal stenosis. You and your doctor can decide when you need to have surgery for your condition. Spinal stenosis symptoms often become worse over time, but this may happen very slowly. Surgery may help when your symptoms become more severe and interfere with your daily life or job.

Laminectomy for spinal stenosis will often provide full or partial relief of symptoms for many patients, but it is not always successful.

Future spine problems are possible for all patients after spine surgery. If you had spinal fusion and laminectomy, the spinal column above and below the fusion are more likely to have problems in the future. If you needed more than one kind of back surgery (such as laminectomy and spinal fusion), you may have more of a chance of future problems.

Some recurrence of back pain and sciatica occurs in half to two-thirds of postoperative patients. Minimally invasive variations are under investigation. For spinal stenosis, the traditional approach is a laminectomy and partial removal of the facet joint. There is controversy whether performing a fusion procedure along with these procedures is needed. Only a few randomized trials have compared this procedure with nonoperative treatment. Their results suggest that surgical treatment is better, at least over the first two years after surgery.

Spinal Fusion

Spinal fusion is surgery to fuse spine bones (vertebrae) that cause you to have back problems. Fusing means two bones are permanently placed together so there is no longer movement between them.

Spinal fusion is usually done along with other surgical procedures of the spine, such as a discectomy, laminectomy, or a foraminotomy. It is done to prevent any movement in a certain area of the spine.

Conditions fusion may be done for include:

- Spinal stenosis

- Injury or fractures to the bones in the spine

- Weak or unstable spine caused by infections or tumors

- Spondylolisthesis, a condition in which one vertebra slips forward on top of another

- Abnormal curvatures, such as those from scoliosis or kyphosis

The surgeon will use a graft (such as bone) to hold (or fuse) the bones together permanently. There are several different ways of fusing vertebrae together:

- Placing strips of bone graft material over the back part of the spine

- Placing bone graft material between the vertebrae

- Placing special cages between the vertebrae. These cages are packed with bone graft material.

The surgeon may get the graft from different places:

- From another part of your body (usually around your pelvic bone). This is called an autograft. Your surgeon will make a small cut over your hip and remove some bone from the back of the rim of the pelvis.

- From a bone bank, in a procedure called an allograft.

- A synthetic bone substitute can also be used, but this is not common yet.

The vertebrae are often also fixed together with screws, plates, or cages. These are used to keep the vertebrae from moving until the bone grafts fully heal.

Future spine problems are possible for all patients after spine surgery. After spinal fusion, the area that was fused together can no longer move. Therefore, the spinal column above and below the fusion is more likely to be stressed when the spine moves, and develop problems later on. Also, if you needed more than one kind of back surgery (such as laminectomy and spinal fusion), you may have more of a chance of future back problems.

There are many video-assisted fusion techniques. These new techniques are less invasive than standard "open" surgical approaches, which use wide incisions. To date, however, the newer procedures have higher complication rates than the open approaches, and some medical centers have abandoned them.

Other Surgical Procedures

Percutaneous vertebroplasty: Percutaneous vertebroplasty involves the injection of a cement-like bone substitute into vertebrae with compression fractures. It is done under endoscopic and x-ray guidance.

Warning: The Food and Drug Administration (FDA) has warned consumers that polymethylmethacrylate bone cement, used during vertebroplasty, could leak. Such leakage could cause damage to soft tissues and nerves. It is extremely important that the patient is sure that the health care provider has had significant experience performing the vertebroplasty procedure.

Percutaneous kyphoplasty: The health care provider injects bone cement into the space surrounding a fractured vertebra. (Vertebroplasty injects the cement directly into the vertebra.) Kyphoplasty is used to stabilize the spine and return spinal height to as normal as possible. Kyphoplasty should only be done if bed rest, medicines, and physical therapy do not relieve back pain. Those with severe fractures or spinal infections should not have kyphoplasty.

Artificial disk replacement: Total disk replacement is an investigative procedure for some patients with severely damaged disks. It is done instead of spinal fusion surgery, but it has not yet been shown to be superior to it. The technique implants artificial disks (such as ProDisc, Link, and SB Charite) consisting of two metal plates and a soft core. The surgery can be performed using a minimally invasive laparoscopic procedure. It is done through tiny cuts using miniature tools and viewing devices. An artificial cushioning device called the prosthetic disk nucleus (PDN) replaces only the inner gel-like core (nucleus pulposus) within the intervertebral space, rather than the entire disk. A possible benefit of these artificial disks is that they would allow more movement of the spine, and therefore prevent disk degeneration below and above the site of surgery (a frequent complication of spinal fusion). This benefit has not yet been proven in large and long-term studies.

In its updated recommendations, the American Pain Society is against vertebral disc replacement in patients with non-radicular (non-radiating or not involving a nerve) low back pain, degenerative spinal changes, and persistent and disabling symptoms.

Intradiscal electrothermal treatment (IDET): Intradiscal electrothermal treatment (IDET) uses electricity to heat a painful disk. Heat is applied for about 15 minutes. Pain may temporarily feel worse, but after healing, the disk shrinks and becomes desensitized to pain. However, healing takes several weeks. While some studies have reported benefit, many consider the evidence to support the use of this procedure weak.

Section 51.2

Minimally Invasive Spine Surgery

Excerpted from "Minimally Invasive Spine Surgery (MIS)," © 2009 American Association of Neurological Surgeons (www.aans.org). Reproduced with permission from the American Association of Neurological Surgeons, 5550 Meadowbrook Dr., Rolling Meadows, IL 60008.

Minimally invasive spine surgery (MIS) was first performed in the 1980s, but has recently seen rapid advances. Technological advances have enabled spine surgeons to expand patient selection and treat an evolving array of spinal disorders, such as degenerative disc disease, herniated disc, fractures, tumors, infections, instability, and deformity.

One potential downside of traditional, open lumbar (back) surgeries is the damage that occurs from the 5- to 6-inch incision. There are many potential sources for damage to normal tissue: the muscle dissection and retraction required to uncover the spine (which contributes to the formation of scar and fibrotic tissue), the need for blood vessel cauterization, and the necessity of bone removal. Disrupting natural spinal anatomy is necessary to facilitate decompression of pinched nerves and the placement of screws and devices to stabilize the spine. This may lead to lengthy hospital stays (up to five days or longer), prolonged pain and recovery periods, the need for postoperative narcotic use, significant operative blood loss, and risk of tissue infection.

MIS was developed to treat disorders of the spine with less disruption to the muscles. This can result in quicker recovery, decrease operative blood loss, and speed patient return to normal function. In some MIS approaches, also called "keyhole surgeries," surgeons use a tiny endoscope with a camera on the end, which is inserted through a small incision in the skin. The camera provides surgeons with an inside view, enabling surgical access to the affected area of the spine.

Not all patients are appropriate candidates for MIS procedures. It is important to keep in mind that there needs to be certainty that the same or better results can be achieved through MIS techniques as with the respective open procedure.

As with all non-emergency spinal surgeries, the patient should undergo an appropriate period of conservative treatment, such as physical therapy, pain medication, or bracing, without showing improvement, before surgery is considered. The time period of this varies depending on the specific condition and procedure, but is generally six weeks to six months. The benefits of surgery should always be weighed carefully against its risks. Although a large percentage of patients report significant symptom and pain relief, there is no guarantee that surgery will help every individual.

Many MIS procedures can be performed on an outpatient basis. In some cases, the surgeon may require a hospital stay, typically less than 24 hours to two days, depending on the procedure.

Benefits

The potential benefits of MIS include:

- Smaller incisions
- Smaller scars/less scar tissue
- Reduced blood loss
- Less pain
- Less soft tissue damage
- Reduced muscle retraction
- Decreased postoperative narcotics
- Shorter hospital stay
- Possibility of performing on outpatient basis
- Faster recovery
- Quicker return to work and activities

Surgery Risks

As with any spinal surgical procedure, there are risks, including:

- Allergic reaction

- Anesthesia reaction
- Bleeding
- Blood vessel damage
- Blood clots
- Bruising
- Death
- Dissatisfactory instrumentation placement; may require re-operation
- Headache
- Incision problems
- Infection
- Need for further surgery
- Pain or discomfort
- Paralysis
- Pneumonia
- Spinal fluid leakage
- Stroke

Conditions Treated Using MIS Procedures

- Degenerative disc disease
- Herniated disc
- Lumbar spinal stenosis
- Spinal deformities such as scoliosis
- Spinal infections
- Spinal instability
- Vertebral compression fractures

Section 51.3

Nerve Blocks

"Nerve Blocks," Copyright © 2013 Regents of the University of California. All rights reserved. Reprinted with permission from the website of University of California, San Francisco Medical Center, at www.ucsfhealth.org.

The sympathetic nerves are part of the autonomic nervous system, which control the body's functions that we don't need to think about, such as blood pressure, digestion, and heart rate. They also help us respond to "fight or flight" situations. Sympathetic nerves do not normally send pain messages to the brain, but may become "switched on" for an unknown cause or due to a condition such as complex regional pain syndrome (CRPS), also known as reflex sympathetic dystrophy (RSD).

A sympathetic nerve block involves injecting local anesthetic around a junction or "crossroads" where many nerves meet. The goal is to decrease or eliminate pain by reducing the pain signals sent to the brain.

Your doctor may suggest a nerve block if other treatments, such as anti-inflammatory medicines, rest and physiotherapy were unsuccessful. Your doctor may also use nerve blocks as a diagnostic tool, to determine if your pain is actually coming from the sympathetic nervous system.

If you experience pain relief after a nerve block, your doctor may recommend additional nerve blocks or other forms of pain therapy to target the sympathetic nerves.

There are various sympathetic nerves located in different parts of the body, which may cause pain in the face, neck, arms, chest, lower back, legs and feet. The University of California, San Francisco (UCSF) Pain Management Center offers the following types of nerve blocks:

- Sympathetic ganglion blockade
- Stellate ganglion blockade
- Lumbar sympathetic blockade

Preparation

Before your nerve block, your doctor will give you specific instructions for preparing for the procedure. These will depend on your condition, current state of health and any medications you are taking.

One Week before the Procedure

Stop taking aspirin. If you take aspirin for your heart or blood vessels as prescribed by your doctor, please get written permission from your doctor to stop and bring that note to your procedure.

If you take Plavix (clopidogrel), you will need to stop taking it. Again, you will need verbal and written permission from your doctor to stop taking Plavix. Please bring the note to your procedure.

Three Days before the Procedure

Stop taking herbal medicines and supplements, fish oil and vitamin E.

24 Hours before the Procedure

Stop taking anti-inflammatory medicines, such as Advil, ibuprofen, etodolac, indomethacin, naproxen, Aleve, Feldene, diclofenac, Mobic, and piroxicam. You do not need to stop taking Celebrex. If you are unsure about any of your medicines, ask your doctor. Call your doctor if you take blood thinners such as heparin or Coumadin (warfarin).

Day of the Procedure

Please arrange to have someone drive you home after the nerve block, as you will not be able to drive or operate machinery for at least 24 hours after the procedure.

You must be healthy on the day of your nerve block. You must:

- Be free of infection and not taking antibiotics

- Be free of cold or flu symptoms

- Be free of any rashes

- Not have a fever greater than 100.4° F

- Be free of any local infection or skin lesion

- If you are feeling sick or have a cold, call us as soon as possible.

Procedure

During the procedure, you will lie on an x-ray table. You will have an intravenous (IV) line in your arm so that, if needed, we can give you medicine to help you relax.

The skin around the injection site will be cleaned, and the area numbed with anesthetic. The doctor will then use x-ray guidance to direct a needle to the targeted area and slowly inject anesthetic.

The procedure takes about 30 minutes.

Recovery

The degree of pain relief you experience will depend in part on whether your pain is actually caused by the sympathetic nerves. In the week after your procedure, it is helpful to keep a "pain diary" to share with your doctor.

Resume taking your regular medications, but please limit your use of pain medications the day of the procedure. This will make it easier to determine whether the nerve block was effective.

You may experience some mild pain around the injection site, which can be treated with ice. You may also experience a sensation of warmth in the targeted area for several hours after the procedure. This will resolve on its own.

On the side of the face that received an injection, you may experience symptoms such as a smaller pupil size, drooping and lack of sweating. You may also have a hoarse voice. These symptoms resolve on their own and are not cause for worry.

On the day of the injection, you should avoid driving and all strenuous activities. On the day after the procedure, you may return to your regular daily activities. If your pain is improved, you may gradually resume regular exercise and more strenuous activities, increasing their frequency over one to two weeks to avoid recurrence of your pain.

Section 51.4

Joint Replacement Surgery

Excerpted from "Joint Replacement Surgery: Information for Multicultural Communities," National Institute of Arthritis and Musculoskeletal and Skin Diseases (www.niams.nih.gov), NIH Pub. No. 09-5149, April 2009.

What is joint replacement surgery?

Joint replacement surgery is removing a damaged joint and putting in a new one. A joint is where two or more bones come together, like the knee, hip, and shoulder. The surgery is usually done by a doctor called an orthopaedic surgeon. Sometimes, the surgeon will not remove the whole joint, but will only replace or fix the damaged parts.

The doctor may suggest a joint replacement to improve how you live. Replacing a joint can relieve pain and help you move and feel better. Hips and knees are replaced most often. Other joints that can be replaced include the shoulders, fingers, ankles, and elbows.

What can happen to my joints?

Joints can be damaged by arthritis and other diseases, injuries, or other causes. Arthritis or simply years of use may cause the joint to wear away. This can cause pain, stiffness, and swelling. Bones are alive, and they need blood to be healthy, grow, and repair themselves. Diseases and damage inside a joint can limit blood flow, causing problems.

What is a new joint like?

A new joint, called a prosthesis, can be made of plastic, metal, or both. It may be cemented into place or not cemented, so that your bone will grow into it. Both methods may be combined to keep the new joint in place.

A cemented joint is used more often in older people who do not move around as much and in people with "weak" bones. The cement holds the new joint to the bone. An uncemented joint is often recommended for younger, more active people and those with good bone quality. It may take longer to heal, because it takes longer for bone to grow and attach to it.

583

New joints generally last at least 10 to 15 years. Therefore, younger patients may need to have the same damaged joint replaced more than once.

Do many people have joints replaced?

Joint replacement is becoming more common. About 773,000 Americans have a hip or knee replaced each year. Research has shown that even if you are older, joint replacement can help you move around and feel better.

Any surgery has risks. Risks of joint surgery will depend on your health before surgery, how severe your arthritis is, and the type of surgery done. Many hospitals and doctors have been replacing joints for several decades, and this experience results in better patient outcomes. For answers to their questions, some people talk with their doctor or someone who has had the surgery. A doctor specializing in joints will probably work with you before, during, and after surgery to make sure you heal quickly and recover successfully.

Do I need to have my joint replaced?

Only a doctor can tell if you need a joint replaced. He or she will look at your joint with an x-ray machine or another machine. The doctor may put a small, lighted tube (arthroscope) into your joint to look for damage. A small sample of your tissue could also be tested.

After looking at your joint, the doctor may say that you should consider exercise, walking aids such as braces or canes, physical therapy, or medicines and vitamin supplements. Medicines for arthritis include drugs that reduce inflammation. Depending on the type of arthritis, the doctor may prescribe corticosteroids or other drugs. However, all drugs may cause side effects, including bone loss.

If these treatments do not work, the doctor may suggest an operation called an osteotomy, where the surgeon "aligns" the joint. Here, the surgeon cuts the bone or bones around the joint to improve alignment. This may be simpler than replacing a joint, but it may take longer to recover. However, this operation is not commonly done today.

Joint replacement is often the answer if you have constant pain and can't move the joint well—for example, if you have trouble with things such as walking, climbing stairs, and taking a bath.

What happens during surgery?

First, the surgical team will give you medicine so you won't feel pain (anesthesia). The medicine may block the pain only in one part of the body (regional), or it may put your whole body to sleep (general). The team will then replace the damaged joint with a prosthesis.

Each surgery is different. How long it takes depends on how badly the joint is damaged and how the surgery is done. To replace a knee or a hip takes about two hours or less, unless there are complicating factors. After surgery, you will be moved to a recovery room for one to two hours until you are fully awake or the numbness goes away.

What happens after surgery?

With knee or hip surgery, you may be able to go home in three to five days. If you are elderly or have additional disabilities, you may then need to spend several weeks in an intermediate-care facility before going home. You and your team of doctors will determine how long you stay in the hospital.

After hip or knee replacement, you will often stand or begin walking the day of surgery. At first, you will walk with a walker or crutches. You may have some temporary pain in the new joint because your muscles are weak from not being used. Also, your body is healing. The pain can be helped with medicines and should end in a few weeks or months.

Physical therapy can begin the day after surgery to help strengthen the muscles around the new joint and help you regain motion in the joint. If you have your shoulder joint replaced, you can usually begin exercising the same day of your surgery! A physical therapist will help you with gentle, range-of-motion exercises. Before you leave the hospital (usually two or three days after surgery), your therapist will show you how to use a pulley device to help bend and extend your arm.

Will my surgery be successful?

The success of your surgery depends a lot on what you do when you go home. Follow your doctor's advice about what you eat, what medicines to take, and how to exercise. Talk with your doctor about any pain or trouble moving.

Joint replacement is usually a success in more than 90 percent of people who have it. When problems do occur, most are treatable. Possible problems include:

- **Infection:** Areas in the wound or around the new joint may get infected. It may happen while you're still in the hospital or after you go home. It may even occur years later. Minor infections in the wound are usually treated with drugs. Deep infections may need a second operation to treat the infection or replace the joint.

- **Blood clots:** If your blood moves too slowly, it may begin to form lumps of blood parts called clots. If pain and swelling develop in your legs after hip or knee surgery, blood clots may be the cause. The doctor may suggest drugs to make your blood thin or special stockings, exercises, or boots to help your blood move faster. If swelling, redness, or pain occurs in your leg after you leave the hospital, contact your doctor right away.

- **Loosening:** The new joint may loosen, causing pain. If the loosening is bad, you may need another operation. New ways to attach the joint to the bone should help.

- **Dislocation:** Sometimes after hip or other joint replacement, the ball of the prosthesis can come out of its socket. In most cases, the hip can be corrected without surgery. A brace may be worn for a while if a dislocation occurs.

- **Wear:** Some wear can be found in all joint replacements. Too much wear may help cause loosening. The doctor may need to operate again if the prosthesis comes loose. Sometimes, the plastic can wear thin, and the doctor may just replace the plastic and not the whole joint.

- **Nerve and blood vessel injury:** Nerves near the replaced joint may be damaged during surgery, but this does not happen often. Over time, the damage often improves and may disappear. Blood vessels may also be injured.

As you move your new joint and let your muscles grow strong again, pain will lessen, flexibility will increase, and movement will improve.

What research is being done?

Scientists are studying replacement joints to find out which are best to improve movement and flexibility. They are also looking at new joint materials and ways to improve surgery. Other researchers are working to find out what causes joint damage, how to prevent it, and how to treat it.

Some scientists are studying a condition called osteolysis, a condition where bone is lost around the implant in response to inflammation. This can cause the prosthesis to loosen and may require a second surgery. In 2008, scientists found that cells called fibroblasts trigger the inflammation that results in osteolysis. This finding could help scientists develop new drugs that prevent osteolysis in joint replacements.

Other scientists are also trying to find out why some people who need surgery don't choose it. They want to know what things make a difference in choosing treatment, in recovery, and in well-being.

There are numerous research studies underway across the country and abroad. To learn more, go to the National Institutes of Health (NIH) Research Portfolio Online Reporting Tool—Expenditures and Results (RePORTER) website at http://projectreporter.nih.gov/reporter.cfm.

Chapter 52

Palliative Care

Improving Quality of Life when You're Seriously Ill

Dealing with the symptoms of any painful or serious illness is difficult. However, special care is available to make you more comfortable right now. It's called palliative care. You receive palliative care at the same time that you're receiving treatments for your illness. Its primary purpose is to relieve the pain and other symptoms you are experiencing and improve your quality of life.

Palliative care is a central part of treatment for serious or life-threatening illnesses. The information in this chapter will help you understand how you or someone close to you can benefit from this type of care.

What Is Palliative Care?

Palliative care is comprehensive treatment of the discomfort, symptoms, and stress of serious illness. It does not replace your primary treatment; palliative care works together with the primary treatment you're receiving. The goal is to prevent and ease suffering and improve your quality of life.

The purpose of palliative care is to address distressing symptoms such as pain, breathing difficulties, or nausea, among others. Receiving palliative care does not necessarily mean you're dying.

From "Palliative Care: The Relief You Need When You're Experiencing the Symptoms of Serious Illness," National Institute of Nursing Research (www .ninr.nih.gov), NIH Pub. No. 11-6415, May 2011.

Palliative care gives you a chance to live your life more comfortably. Palliative care provides relief from distressing symptoms including pain, shortness of breath, fatigue, constipation, nausea, loss of appetite, problems with sleep, and many other symptoms. It can also help you deal with the side effects of the medical treatments you're receiving. Perhaps, most important, palliative care can help improve your quality of life.

Palliative care also provides support for you and your family and can improve communication between you and your health care providers. Palliative care strives to provide you with these benefits:

- Expert treatment of pain and other symptoms so you can get the best relief possible.

- Open discussion about treatment choices, including treatment for your disease and management of your symptoms.

- Coordination of your care with all of your health care providers.

- Emotional support for you and your family.

Researchers have studied the positive effects palliative care has on patients. Recent studies show that patients who receive palliative care report improvement in these areas:

- Pain and other distressing symptoms, such as nausea or shortness of breath.

- Communication with their health care providers and family members.

- Emotional support.

Other studies also show that palliative care ensures that care is more in line with patients' wishes and meets the emotional and spiritual needs of patients.

Palliative Care Is Different from Hospice Care

Palliative care is available to you at any time during your illness. Remember that you can receive palliative care at the same time you receive treatments that are meant to cure your illness. Its availability does not depend upon whether or not your condition can be cured. The goal is to make you as comfortable as possible and improve your quality of life.

You don't have to be in hospice or at the end of life to receive palliative care. People in hospice always receive palliative care, but hospice focuses on a person's final months of life. To qualify for some hospice programs, patients must no longer be receiving treatments to cure their illness.

Palliative Care Is Comprehensive

Palliative care can improve your quality of life in a variety of ways. Together with your primary health care provider, your palliative care team combines vigorous pain and symptom control into every part of your treatment. Team members spend as much time with you and your family as it takes to help you fully understand your condition, care options and other needs. They also make sure you experience a smooth transition between the hospital and other services, such as home care or nursing facilities.

This results in well-planned, complete treatment for all of your symptoms throughout your illness—treatment that takes care of you in your present condition and anticipates your future needs.

Palliative care is provided by a team of specialists that may include palliative care doctors, palliative care nurses, social workers, chaplains, pharmacists, nutritionists, counselors, and others.

Palliative care supports you and those who love you by maximizing your comfort. It also helps you set goals for the future that lead to a meaningful, enjoyable life while you get treatment for your illness.

How Do You Know If You Need Palliative Care?

Many adults and children living with illnesses such as cancer, heart disease, lung disease, kidney failure, AIDS, and cystic fibrosis, among others, experience physical symptoms and emotional distress related to their diseases. Sometimes these symptoms are related to the medical treatments they are receiving. You may want to consider palliative care if you or your loved one suffers from pain or other symptoms due to ANY serious illness, experiences physical or emotional pain that is NOT under control, or needs help understanding your situation and coordinating your care.

Start palliative care as soon as you need it. It's never too early to start palliative care. In fact, palliative care occurs at the same time as all other treatments for your illness and does not depend upon the course of your disease. There is no reason to wait. Serious illnesses and their treatments can cause exhaustion, anxiety, and depression.

Palliative care teams understand that pain and other symptoms affect your quality of life and can leave you lacking the energy or motivation to pursue the things you enjoy. They also know that the stress of what you're going through can have a big impact on your family. And they can assist you and your loved ones as you cope with the difficult experience.

Working Together as a Team

Patients who are considering palliative care often wonder how it will affect their relationships with their current health care providers. These are some of their questions:

- Will I have to give up my primary health care provider?
- What do I say if there is resistance to referring me for palliative care services?
- Will I offend my health care provider if I ask questions?

Most important, you do NOT give up your own health care provider in order to get palliative care. The palliative care team and your health care provider work together. Most clinicians appreciate the extra time and information the palliative care team provides to their patients. Occasionally a clinician may not refer a patient for palliative care services. If this happens to you, ask for an explanation. Let your health care provider know why you think palliative care could help you.

Getting Palliative Care

In most cases, palliative care is provided in the hospital. The process begins when either your health care provider refers you to the palliative care team or you ask your health care provider for a referral. In the hospital, palliative care is provided by a team of professionals, including medical and nursing specialists, social workers, pharmacists, nutritionists, clergy, and others.

Most insurance plans cover all or part of the palliative care treatment you receive in the hospital, just as they would other services. Medicare and Medicaid also typically cover palliative care. If you have concerns about the cost of palliative care treatment, a social worker from the palliative care team can help you.

When you leave the hospital, your palliative care team will help you make a successful move to your home, hospice, or other health care setting.

About Morphine

If you have an illness causing pain that is not relieved by drugs such as acetaminophen or ibuprofen, the palliative care team may recommend trying stronger medicines such as morphine. Simply stated, morphine is an opiate—a strong medicine for treating pain. Like other similar opiate medicines (hydrocodone, oxycodone), it provides safe and effective pain treatment. In fact, almost all pain can be relieved with morphine and similar strong drugs that are available today. So no one should suffer because they or their health care provider have concerns about morphine or other drugs in the opiate family.

In fact, very few people who use opiates for pain relief ever become addicted or dependent on these medicines. However, it is important to be aware that anyone taking opiates for more than two weeks should not stop doing so abruptly. You should ask your health care provider about gradually reducing your dose so that your body is able to adjust.

There is no reason to wait until your pain is unbearable before you begin taking morphine. As your pain increases, your morphine dose can be safely increased to provide the relief you need over time.

All opiates can cause nausea, drowsiness and constipation. However, as your body adjusts to the medicine, side effects will generally decrease. Also, side effects such as constipation can easily be managed.

As always, if you have concerns about taking these or any medications, talk to your palliative care team. They can tell you about how various medications work, what their side effects are and how to get the most effective pain relief.

Don't Wait to Get the Help You Deserve

If you think you need palliative care, ask for it now. Tell your health care provider that you'd like to add palliative care specialists to your treatment team and request a consultation.

If you want to find a hospital in your area that offers a palliative care program, you can go to the Palliative Care Provider Directory of Hospitals at www.getpalliativecare.org to search by state and city.

Part Five

Additional Help and Information

Chapter 53

Terms Related to Pain and Pain Management

acetaminophen: The basic ingredient found in Tylenol and its many generic equivalents. It is sold over the counter, in a prescription-strength preparation, and in combination with codeine (also by prescription).[1]

acupuncture: A form of complementary and alternative medicine that involves inserting thin needles through the skin at specific points on the body to control pain and other symptoms.[2]

acute pain: Pain that has a known cause and occurs for a limited time. Acute pain usually responds to treatment with analgesic medications and treatment of the cause of the pain.[3]

advance medical directives: Advance directives are used to give other people, including health care providers, information about your wishes for medical care. Advance directives are important in case there is ever a time when you are not physically or mentally able to speak for yourself and make your wishes known. The most common

---

Terms marked [1] are excerpted and adapted from "Pain: Hope Through Research," National Institute of Neurological Disorders and Stroke (NINDS), January 10, 2013. Terms marked [2] are excerpted from "Glossary," produced by the Office on Women's Health, U.S. Department of Health and Human Services (www.womenshealth.gov). Terms marked [3] are from "Glossary," reprinted with permission from www.StopPain.org, the website of the Department of Pain Medicine and Palliative Care at Beth Israel Medical Center, New York, New York. © Continuum Health Partners, Inc., reviewed 2013.

types of advance directives are the living will and the durable power of attorney for health care.[3]

allodynia: When pain is caused by something that does not normally cause pain (such as clothing touching the skin).[3]

analgesic medications: Medications used to prevent or treat pain.[3]

anesthesia: The use of medicine to prevent the feeling of pain or another sensation during surgery or other procedures that might be painful.[2]

angina: A recurring pain or discomfort in the chest that happens when some part of the heart does not receive enough blood. It is a common symptom of coronary heart disease, which occurs when vessels that carry blood to the heart become narrowed and blocked due to atherosclerosis. Angina feels like a pressing or squeezing pain, usually in the chest under the breast bone, but sometimes in the shoulders, arms, neck, jaws, or back. Angina is usually is brought on by exertion, and relieved within a few minutes by resting or by taking prescribed angina medicine.[2]

anticonvulsants: Used for the treatment of seizure disorders but are also sometimes prescribed for the treatment of pain. Carbamazepine in particular is used to treat a number of painful conditions, including trigeminal neuralgia. Another antiepileptic drug, gabapentin, is being studied for its pain-relieving properties, especially as a treatment for neuropathic pain.[1]

antidepressant: Medications used to treat depression, and also used to treat chronic pain. Antidepressants can also be helpful for pain-related symptoms, like sleep problems and muscle spasms.[3]

anxiolytic: Medications used to treat anxiety, and also used to treat chronic pain. Anxiolytics reduce pain-related anxiety, help relax muscles and can help a person cope with pain.[3]

aromatherapy: A form of complementary and alternative medicine in which the scent of essential oils from flowers, herbs, and trees is inhaled to promote health and well-being.[2]

aspirin: May be the most widely used pain-relief agent and has been sold over the counter since 1905 as a treatment for fever, headache, and muscle soreness.[1]

bereavement: The act of grieving someone's death.[3]

biofeedback: Used for the treatment of many common pain problems, most notably headache and back pain. Using a special electronic machine, the patient is trained to become aware of, to follow, and to gain control over certain bodily functions, including muscle tension, heart rate, and skin temperature. The individual can then learn to effect a change in his or her responses to pain, for example, by using relaxation techniques. Biofeedback is often used in combination with other treatment methods, generally without side effects. Similarly, the use of relaxation techniques in the treatment of pain can increase the patient's feeling of well-being.[1]

capsaicin: A chemical found in chili peppers that is also a primary ingredient in pain-relieving creams.[1]

caregiver: Any person who provides care for the physical and emotional needs of a family member or friend.[3]

causalgia (complex regional pain syndrome II): Pain, usually burning, that is associated with autonomic changes—change in color of the skin, change in temperature, change in sweating, swelling. Causalgia occurs after a nerve injury.[3]

central nervous system: The brain and the spinal cord.[3]

chemonucleolysis: A treatment in which an enzyme, chymopapain, is injected directly into a herniated lumbar disc in an effort to dissolve material around the disc, thus reducing pressure and pain. The procedure's use is extremely limited, in part because some patients may have a life-threatening allergic reaction to chymopapain.[1]

chickenpox: A disease caused by the varicella-zoster virus, which results in a blister-like rash, itching, tiredness, and fever.[2]

chiropractic: An alternative medical system that takes a different approach from standard medicine in treating health problems. The goal of chiropractic therapy is to normalize this relationship between your body's structure (mainly the spine) and its function. Chiropractic professionals use a type of hands-on therapy called spinal manipulation or adjustment.[2]

chronic fatigue syndrome (CFS): A complex disorder characterized by extreme fatigue that lasts six months or longer, and does not improve with rest or is worsened by physical or mental activity. Other symptoms can include weakness, muscle pain, impaired memory and/or mental concentration, and insomnia. The cause is unknown.[2]

chronic pain: Pain that occurs for more than one month after healing of an injury, that occurs repeatedly over months, or is due to a lesion that is not expected to heal.[3]

clinical trials: Carefully planned and monitored experiments to test a new drug or treatment.[3]

complementary medicine: Approaches to medical treatment that are outside of mainstream medical training. Complementary medicine treatments used for pain include: acupuncture, low-level laser therapy, meditation, aroma therapy, Chinese medicine, dance therapy, music therapy, massage, herbalism, therapeutic touch, yoga, osteopathy, chiropractic treatments, naturopathy, and homeopathy.[3]

computed tomography (CT/CAT) scanning: A painless technique used to produce a picture of a cross-section, or "slice," of a part of the body. X-rays are used to produce this picture.[3]

constipation: Difficulty having a bowel movement.[3]

cordotomy: A surgical procedure in which bundles of nerves within the spinal cord are severed. Cordotomy is generally used only for the pain of terminal cancer that does not respond to other therapies.[1]

deep brain (or intracerebral) stimulation: Considered an extreme treatment and involves surgical stimulation of the brain, usually the thalamus. It is used for a limited number of conditions, including severe pain, central pain syndrome, cancer pain, phantom limb pain, and other neuropathic pains.[1]

delirium: A disturbance of the brain function that causes confusion and changes in alertness, attention, thinking and reasoning, memory, emotions, sleeping patterns, and coordination. These symptoms may start suddenly, are due to some type of medical problem, and they may get worse or better multiple times.[3]

discectomy: A procedure in which an entire vertebral disc is removed by a surgeon; when microsurgical techniques are used it is called microdiscectomy.[1]

do-not-resuscitate (DNR) orders: Instructions written by a doctor telling other healthcare providers not to try to restart a patient's heart, using cardiopulmonary resuscitation (CPR) or other related treatments, if his/her heart stops beating. Usually, DNR orders are written after a discussion between a doctor and the patient and/or family members. DNR orders are written for people who are very unlikely to have a successful result from CPR—those who are terminally ill or those who are elderly and frail.[3]

dorsal root entry zone operation (DREZ): A surgical procedure in which spinal neurons corresponding to the patient's pain are destroyed surgically. Because surgery can result in scar tissue formation that may cause additional problems, patients are well advised to seek a second opinion before proceeding.[1]

durable power of attorney for health care (DPOAHC): A legal document that specifies one or more individuals (called a health care proxy) you would like to make medical decisions for you if you are unable to do so yourself.[3]

dyspnea: Difficulty in breathing.[3]

end-of-life care: Doctors and caregivers provide care to patients approaching the end of life that is focused on comfort, respect for decisions, support for the family, and treatments to help psychological and spiritual concerns.[3]

entitlement: A federal program (such as Social Security or unemployment benefits) that guarantees a certain level of benefits to those who meet requirements set by law.[3]

EPEC (Education for Physicians on End-of-Life Care): A project designed to educate physicians across the United States about providing good end-of-life care for patients. EPEC includes a curriculum used to train doctors in clinical knowledge and skills they need to care for dying patients.[3]

epidural: During labor a woman may be offered an epidural, where a needle is inserted into the epidural space at the end of the spine, to numb the lower body and reduce pain. This allows a woman to have more energy and strength for the end stage of labor, when it is time to push the baby out of the birth canal.[2]

ethics: A system of moral principles and rules that are used as standards for professional conduct. Many hospitals and other health care facilities have ethics committees that can help doctors, other healthcare providers, patients and family members in making difficult decisions regarding medical care.[3]

fatigue: A feeling of becoming tired easily, being unable to complete usual activity, feeling weak, and difficulty concentrating.[3]

fibromyalgia: A pain disorder in which a person feels widespread pain and stiffness in the muscles, fatigue, and other symptoms.[3]

gallstone: Solid material that forms in the gallbladder or common bile duct. Gallstones are made of cholesterol or other substances found in the gallbladder. They may occur as one large stone or as many small ones, and they may vary from the size of a grain of sand to a golf ball.[2]

hemorrhoids: Veins around the anus or lower rectum that are swollen and inflamed.[2]

hospice: A special way of caring for people with terminal illnesses and their families by meeting the patient's physical, emotional, social, and spiritual needs, as well as the needs of the family. The goals of hospice are to keep the patient as comfortable as possible by relieving pain and other symptoms; to prepare for a death that follows the wishes and needs of the patient; and to reassure both the patient and family members by helping them to understand and manage what is happening.[3]

hospice home care: Most hospice patients receive care while living in their homes. Home hospice patients have family members or friends who provide most of their care, with help and support from the trained hospice team. The hospice team visits at the house to provide medical and nursing care, emotional support, counseling, information, instruction and practical help. A home care aide may also be available to help with daily care, if needed.[3]

hyperalgesia: Extreme sensitivity to pain.[3]

hyperpathia: An exaggerated response to something that causes pain, with continued pain after the cause of the pain is no longer present.[3]

hypnosis: A focused state of concentration used to reduce pain. With self-hypnosis, you repeat a positive statement over and over. With guided imagery, you create relaxing images in your mind.[2]

ibuprofen: A member of the aspirin family of analgesics, the so-called nonsteroidal anti-inflammatory drugs. It is sold over the counter and also comes in prescription-strength preparations.[1]

inflammation: Used to describe an area on the body that is swollen, red, hot, and in pain.[2]

inflammatory bowel disease: Long-lasting problems that cause irritation and ulcers in the gastrointestinal tract. The most common disorders are ulcerative colitis and Crohn disease.[2]

informed consent: The process of making decisions about medical care that are based on open, honest communication between the health care provider and the patient and/or the patient's family members.[3]

interstitial cystitis: A long-lasting condition also known as painful bladder syndrome or frequency-urgency-dysuria syndrome. The wall of the bladder becomes inflamed or irritated, which affects the amount of urine the bladder can hold and causes scarring, stiffening, and bleeding in the bladder.[2]

kidney stone: Hard mass developed from crystals that separate from the urine and build up on the inner surfaces of the kidney.[2]

Lamaze: A philosophy of giving birth developed by Dr. Ferdinand Lamaze. The goal of Lamaze classes is to increase women's confidence in their ability to give birth. Lamaze classes teach women simple coping strategies for labor, including focused breathing. But Lamaze also teaches that breathing techniques are just one of the many things that help women in labor. Movement, positioning, labor support, massage, relaxation, hydrotherapy and the use of heat and cold are some others.[2]

laminectomy: A procedure in which a surgeon removes only a disc fragment, gaining access by entering through the arched portion of a vertebra.[1]

living will: A legal document which outlines the kinds of medical care a patient wants and doesn't want. The living will is used only if the patient becomes unable to make decisions for him/herself.[3]

magnetic resonance imaging (MRI): A painless technique that uses magnetic fields and radio waves (without radiation) to create clear cross-sectional pictures of the body.[3]

migraine: A medical condition that usually involves a very painful headache, usually felt on one side of the head. Besides intense pain, migraine also can cause nausea and vomiting and sensitivity to light and sound. Some people also may see spots or flashing lights or have a temporary loss of vision.[2]

myofascial pain: Muscle pain and tenderness.[3]

nerve blocks: Injections of anesthetic (or numbing) substances into nerves in order to reduce pain.[3] Nerve blocks may employ the use of drugs, chemical agents, or surgical techniques to interrupt the relay of pain messages between specific areas of the body and the brain. There are many different names for the procedure, depending on the technique or agent used. Types of surgical nerve blocks include neurectomy; spinal dorsal, cranial, and trigeminal rhizotomy; and sympathectomy, also called sympathetic blockade.[1]

nerves: Cells in the human body that are the building blocks of the nervous system (the system that records and transmits information chemically and electrically within a person). Nerve cells, or neurons, are made up of a nerve cell body and various extensions from the cell body that receive and transmit impulses from and to other nerves and muscles.[2]

nonsteroidal anti-inflammatory drugs (NSAIDs): Including aspirin and ibuprofen; are widely prescribed and sometimes called non-narcotic or non-opioid analgesics. They work by reducing inflammatory responses in tissues. Many of these drugs irritate the stomach and for that reason are usually taken with food. Although acetaminophen may have some anti-inflammatory effects, it is generally distinguished from the traditional NSAIDs.[1]

nutrition/hydration: Intravenous (IV) fluid and nutritional supplements given to patients who are unable to eat or drink by mouth, or those who are dehydrated or malnourished.[3]

opioid: A type of medication related to opium. Opioids are strong analgesics. Opioids include morphine, codeine, and a large number of synthetic (man-made) drugs like methadone and fentanyl.[3]

osteoarthritis: A joint disease that mostly affects cartilage, the slippery tissue that covers the ends of bones in a joint. The top layer of cartilage breaks down and wears away. This allows bones under the cartilage to rub together, which causes pain, swelling, and loss of motion of the joint.[2]

osteoporosis: A bone disease that is characterized by progressive loss of bone density and thinning of bone tissue, causing bones to break easily.[2]

pain: An unpleasant feeling that may or may not be related to an injury, illness, or other bodily trauma. Pain is complex and differs from person to person.[3]

pain due to nerve injury: Pain caused by an injury or other problem in the nervous system.[3]

palliative care: The total care of patients with progressive, incurable illness. In palliative care, the focus of care is on quality of life. Control of pain and other physical symptoms, and psychological, social, and spiritual problems is considered most important.[3]

patient-controlled analgesia (PCA): Pain medication given through an IV or epidural catheter. Patients control the dose of medication they take, depending on how much is needed to control the pain. PCA is usually used for patients recovering from intra-abdominal, major orthopedic, or thoracic surgery, and for chronic pain states, such as those due to cancer.[3]

peripheral nervous system: The nerves throughout the body that send messages to the central nervous system.[3]

peripheral neuropathy: Pain caused by an injury or other problem with the peripheral nervous system.[3]

phantom pain: Pain that develops after an amputation. To the patient, the pain feels like it is coming from the missing body part.[3]

pharmacotherapy: The treatment of diseases and symptoms with medications.[3]

physician assisted suicide: Actions by a doctor that help a patient commit suicide. Though the doctor may provide medication, a prescription, or take other steps, the patient takes his/her own life (for instance, by swallowing the pills that are expected to bring about death).[3]

placebos: Inactive substances, such as sugar pills, or harmless procedures, such as saline injections or sham surgeries, generally used in clinical studies as control factors to help determine the efficacy of active treatments. Although placebos have no direct effect on the underlying causes of pain, evidence from clinical studies suggests that many pain conditions such as migraine headache, back pain, post-surgical pain, rheumatoid arthritis, angina, and depression sometimes respond well to them. This positive response is known as the placebo effect, which is defined as the observable or measurable change that can occur in patients after administration of a placebo. Some experts believe the effect is psychological and that placebos work because the patients believe or expect them to work. Others say placebos relieve pain by stimulating the brain's own analgesics and setting the body's self-healing forces in motion. A third theory suggests that the act of taking placebos relieves stress and anxiety—which are known to aggravate some painful conditions—and, thus, cause the patients to feel better. Still, placebos are considered controversial because by definition they are inactive and have no actual curative value.[1]

postherpetic neuralgia (PHN): Painful condition following shingles (herpes zoster).[3]

psychological approaches: Techniques used to help patients cope with over their pain and deal with emotional factors that can increase pain. Such strategies include biofeedback, imagery, hypnosis, relaxation training, stress management, cognitive-behavioral therapy, and family counseling.[3]

reflex sympathetic dystrophy (complex regional pain syndrome I): Pain, usually burning, that is associated with "autonomic changes"—change in color of the skin, change in temperature, change in sweating, swelling. Reflex sympathetic dystrophy is caused by injury to bone, joint, or soft tissues.[3]

rehabilitation: Treatment for an injury, illness, or pain with the goal of restoring function.[3]

rheumatoid arthritis: A form of arthritis that causes pain, swelling, stiffness and loss of function in your joints. It can affect any joint but is common in the wrist and fingers. If one hand has RA, the other one usually does too. It is an autoimmune disease. This means the arthritis is caused by your immune system attacking your body's own tissues. RA can affect body parts besides joints, such as your eyes, mouth and lungs.[2]

rhizotomy: A surgical procedure in which a nerve close to the spinal cord is cut.[1]

RICE (rest, ice, compression, and elevation): Four components prescribed by many orthopedists, coaches, trainers, nurses, and other professionals for temporary muscle or joint conditions, such as sprains or strains. While many common orthopedic problems can be controlled with these four simple steps, especially when combined with over-the-counter pain relievers, more serious conditions may require surgery or physical therapy, including exercise, joint movement or manipulation, and stimulation of muscles.[1]

shingles: A disease that occurs when the same virus that causes chicken pox becomes active again. After a person has chicken pox, the virus stays in the body. It may not cause problems for many years. As a person gets older, the virus may come back as shingles. It can cause mild to severe pain, usually on one side of the body or face.[2]

sickle cell anemia: A blood disorder passed down from parents to children. It involves problems in the red blood cells. Normal red blood cells are round and smooth and move through blood vessels easily. Sickle cells are hard and have a curved edge. These cells cannot squeeze through small blood vessels. They block the organs from getting blood. Your body destroys sickle red cells quickly, but it can't make new red blood cells fast enough—a condition called anemia.[2]

spinal cord stimulation: uses electrodes surgically inserted within the epidural space of the spinal cord. The patient is able to deliver a pulse of electricity to the spinal cord using a small box-like receiver and an antenna taped to the skin.[1]

spinal fusion: A procedure where the entire disc is removed and replaced with a bone graft. In a spinal fusion, the two vertebrae are then fused together. Although the operation can cause the spine to stiffen, resulting in lost flexibility, the procedure serves one critical purpose: protection of the spinal cord.[1]

transcutaneous electrical nerve stimulation (TENS): Uses tiny electrical pulses, delivered through the skin to nerve fibers, to cause changes in muscles, such as numbness or contractions. This in turn produces temporary pain relief. There is also evidence that TENS can activate subsets of peripheral nerve fibers that can block pain transmission at the spinal cord level, in much the same way that shaking your hand can reduce pain.[1]

treatment withdrawal: A syndrome that might occur when a medication that has been used regularly to treat pain is no longer used, or when the dose is decreased. Showing symptoms of withdrawal does not mean that a patient is addicted to his/her pain medication.[3]

trigeminal neuralgia: A disorder of the trigeminal nerve that causes brief attacks of severe pain in the lips, cheeks, gums, or chin on one side of the face.[3]

uric acid: A chemical created when the body breaks down substances called purines. Purines are found in some foods and drinks, such as liver, anchovies, mackerel, dried beans and peas, beer, and wine. Most uric acid dissolves in blood and passes out of the body in urine. If your body produces too much uric acid or doesn't remove enough of it, you can get sick.[2]

uterine fibroids: Common, benign (noncancerous) tumors that grow in the muscle of the uterus, or womb. Fibroids often cause no symptoms and need no treatment, and they usually shrink after menopause. But sometimes fibroids cause heavy bleeding or pain, and require treatment.[2]

Chapter 54

Resources for More Information about Pain Management

Agency for Healthcare Research and Quality
Office of Communications and Knowledge Transfer
540 Gaither Road, Suite 2000
Rockville, MD 20850
Phone: 301-427-1104
Website: www.ahrq.gov

American Burn Association
311 South Wacker Drive
Suite 4150
Chicago, IL 60606
Phone: 312-642-9260
Fax: 312-642-9130
Website: www.ameriburn.org
E-mail: info@ameriburn.org

American Academy of Orthopaedic Surgeons
6300 North River Road
Rosemont, IL 60018-4262
Phone: 847-823-7186
Fax: 847-823-8125
Website: www.aaos.org
E-mail: pemr@aaos.org

American Academy of Pain Management
975 Morning Star Drive, Suite A
Sonora, CA 95370
Phone: 209-533-9744
Fax: 209-533-9750
Website: www.aapainmanage.org
E-mail: info@aapainmanage.org

Information in this chapter was compiled from many sources deemed reliable. Inclusion does not constitute endorsement, and there is no implication associated with omission. All contact information was verified in March 2013.

American Academy of Pain Medicine
4700 West Lake Avenue
Glenview, IL 60025
Phone: 847-375-4731
Fax: 847-375-6477
Website: www.painmed.org
E-mail: info@painmed.org

American Academy of Pediatrics
141 Northwest
Point Boulevard
Elk Grove Village,
IL 60007-1098
Toll-Free: 800-433-9016
Phone: 847-434-4000
Fax: 847-434-8000
Website: www.aap.org

American Association of Endodontists
211 East Chicago Avenue
Suite 1100
Chicago, IL 60611-2691
Toll-Free: 800-872-3636
Phone: 312-266-7255
Toll-Free Fax: 866-451-9020
Fax: 312-266-9867
Website: www.aae.org
E-mail: info@aae.org org

American Association of Neurological Surgeons
5550 Meadowbrook Drive
Rolling Meadows,
IL 60008-3852
Toll-Free: 888-566-AANS
(888-566-2267)
Phone: 847-378-0500
Fax: 847-378-0600
Website: www.aans.org

American Board of Pain Medicine
4700 West Lake Avenue
Glenview, IL 60025
Phone: 847-375-4726
Fax: 847-375-6747
Website: www.abpm.org
E-mail: info@abpm.org

American Chiropractic Association
1701 Clarendon Boulevard
Arlington, VA 22209
Toll-Free: 800-986-4636
Phone: 703-276-8800
Fax: 703-243-2593
Website: www.acatoday.org

American Chronic Pain Association
P.O. Box 850
Rocklin, CA 95677-0850
Toll-Free: 800-533-3231
Phone: 916-632-0922
Fax: 916-632-3208
Website: www.theacpa.org
E-mail: ACPA@theacpa.org

American College of Rheumatology
2200 Lake Boulevard NE
Atlanta, GA 30319
Phone: 404-633-3777
Fax: 404-633-1870
Website:
www.rheumatology.org
E-mail: acr@rheumatology.org

**American College
of Sports Medicine**
401 West Michigan Street
Indianapolis, IN 46206-3233
Phone: 317-637-9200
Fax: 317-634-7817
Website: www.acsm.org
E-mail: publicinfo@acsm.org

**American Diabetes
Association**
Center for Information
1701 North Beauregard Street
Alexandria, VA 22311
Toll-Free: 800-DIABETES
(800-342-2383)
Phone: 703-549-1500
Website: www.diabetes.org
E-mail: askada@diabetes.org

**American
Gastroenterological
Association**
4930 Del Ray Avenue
Bethesda, MD 20814
Phone: 301-654-2055
Fax: 301-654-5920
Website: www.gastro.org

**American Headache
Society Committee for
Headache Education
(ACHE)**
19 Mantua Road
Mt. Royal, NJ 08061
Phone: 856-423-0043
Fax: 856-423-0082
Website: www.achenet.org

**American Industrial
Hygiene Association**
3141 Fairview Park Drive
Suite 777
Falls Church, VA 22042
Phone: 703-849-8888
Fax: 703-207-3561
Website: www.aiha.org
E-mail: infonet@aiha.org

**American Medical Society
for Sports Medicine**
4000 West 114th Street
Suite 100
Leawood, KS 66211
Phone: 913-327-1415
Fax: 913-327-1491
Website: www.amssm.org
E-mail: office@amssm.org

**American
Orthopaedic Society for
Sports Medicine**
6300 North River Road
Suite 500
Rosemont, IL 60018
Toll-Free: 877-321-3500
Phone: 847-292-4900
Fax: 847-292-4905
Website: www.sportsmed.org
E-mail: info@aossm.org

**American Osteopathic
Association**
142 East Ontario Street
Chicago, IL 60611
Toll-Free: 800-621-1773
Phone: 312-202-8000
Fax: 312-202-8200
Website: www.osteopathic.org
E-mail: info@osteopathic.org

American Physical Therapy Association
1111 North Fairfax Street
Alexandria, VA 22314-1488
Toll-Free: 800-999-APTA
(800-999-2782)
Phone: 703-684-APTA
(703-684-2782)
TDD: 703-683-6748
Fax: 703-684-7343
Website: www.apta.org
E-mail:
memberservices@apta.org

American Podiatric Medical Association
9312 Old Georgetown Road
Bethesda, MD 20814-1621
Toll-Free: 800-FOOTCARE
(800-366-8227)
Phone: 301-581-9200
Fax: 301-530-2752
Website: www.apma.org
E-mail: askapma@apma.org

American Psychological Association
750 First Street NE
Washington, DC 20002-4242
Toll-Free: 800-374-2721
Phone: 202-336-5500
TDD/TTY: 202-336-6123
Website: www.apa.org
E-mail:
public.affairs@apa.org

American Society for Bone and Mineral Research
2025 M Street NW
Suite 800
Washington, DC 20036-3309
Phone: 202-367-1161
Fax: 202-367-2161
Website: www.asbmr.org
E-mail: asbmr@asbmr.org

American Society of Interventional Pain Physicians
81 Lakeview Drive
Paducah, KY 42001
Phone 270-554-9412
Fax 270-554-5394
Website: www.asipp.org
E-mail: asipp@asipp.org

Anxiety and Depression Association of America
8701 Georgia Avenue #412
Silver Spring, MD 20910
Phone: 240-485-1001
Fax: 240-485-1035
Website: www.adaa.org

Arthritis Foundation
1330 West Peachtree Street
Suite 100
Atlanta, GA 30309
Toll-Free: 800-283-7800
Phone: 404-872-7100
or 404-965-7888
Fax: 404-872-0457
Website: www.arthritis.org
E-mail: help@arthritis.org

Beth Israel Medical Center
Department of Pain Medicine
and Palliative Care
First Avenue at 16th Street
New York, NY 10003
Toll-Free: 877-620-9999
Fax: 212-844-1503
Website: www.stoppain.org
E-mail: stoppain@chpnet.org

British Psychological Society
Website:
www.thepsychologist.org.uk

Centers for Disease Control and Prevention (CDC)
1600 Clifton Road
Atlanta, GA 30333
Toll-Free: 800-CDC-INFO
(800-232-4636)
Toll-Free TTY: 888-232-6348
Phone: 404-639-3311
or 404-639-3543
Website: www.cdc.gov
E-mail: inquiry@cdc.gov

Charcot-Marie-Tooth Association
P.O. Box 105
Glenolden, PA 19036
Toll-Free: 800-606-CMTA
(800-606-2682)
Phone: 610-499-9264
Fax: 610-499-9267
Website: www.cmtausa.org
E-mail: info@cmtausa.org

Cleveland Clinic
9500 Euclid Avenue
Cleveland, OH 44195
Toll-Free: 800-223-2273
TTY: 216-444-0261
Website: http://
my.clevelandclinic.org

Ehlers-Danlos National Foundation
1760 Old Meadow Road
Suite 500
McLean, VA 22102
Phone: 703-506-2892
Fax: 703-506-3266
Website: www.ednf.org
E-mail: ednfstaff@ednf.org

Fibrocentre.ca
Website: www.fibrocentre.ca

Fibromyalgia Network
P.O. Box 31750
Tucson, AZ 85751
Toll-Free: 800-853-2929
Phone: 520-290-5508
Website: www.fmnetnews.com

Foundation for Peripheral Neuropathy
485 Half Day Road, Suite 200
Buffalo Grove, IL 60089
Toll-Free: 877-883-9942
Fax: 847-883-9960
Website: www.foundationforpn.org
E-mail: info@tffpn.org

Hip Society
6300 North River Road
Suite 727
Rosemont, IL 60018-4226
Phone: 847-698-1638
Fax: 847-823-0536
Website: www.hipsoc.org
E-mail: hip@aaos.org

International RadioSurgery Association
P.O. Box 5186
Harrisburg, PA 17110
Phone: 717-260-9808
Fax: 717-260-9809
Website: www.irsa.org

International Research Foundation for RSD/CRPS
1910 East Busch Boulevard
Tampa, FL 33612
Phone: 813-907-2312
Website: www.rdsfoundation.org
E-mail: info@rdsfoundation.org

Interstitial Cystitis Association
1760 Old Meadow Road
Suite 500
McLean, VA 22102
Toll-Free: 800-435-7422
Phone: 703-442-2070
Fax: 703-506-3266
Website: www.ichelp.org
E-mail: ICAmail@ichelp.org

Juvenile Diabetes Research Foundation
26 Broadway
New York, NY 10004
Toll-Free: 800-533-CURE
(800-533-2873)
Fax: 212-785-9595
Website: www.jdrf.org
E-mail: info@jdrf.org

Lower Extremity Amputation Prevention Program
Health Resources and Services
Administration
5600 Fishers Lane
Rockville, MD 20857
Toll-Free: 888-ASK-HRSA
(888-275-4772)
Toll-Free TTY: 877-489-4772
Website: www.hrsa.gov/leap
E-mail: ask@hrsa.gov

Model Systems Knowledge Translation Center
American Institutes for Research
1000 Thomas Jefferson Street NW
Washington, DC 20007
Phone: 202-403-5600
Toll-Free TTY: 877-334-3499
Website: www.msktc.org
E-mail: msktc@air.org

Muscular Dystrophy Association
3300 East Sunrise Drive
Tucson, AZ 85718-3208
Toll-Free: 800-572-1717
Phone: 520-529-2000
Fax: 520-529-5300
Website: www.mda.org
E-mail: mda@mdausa.org

MyDr
1 Chandos Street, 2nd Floor
St Leonards, NSW 2065
Australia
Website: MyDr.com.au

National Athletic Trainers Association
2952 Stemmons Freeway #200
Dallas, TX 75247
Toll-Free: 800-TRY-NATA
(800-879-6282)
Phone: 214-637-6282
Fax: 214-637-2206
Website: www.nata.org

National Cancer Institute
6116 Executive Boulevard
Suite 300
Bethesda, MD 20892-8322
Toll-Free: 800-4-CANCER
(800-422-6237)
Website: www.cancer.gov

National Center for Chronic Disease Prevention and Health Promotion
4770 Buford Highway NE
Mail Stop K-10
Atlanta, GA 30341-3717
Toll-Free: 1-800-CDC-INFO
(800-232-4636)
Phone: 770-488-5000
Website: www.cdc.gov
E-mail: cdcinfo@cdc.gov

National Center for Complementary and Alternative Medicine
P.O. Box 7923
Gaithersburg, MD 20898-7923
Toll-Free: 888-644-6226
Toll-Free TTY: 866-464-3615
Toll-Free Fax: 866-464-3616
Website: http://nccam.nih.gov
E-mail: info@nccam.nih.gov

National Diabetes Education Program
1 Diabetes Way
Bethesda, MD 20814-9692
Toll-Free: 888-693-NDEP
(888-693-6337)
Phone: 301-496-3583
Website: www.ndep.nih.gov
E-mail: ndep@mail.nih.gov

National Diabetes Information Clearinghouse
1 Information Way
Bethesda, MD 20892-3560
Toll-Free: 800-860-8747
Toll-Free TTY: 866-569-1162
Fax: 703-738-4929
Website:
www.diabetes.niddk.nih.gov
E-mail: ndic@info.niddk.nih.gov

National Digestive Diseases Information Clearinghouse
2 Information Way
Bethesda, MD 20892-3570
Toll-Free: 800-891-5389
Toll-Free TTY: 866-569-1162
Fax: 703-738-4929
Website:
www.digestive.niddk.nih.gov
E-mail: nddic@info.niddk.nih.gov

National Fibromyalgia Association
1000 Bristol Street N
Suite 17-247
Newport Beach, CA 92660
Phone: 714-921-0150
Fax: 714-921-6920
Website: www.fmaware.org

National Fibromyalgia Partnership, Inc.
140 Zinn Way
Linden, VA 22642-5609
Toll-Free: 866-725-4404
Website:
www.fmpartnership.org

National Headache Foundation
820 North Orleans, Suite 411
Chicago, IL 60610
Toll-Free: 888-NHF-5552
(888-643-5552)
Phone: 312-274-2650
Website: www.headaches.org
E-mail: info@headaches.org

National Heart, Lung, and Blood Institute Information Center
P.O. Box 30105
Bethesda, MD 20824-0105
Phone: 301-592-8573
Fax: 240-629-3246
Website: www.nhlbi.nih.gov
E-mail:
nhlbiinfo@nhlbi.nih.gov

National Institute for Occupational Safety and Health
4676 Columbia Parkway
Cincinnati, OH 45226
Toll-Free: 800-CDC-INFO
(800-232-4636)
Toll-Free TTY: 888-232-6348
Phone: 513-533-8328
Fax: 513-533-8347
Website: www.cdc.gov/niosh
E-mail: cdcinfo@cdc.gov

National Institute of Allergy and Infectious Diseases
6610 Rockledge Drive, MSC 6612
Bethesda, MD 20892-6612
Toll-Free: 866-284-4107
Toll-Free TDD: 800-877-8339
Phone: 301-496-5717
Fax: 301-402-3573
Website: www.niaid.nih.gov
E-mail: ocpostoffice@niaid.nih.gov

National Institute of Arthritis and Musculoskeletal and Skin Diseases
1 AMS Circle
Bethesda, MD 20892-3675
Toll-Free: 877-22-NIAMS
(877-226-4267)
Phone: 301-495-4484
TTY: 301-565-2966
Fax: 301-718-6366
Website: www.niams.nih.gov
E-mail: NIAMSinfo@mail.nih.gov

National Institute of Child Health and Human Development

31 Center Drive
Building 31, Room 2A32
Bethesda, MD 20892-2425
Toll-Free: 800-370-2943
Toll-Free TTY: 888-320-6942
Toll-Free Fax: 866-760-5947
Website: www.nichd.nih.gov
E-mail: NICHDInformation
ResourceCenter@mail.nih.gov

National Institute of Dental and Craniofacial Research

Public Information
and Liaison Branch
31 Center Drive, MSC 2190
Building 31, Room 5B55
Bethesda, MD 20892-2190
Toll-Free: 866-232-4528
Phone: 301-496-4261
Fax: 301-480-4098
Website: www.nidcr.nih.gov
E-mail: nidcrinfo@mail.nih.gov

National Institute of Mental Health

6001 Executive Boulevard
Room 6200, MSC 9663
Bethesda, MD 20892-9663
Toll-Free: 866-615-6464
Toll-Free TTY: 866-415-8051
Phone: 301-443-4513
TTY: 301-443-8431
Fax: 301-443-4279
Website: www.nimh.nih.gov
E-mail: nimhinfo@nih.gov

National Institute of Neurological Disorders and Stroke

P.O. Box 5801
Bethesda, MD 20824
Toll-Free: 800-352-9424
Phone: 301-496-5751
TTY: 301-468-5981
Website: www.ninds.nih.gov

National Institute of Nursing Research

31 Center Drive, Room 5B10
Bethesda, MD 20892-2178
Phone: 301-496-0207
Fax: 301-496-8845
Website: www.ninr.nih.gov
E-mail: info@ninr.nih.gov

National Institute on Aging

Building 31, Room 5C27
31 Center Drive, MSC 2292
Bethesda, MD 20892
Toll-Free: 800-222-2225
Toll-Free TTY: 800-222-4225
Website: www.nia.nih.gov
E-mail: niaic@nia.nih.gov

National Kidney and Urologic Diseases Information Clearinghouse

3 Information Way
Bethesda, MD 20892-3580
Toll-Free: 800-891-5390
Toll-Free TTY: 866-569-1162
Phone: 301-654-4415
Fax: 703-738-4929
Website: www.kidney.niddk.nih.gov
E-mail: nkudic@info.niddk.nih.gov

National Osteonecrosis Foundation
Good Samaritan Professional
Building, Suite 201
5601 Loch Raven Boulevard
Baltimore, MD 21239
Phone: 443-444-5985
Fax: 443-444-5908
Website: www.nonf.org

National Women's Health Information Center
Office on Women's Health
Department of Health
and Human Services
200 Independence Avenue SW
Room 712E
Washington, DC 20201
Toll-Free: 800-994-9662
Phone: 202-690-7650
Fax: 202-205-2631
Website:
www.womenshealth.gov

Neuropathy Association
60 East 42nd Street
Suite 942
New York, NY 10165
Phone: 212-692-0662
Fax: 212-692-0668
Website: www.neuropathy.org
E-mail: info@neuropathy.org

New Zealand Dermatological Society
Website: http://dermnetnz.org

NIH Osteoporosis and Related Bone Diseases— National Resource Center
2 AMS Circle
Bethesda, MD 20892-3676
Toll-Free: 800-624-BONE
(800-624-2663)
Phone: 202-223-0344
TTY: 202-466-4315
Fax: 202-293-2356
Website: www.bones.nih.gov
E-mail:
NIHBoneInfo@mail.nih.gov

NIH Pain Consortium
Website:
http://painconsortium.nih.gov
E-mail: NIHPainInfo@mail.nih.gov

North American Spine Society
7075 Veterans Boulevard
Burr Ridge, IL 60527
Toll-Free: 866-960-NASS
(866-960-6277)
Phone: 630-230-3600
Fax: 630-230-3700
Website:
www.knowyourback.org
Website: www.spine.org
E-mail: info@spine.org

Occupational Safety and Health Administration
U.S. Department of Labor
200 Constitution Avenue NW
Washington, DC 20210
Phone: 800-321-OSHA
(800-321-6742)
Toll-Free TTY: 877-889-5627
Website: www.osha.gov

Paget Foundation
(Paget's Disease of Bone
and Related Disorders)
P.O. Box 24432
Brooklyn, NY 11202
Toll-Free: 800-23-PAGET
(800-237-2438)
Website: www.paget.org
E-mail:PagetFdn@aol.com

Partners Against Pain
Purdue Pharma L.P.
One Stamford Forum
201 Tresser Boulevard
Stamford, CT 06901-3431
Toll-Free: 888-726-7535
Fax: 203-588-6254
Website:
www.partnersagainstpain.com
E-mail:
medical_services@pharma.com

**Pedorthic Footwear
Association**
8400 Westpark Drive
2nd Floor
McLean, VA 22102
Phone: 703-610-9035
Fax: 703-995-4456
Website: www.pedorthics.org
E-mail: info@pedorthics.org

**Phoenix Society for Burn
Survivors**
1835 R W Berends Drive SW
Grand Rapids, MI 49519-4955
Toll-Free: 800-888-2876
Phone: 616-458-2773
Fax: 616-458-2831
Website: www.phoenix-society.org
E-mail: info@phoenix-society.org

**Reflex Sympathetic Dystrophy
Syndrome Association**
P.O. Box 502
Milford, CT 06460
Toll-Free: 877-662-7737
Phone: 203-877-3790
Fax: 203-882-8362
Website: www.rsds.org
E-mail: info@rsds.org

**Sickle Cell Disease
Association of America**
231 East Baltimore St., Suite 800
Baltimore, MD 21202
Toll-Free: 800-421-8453
Phone: 410-528-1555
Fax: 410-528-1495
Website: www.sicklecelldisease.org
E-mail: scdaa@sicklecelldisease.org

Sleep HealthCenters
1505 Commonwealth Avenue
Brighton, MA 02135
Toll-Free: 877-SLEEP-HC
(877-753-3742)
Website: www.sleepandyou.com
E-mail: info@sleephealth.com

**Spine Care Treatment
Centers**
Website: www.spinecarehelp.com

**Spondylitis Association of
America**
P.O. Box 5872
Sherman Oaks, CA 91413
Toll-Free: 800-777-8189
Phone: 818-892-1616
Fax: 818-892-1611
Website: www.spondylitis.org
E-mail: info@spondylitis.org

TNA—Facial Pain Association
Formerly the Trigeminal
Neuralgia Association
408 West University Avenue
Suite 602
Gainesville, FL 32601
Toll-Free: 800-923-3608
Phone: 352-384-3600
Fax: 352-384-3606
Website: www.fpa-support.org
E-mail: info@fpa-support.org

University of California, San Diego
Student Health Services
9500 Gilman Drive
La Jolla, CA 92093-0039
Phone: 858-534-3300
Fax: 858-246-0256
Website:
http://studenthealth.ucsd.edu
E-mail:
studenthealth@ucsd.edu

University of California, San Francisco
Medical Center
505 Parnassus Avenue
San Francisco, CA 94143-0296
Toll-Free: 888-689-UCSF
(888-689-8273)
Phone: 415-476-1000
Website: www.ucsfhealth.org
E-mail: referral.center
@ucsfmedctr.org

University of Michigan Health System
Your Child Development
and Behavior Resources
1500 East Medical Center Drive
Ann Arbor, MI 48109
Toll-Free: 800-211-8181
Phone: 734-936-6641
Website: www.med.umich.edu

Urology Care Foundation
Formerly American Urological
Association Foundation
1000 Corporate Boulevard
Linthicum, MD 21090
Toll-Free: 800-828-7866
Phone: 410-689-3700
Fax: 410-689-3998
Website:
www.urologyhealth.org
E-mail:
info@urologycarefoundation.org

U.S. Department of Veterans Affairs
810 Vermont Avenue NW
Washington, DC 20420
Website: www.va.gov
Toll-Free: 800-827-1000

U.S. Food and Drug Administration (FDA)
10903 New Hampshire Avenue
Silver Spring, MD 20993-0002
Toll-Free: 888-INFO-FDA
(888-463-6332)
Website: www.fda.gov

Index

Index

Page numbers followed by 'n' indicate a footnote. Page numbers in *italics* indicate a table or illustration.

A

AANS *see* American Association of Neurological Surgeons
AAOS *see* American Academy of Orthopaedic Surgeons
"AAPM Facts and Figures on Pain" (American Academy of Pain Medicine) 9n
abdominal adhesions 286–87
"Abdominal Adhesions" (NDDIC) 286n
abdominal pain, gas 301
About Inc., corticosteroid injections publication 559n
acetaminophen
  back pain 117
  cancer pain 247
  defined 597
  described 510, 511–12, 519, 523
  drug interactions 432, 520
  intravenous 521
  older adults and children 7
  opioids containing 428–29, 532–37
  osteoarthritis 101

Achilles tendinitis 154–55, 203–4
Achilles tendon injuries 225
acid reflux, described 302
ACPA *see* American Chronic Pain Association
"ACPA Resource Guide to Chronic Pain Medication and Treatment" (ACPA) 44n, 46n, 47n, 513n, 519n, 528n, 543n, 563n
ACSM *see* American College of Sports Medicine
Actiq (fentanyl) 533
acupuncture
  back pain 119–20
  cancer pain 251
  defined 597
  described 482, 492–96
  spinal stenosis 129
"Acupuncture for Pain" (NCCAM) 492n

acute pain
  back 115–16, 500
  burns 239
  cancer 244
  versus chronic pain 10, 20, 52
  defined 597
  rating scales 457–61
ADAA *see* Anxiety and Depression
  Association of America
A.D.A.M., Inc., publications
  back and spinal pain 120n
  back surgery 572n
  foot pain 145n
  neck pain 190n
  somatoform pain disorder 415n
addiction,
  pain medication 250, 431
adenoids
  described 281
  removal 409
adhesive capsulitis,
  described 220–21
adjuvant analgesics, types 475
advance medical directives,
  defined 597–98
Advil (ibuprofen) 523–24
aerobics *see* exercise(s)
Agency for Healthcare Research
  and Quality (AHRQ)
  chronic pelvic pain
    publication 318n
  contact information 609
AIHA *see* American Industrial
  Hygiene Association
air travel, sinusitis 410
alcohol use
  chronic pain 46–47
  stress management 64
Aleve (naproxen sodium) 524
algiatry, defined 450
allodynia
  defined 5, 598
  peripheral neuropathy 386
alpha-galactosidase 301
alternative therapies
  see complementary
  and alternative medicine
Ambien
  (zolpidem tartrate) 550–51

American Academy of
  Orthopaedic Surgeons (AAOS)
  contact information 609
  muscle cramp publication 184n
American Academy of Pain
  Management,
  contact information 609
American Academy
  of Pain Medicine
  contact information 610
  pain data publication 9n
American Academy of Pediatrics,
  contact information 610
American Association
  of Endodontists
  contact information 610
  tooth pain publication 268n
American Association of
  Neurological Surgeons (AANS)
  contact information 610
  spinal surgery
    publication 577n
American Board of Pain
  Medicine
  contact information 610
  pain medicine specialists
    publication 450n
American Burn Association,
  contact information 609
American Chiropractic
  Association, contact
  information 610
American Chronic Pain
  Association (ACPA)
  contact information 55, 366, 610
  publications
    alcohol and chronic pain 46n
    cigarette smoke and pain 44n
    illegal drugs and pain 47n
    invasive and implanted pain
      interventions 563n
    nerve pain 364n
    non-opioid analgesics 519n
    opioid medications 528n
    other medications 543n
    pain management
      programs 451n
    Quality of Life Scale 55n
    topical pain relievers 513n

American College of
Rheumatology
contact information 610
publications
giant cell arteritis 355n
polymyalgia
rheumatica 110n
American College of Sports
Medicine (ACSM)
contact information 611
muscle soreness
publication 179n
American Diabetes Association,
contact information 611
American Gastroenterological
Association,
contact information 611
American Geriatrics Society,
pain management
guidelines 6–7
American Headache Society
Committee for Headache
Education (ACHE),
contact information 611
American Industrial Hygiene
Association (AIHA)
contact information 83, 611
ergonomics publication 73n
American Medical Society
for Sports Medicine,
contact information 611
American Orthopaedic
Society for Sports Medicine,
contact information 611
American Osteopathic Association,
contact information 611
American Pain Foundation,
chronic pain survey 12–13
American Physical
Therapy Association,
contact information 612
American Podiatric Medical
Association,
contact information 612
American Psychological
Association (APA)
chronic pain management
publication 50n
contact information 612

American Society for Bone
and Mineral Research,
contact information 612
American Society of
Interventional Pain Physicians,
contact information 612
American Urological
Association Foundation,
contact information 620
Amitiza (lubiprostone) 308
amitriptyline, topical 517
amputation, phantom
and stump pain 395–98
Amputee Coalition of America,
website address 398
Amrix (cyclobenzaprine) 552, 553
ANA (antinuclear antibody),
rheumatic diseases 92
"Analgesic Rebound" (National
Headache Foundation) 352n
analgesics
back pain 117
defined 598
labor pain 316
migraine 345
non-opioid
cancer pain 247–48
described 519–25
surgical pain 429
over-the-counter 509–12, 519
overuse headache 345–46, 354
patient-controlled 426–27, 604
topical 513–17
types 475
see also acetaminophen;
aspirin; nonsteroidal anti-
inflammatory drugs; opioids
Anaprox (naproxen sodium) 524
"An Ergonomics Approach
to Avoiding Workplace Injury"
AIHA 73n
anesthesia
approaches 475, 483–84
defined 598
labor pain 316
peripheral neuropathy 388
postherpetic neuralgia 379
topical 514–16
see also nerve blocks

angina
  defined 598
  described 254, 256–64
angioplasty, angina 263
ankylosing spondylitis
  back pain 124
  described 90
annular ring, abnormalities 122
antacids
  gastrointestinal protection 522
  GERD 303, 304
anti-anxiety medications 551–52
anti-arrhythmic agents 549–50
antibiotics
  ear infections 282, 283
  reactive arthritis 106
anticonvulsants
  burn pain 240
  cancer pain 249
  defined 598
  diabetic neuropathy 392
  neuropathic pain 387–88, 547–49
  postherpetic neuralgia 379
  trigeminal neuralgia 276
antidepressants
  back pain 118
  burn pain 240
  cancer pain 249
  defined 598
  depression 36
  described 543–47
  diabetic neuropathy 392
  irritable bowel syndrome 307–8
  migraine 556–57
  peripheral neuropathy 388
  somatoform pain disorder 416
  see also tricyclic
    antidepressants
antidiarrheals, irritable
  bowel syndrome 307
anti-hypertensive
  medications 554
antinuclear antibody (ANA),
  rheumatic diseases 92
anti-psychotic medications 553–54
antiseizure drugs
  see anticonvulsants
antispasmodics,
  irritable bowel syndrome 307

antiviral drugs, shingles 377
anxiety
  benzodiazepines 551
  chronic pain 37–39
Anxiety and Depression
    Association of America (ADAA)
    anxiety and chronic pain
      publication 37n
    contact information 612
anxiolytics
  defined 598
  examples 551–52
APA *see* American
    Psychological Association
appendectomy 290
appendiceal abscess,
  drainage 290
appendicitis 288–91
"Appendicitis" (NDDIC) 288n
Applegate, Katherine 29–30
arachnoiditis 21, 367–68
"Arachnoiditis Information
    Page" (NINDS) 367n
aromatherapy, defined 598
arthritis
  anxiety disorders 37
  back pain 124–25
  CAM therapies 490
  cure 93–94
  defined 88
  described 21
  diagnosis 91–93
  gouty 107–8
  knee 167
  reactive 90, 104–7, 124–25
  shoulder 222
  temporomandibular
    joint 271, 272
  types 88–91
  see also osteoarthritis;
    rheumatoid arthritis
Arthritis Foundation,
  contact information 612
arthrodesis
  rheumatoid arthritis 97
  toe 149
arthrogram, shoulder pain 215
Arthropan
  (choline salicylate) 523

arthroplasty, toe 149, 151
see also joint replacement surgery
arthroscopy, sports
injuries 232
aspirin
back pain 117
chronic pain 53
defined 598
described 519
history 4
NSAID interaction 520
opioids containing 533, 534,
535, 537
prostaglandins 323
rheumatoid arthritis 96
aura, migraine 343–44
autogenic training,
described 504
autonomic neuropathy
described 385, 386
diabetic 391
avascular necrosis 136–38

B

back pain
anxiety disorders 38
CAM therapies 53, 489–90, 494,
499–500
described 21, 114–20
ergonomics 79–81
exercises 65–72
magnetic resonance
imaging 465–67
survey data 11–12
symptoms and causes 120–26
x-rays 462–64
"Back Pain and Sciatica"
(A.D.A.M., Inc.) 120n, 572n
back surgery, types 572–77
baclofen 553
balloon dilatation, pancreatic
or bile ducts 312
ball/wall stand exercise 72
Bayer *see* aspirin
Beano (alpha-galactosidase) 301
behavioral therapies
see cognitive behavioral therapy;
psychological approaches
BenGay patch 514

benzodiazepines 551–52
bereavement, defined 598
"Best Way to Take
Your Over-the-Counter
Pain Reliever? Seriously"
(FDA) 509n
Beth Israel Medical Center,
Department of Pain Medicine
and Palliative Care
contact information 613
publications
pain management
therapies 476n
pain treatment plans 474n
phantom and
stump pain 395n
rehabilitation
approaches 485n
biofeedback
cancer pain 251
defined 598–99
described 480, 504
biologic response modifiers,
arthritis 96, 106
birth control pills
see contraceptives
bisphosphonates
giant cell arteritis 357
jaw osteonecrosis 136
bladder distention 439
bladder instillation 439–40
bladder surgery,
interstitial cystitis 442–43
bladder training 442
bloating, gas 300
blood glucose, control 391
blood tests
angina 261
back pain 115
body mechanics, whiplash 197
"Bone Cancer" (National
Cancer Institute) 132n
bone cancer, described 132–34
bone grafting,
osteonecrosis 138
bone spur, neck pain 195
borderline personality
disorder, pain experience 30
botanical, described 497

botulinum toxins
    described 554–55
    FDA warning 555–56
    heel pain 159
    migraine 556
    TMJ disorders 273
Boyse, Kyla 399n
braces
    back pain 118
    spinal stenosis 129
Bradley birthing method 315
brain, pain reception 3, 4
brain freeze, described 349
Braun, William 179n
breakthrough pain
    burns 239
    cancer 244
British Psychological Society
    pain experience publication 25n
    website address 613
bruises, sports injuries 224
Bufferin *see* aspirin
bunionectomy, described 149
bunions, described 148–49
buprenorphine 536
buprenorphine/naloxone 537
bupropion 45
burn pain, described 21, 238–42
burns, facts 236–37
"Burns Fact Sheet" (National
    Institute of General Medical
    Sciences) 236n
burping, described 300
bursitis
    described 91, 201–6
    heel 155
    shoulder 202–3, 218
butorphanol 6, 537

C

CABG (coronary artery
    bypass grafting) 263
caffeine 64, 345
calcium stones, types 444
Caldolor (ibuprofen) 521
calf muscle stretch 187
calluses, described 146–48
CAM *see* complementary
    and alternative medicine

Campbell, Andrew D. 399n
Campbell, Claudia 28
cancer
    back pain 125–26
    incidence 11
    paranasal sinus and
        nasal cavity 411–13
cancer pain
    described 22
    treatment 243–44, 246–52
    types and causes 244–45
capsaicin
    defined 599
    topical 379, 515
Carafate (sucralfate) 521, 522
carbamazepine 547, 548, 598
cardiac catheterization 260–61
cardiac rehabilitation 263
caregiver, defined 599
carisoprodol 552
carpal tunnel syndrome
    acupuncture 493
    described 23, 206–11
    ergonomics 74, 75
"Carpal Tunnel Syndrome
    Fact Sheet" (NINDS) 206n
casts, sports injuries 230
Catapres (clonidine) 554
catastrophizing
    described 481
    gender differences 27
cat/camel exercise *71*
CAT scan *see* computed
    tomography (CT/CAT) scan
cauda equina syndrome
    back pain 122–23
    spinal manipulation 499
    spinal stenosis 127
causalgia, defined 599
    see also complex regional
        pain syndrome
CBC (complete blood count),
    rheumatic diseases 93
CBT *see* cognitive
    behavioral therapy
CCP (or anti-CCP)
    antibody test,
    rheumatic diseases 92
celecoxib 520, 524–25

Centers for Disease Control
and Prevention (CDC)
   contact information 613
   opioid overdose death
      statistics 17–18
   pain data 16
central nervous system,
   defined 599
central pain syndrome
   described 21, 368–69
   post-stroke 419
   post-trauma 24–25
"Central Pain Syndrome
   Information Page"
   (NINDS) 368n
cervical radiculopathy,
   electrodiagnostic tests 470–71
CFS *see* chronic fatigue syndrome
chair, ergonomic 80–81
chair stand exercise *71*
Chantix (varenicline) 45
Charcot-Marie-Tooth Association,
   contact information 613
chemonucleolysis, defined 599
chemotherapy
   bone cancer 133
   cancer pain 251
chest pain
   angina 256–64
   heart attack 254
   incidence 11
chickenpox
   defined 599
   shingles 376
childbirth, pain 314–17
children
   codeine 7, 434–36
   ear infections 280–84
   pain experience 6–7
   pain scales 401–2, 458–61
   sickle cell pain 399–404
   treatment plans 476
chiropractic
   defined 599
   spinal stenosis 129
   see also spinal manipulation
chlorzoxazone 553
cholecystectomy, gallstones 298–99
choline magnesium trisalicylate 523

choline salicylate 523
chondromalacia (patellae),
   described 167–68
chondrosarcoma, described 132
chronic daily headache, types 348–49
chronic fatigue syndrome (CFS)
   defined 599
   versus fibromyalgia 143–44
"Chronic Myofascial Pain"
   (Cleveland Clinic) 176n
chronic myofascial pain
   (CMP) 176–79
chronic pain
   versus acute pain 10, 20, 52
   alcohol use 46–47
   anxiety 37–39
   back 115, 116, 500
   burns 239
   CAM therapies 488–92
   cancer 244
   costs 9–10
   defined 10, 599
   depression 34–36
   diagnosis 456–61
   incidence 10–11
   learning to control 52–54
   opioid use 528–29, 541–42
   personality profile 29–30
   Quality of Life Scale 55–56
   risk factors 31–32
   statistics 15–17
   stress management 50, 57–64
   survey data 12–14
   tips for managing 50–51
"Chronic Pain" (ADAA) 37n
"Chronic Pain and CAM:
   At a Glance" (NCCAM) 488n
chronic pelvic pain (CPP) 318–20
cigarette smoking *see* smoking
Cleveland Clinic
   contact information 613
   publications
      chronic myofascial pain 176n
      pain control after surgery 424n
clinical trials, defined 600
clonazepam 548, 552
clonidine 554
Cloninger, Robert 29
Cluett, Jonathan 559n

cluster headaches,
  described 22, 348
CMP (chronic myofascial
  pain) 176–79
codeine
  children 7, 434–36
  described 532
cognitive behavioral therapy (CBT)
  anxiety disorders 38
  depression 36
  irritable bowel syndrome 308
  somatoform pain disorder 416
  techniques 479–81
colchicine, gout 109
cold temperature, ergonomics 77
cold therapy
  back pain 116
  cancer pain 251
  described 478
  neck pain 191
  osteoarthritis 101
  rehabilitation 485, 486
  sports injuries 231
  surgical pain 430
collateral ligaments, knee
  described *166*, 167
  injuries 170
colon resection, diverticulitis 296
colostomy, diverticulitis 296
compartment syndrome, sports
  injuries 224–25
complement, rheumatic diseases 93
complementary and alternative
  medicine (CAM)
  anxiety disorders 38
  approaches 482–83
  back pain 119–20
  cancer pain 251–52
  carpal tunnel syndrome 210
  chronic pain 53, 488–92
  fibromyalgia 142
  osteoarthritis 101
  post-stroke pain 421
  rheumatoid arthritis 97–98
  spinal stenosis 129
complementary medicine,
  defined 600
complete blood count (CBC),
  rheumatic diseases 93

complex regional
  pain syndrome (CRPS)
  described 23, 370
  phantom pain 395
  type I, defined 605–6
  type II, defined 599
"Complex Regional Pain
  Syndrome Information Page"
  (NINDS) 370n
compounded medications,
  topical 514–15, 517
compression fractures,
  vertebral 125, 467
compression neuropathies,
  described 23
computed tomography
  angiography, angina 261
computed tomography (CT/CAT) scan
  back pain 115
  defined 600
  whiplash 197
computer, ergonomics 74, 77–83
Conrad, Rupert 30, 31–32
constipation
  defined 600
  opioid-induced 249, 538–39
Continuum Health Partners
  see Beth Israel Medical Center
contraceptives
  endometriosis 330
  migraine 353
  prostaglandins 323
  uterine fibroids 332–33
Cooke, David A. 55n, 132n, 331n,
  364n, 375n, 380n, 456n, 541n
coping strategies
  burn pain 241–42
  chronic pain 50–51
"Coping with chronic pain" (APA) 50n
cordotomy, defined 600
core decompression,
  osteonecrosis 138
corns, described 146–48
coronary angiography 260–61
coronary artery bypass
  grafting (CABG) 263
coronary heart disease
  angina 256, 257
  incidence 11

corsets
  back pain 118
  spinal stenosis 129
corticosteroid injections
  back pain 118–19
  bursitis and tendinitis 205
  carpal tunnel syndrome 209–10
  described 559–61
  epidural 483, 568–69
  intra-articular 563
  osteoarthritis 102
  plantar fasciitis 157
  reactive arthritis 105–6
  spinal stenosis 128
corticosteroids
  cancer pain 249
  giant cell arteritis 356–57
  gout 108–9
  polymyalgia
    rheumatica 111, 112
  sinusitis 409
cortisone, injectable 559–61
costochondritis 264–66
"Costochondritis"
  (Nemours Foundation) 264n
counterirritants, topical 513–14
COX-2 (cyclooxygenase-2)
  inhibitors 520, 524–25
CPP (chronic pelvic pain) 318–20
C-reactive protein
  angina 261
  rheumatic diseases 92
creatinine, rheumatic diseases 93
CRIES Pain Scale 458–60
Crohn disease 291–93
"Crohn's Disease" (NDDIC) 291n
CRPS *see* complex
  regional pain syndrome
cruciate ligaments, knee
  described *166*, 167
  injuries 169–70
cryosurgery, bone cancer 133
cryotherapy *see* cold therapy
CT scan *see* computed
  tomography (CT/CAT) scan
culture, pain experience 28, 29
cumulative trauma disorders
  see repetitive motion disorders
curl up exercise *71*

cyclobenzaprine 552, 553
cyclooxygenase-2 (COX-2)
  inhibitors 520, 524–25
Cymbalta (duloxetine)
  diabetic neuropathy 392
  fibromyalgia 141
cystectomy, interstitial cystitis 443
cystine stones, described 445
cytokines 35
cytoprotective medications 521–22
Cytotec (misoprostol) 521, 522

D

danazol, endometriosis 330
dantrolene 553
Darvon, Darvocet
  (propoxyphene) 537–38
da Vinci, Leonardo 3
"Dealing with Pain
  during Childbirth"
  (Nemours Foundation) 314n
deep brain stimulation
  defined 600
  described 484
deep breathing,
  described 479, 504
degenerative joint disease
  see osteoarthritis
delayed onset muscle
  soreness 179–84
"Delayed Onset Muscle
  Soreness (ACSM) 179n
delirium, defined 600
Demerol (meperidine) 403, 534
Depakote (valproic acid) 548
depression
  chronic pain 34–36, 456
  signs and symptoms 34–35
"Depression and Chronic Pain"
  (NIMH) 34n
Descartes, René 3
De Simone, Laura Lee 26
desipramine 544–45
diabetes, incidence 10
diabetic neuropathies 389–94
"Diabetic Neuropathies: The
  Nerve Damage of Diabetes"
  (National Diabetes Information
  Clearinghouse) 389n

diagnosis
  chronic pain 456–61
  technologies 7–8
diathermy, described 486
diazepam 552, 553
Dickinson, Emily 4
diclofenac, topical 520–21
diet and nutrition
  anxiety disorders 39
  diverticulosis 295
  fibromyalgia 143
  gas-forming foods 301
  gout 109
  interstitial cystitis 441
  irritable bowel syndrome 307
  pancreatitis 310, 311
  rheumatoid arthritis 96
  stress management 63–64
Dietary Supplement Health and
  Education Act (DSHEA) 496
dietary supplements 496–98
diffuse noxious inhibitory
  controls, described 28
dihydrocodeine bitartrate,
  aspirin, caffeine 533
Dilantin (phenytoin) 548
Dilaudid (hydromorphone) 534
dimethyl sulfoxide (DMSO) 439–40
Dionne, Raymond 53
disability insurance,
  fibromyalgia 144
discectomy
  defined 600
  described 572–74
discography, whiplash 196
discs, spinal
  artificial replacement 576
  degeneration and herniation
    back pain 21, 122
    electrodiagnostic tests 470–71
    magnetic resonance
      imaging 465–66
    neck pain 195
disease-modifying
  antirheumatic drugs
  (DMARDs) 96
dislocations
  shoulder 216–17
  sports injuries 227

distraction
  cancer pain 251
  described 480
diverticulosis and
  diverticulitis 294–96
"Diverticulosis and
  Diverticulitis" (NDDIC) 291n
DMARDs (disease-modifying
  antirheumatic drugs) 96
DMSO (dimethyl sulfoxide) 439–40
Dolophine (methadone) 534
do-not-resuscitate (DNR) orders,
  defined 600
dopamine 45
dorsal root entry zone operation
  (DREZ), defined 600–601
DPOAHC (durable power
  of attorney for health care),
  defined 601
drug abuse
  illegal drugs 47–48
  prescription 14–15, 17–18
  stress management 64
duloxetine
  diabetic neuropathy 392
  fibromyalgia 141
durable power of attorney
  for health care (DPOAHC),
  defined 601
Duragesic (fentanyl) 533
dysmenorrhea
  acupuncture 494
  described 321–23
dyspareunia 324–27
dyspnea, defined 601

E

ear, function 279–80
ear pain 279–84
eccentric muscle action,
  examples 181
economics of pain,
  statistics 9–10, 11, 13, 16
Ehlers-Danlos National
  Foundation,
  contact information 613
electrical nerve stimulation
  see transcutaneous electrical
  nerve stimulation

electrocardiogram (EKG),
  angina 260
electrodiagnostic procedures
  carpal tunnel syndrome 209
  types 7–8, 469
Electrodiagnostic Testing (NASS) 469n
electromagnetic radiation and
  electrostatic fields, computers 82
electromyography (EMG)
  described 7, 469–72
  whiplash 197
electrostimulation, sports injuries 231
Elmiron (pentosan
  polysulfate sodium) 440
EMG *see* electromyography
EMLA (Eutectic Mixture of
  Local Anesthetic) cream 515–16
end-of-life care, defined 601
endometrial ablation,
  uterine fibroids 334
endometriosis
  chronic pelvic pain 318, 319
  described 328–30
"Endometriosis Fact Sheet"
  (Office on Women's Health) 328n
endorphins 5, 529, 530
endoscopic retrograde
  cholangiopancreatography (ERCP)
  gallstones 299
  pancreatitis 311–12
endoscopic techniques, GERD 304–5
enhanced external counterpulsation
  therapy, angina 264
enkephalins 5
enteropathic arthritis, back pain 125
entitlement, defined 601
entrapment neuropathies,
  described 23
EPEC (Education for Physicians
  on End-of-Life Care), defined 601
epidural
  defined 601
  described 568–69
  labor pain 316
  patient-controlled 427
  steroid injections 483
  whiplash 197–98
ERCP *see* endoscopic retrograde
  cholangiopancreatography

erectile dysfunction,
  diabetic neuropathy 393
ergonomics, workplace 73–84
ergot derivatives, migraine 345
erythrocyte sedimentation rate,
  (ESR) rheumatic diseases 93
estrogen
  migraine 352–53
  pain response 5, 6
ESWT (extracorporeal shock
  wave therapy), heel pain 158
eszopiclone 551
ethics, defined 601
ethmoid sinuses,
  location 407, *407*, 411
ethnicity
  codeine metabolism 435
  pain experience 27–29, 32
eustachian tube, function 280, 281
Evista (raloxifene) 318
Ewing sarcoma family
  of tumors, described 132
EXALGO (hydromorphone) 534
exercise(s)
  Achilles tendinitis 155
  anxiety disorders 39
  back/spinal pain 65–72, 116–17
  cardiac rehabilitation 263
  carpal tunnel syndrome 210
  delayed onset muscle
    soreness 179–84
  fibromyalgia 143
  interstitial cystitis 442
  knee problems 168, 169, 171
  labor pain 315
  muscle cramps 187
  neck pain 191, 192
  osteoarthritis 99–100
  Paget's disease 135
  plantar fasciitis 157
  post-stroke pain 420
  reactive arthritis 106
  rehabilitation 485–86
  rheumatoid arthritis 95–96
  spinal stenosis 128
  sports injuries 230–31
  stress management 63
  therapeutic 477–78
  whiplash 197

Exercise: The Backbone of Spine Treatment (North American Spine Society) 65n
exostosectomy, toe 149
extracorporeal shock wave therapy (ESWT), heel pain 158
eyestrain, ergonomics 78–79

F

face-down extension exercises 66–67, *67*, 70, *70*
facet blocks
  back pain 119
  described 569
facet joint pain
  described 195
  medial branch block 560
facial pain, described 22
fatigue
  defined 601
  workplace 74
FDA *see* US Food and Drug Administration
fentanyl 533
FeverAll *see* acetaminophen
fiber
  diverticulosis 295
  irritable bowel syndrome 307
Fibrocentre.ca, website address 613
fibromyalgia
  acupuncture 493–94
  anxiety disorders 37
  versus chronic myofascial pain 176–77
  defined 601
  depression 35–36
  described 22, 90, 139–44
  relaxation techniques 506
  tai chi 53
"Fibromyalgia Fact Sheet" (Office on Women's Health) 139n
Fibromyalgia Network, contact information 613
Fillingim, Roger 26, 28, 29, 31, 32
5-aminosalicylic acid (5-ASA) agents, Crohn disease 293

FLACC Scale 460
flatus/flatulence, described 299, 300
flecainide 549–50
Flector (diclofenac) 521
Flexeril (cyclobenzaprine) 552, 553
focal neuropathies, electrodiagnostic tests 471
Food and Drug Administration *see* US Food and Drug Administration
foot care, diabetic neuropathy 393–94
foot pain
  forefoot 152–54
  heel 154–59
  injuries 160
  locations 145–46
  toe 146–52
"Foot Pain" (A.D.A.M., Inc.) 145n
forefoot pain
  bone groups 146
  causes 152–54
Foundation for Peripheral Neuropathy, contact information 613
Four A's of stress management 59–62
fractures
  foot 153–54, 160
  shoulder 221–22
  skull 225–26
  sports injuries 226–27
  vertebral 125, 467
frequency-urgency-dysuria syndrome *see* interstitial cystitis
"Frequently Asked Questions" (Beth Israel Medical Center) 474n
frontal sinuses, location 406, *407*, 411
frozen shoulder, described 220–21
fulguration, interstitial cystitis 442
fundoplication, GERD 304

G

gabapentin 547–48, 598
Gabitril (tiagabine) 548
gadolinium-enhanced MRI,
   disc herniation 466
gallstones
   defined 601
   described 297–99
   pancreatitis 309, 312
"Gallstones" (NDDIC) 297n
gas, digestive tract 299–301
"Gas in the Digestive Tract"
   (NDDIC) 299n
gastroesophageal
   reflux (GER) 302
gastroesophageal
   reflux disease (GERD)
   described 302–5
   symptoms 300
gastrointestinal problems,
   diabetic neuropathy 392–93
gastrointestinal protective
   medications 521–22
Gas-X (simethicone) 301
GCA (giant cell arteritis),
   described 91, 355–57
gender, pain
   perception 5–6, 26–27
genetics, pain perception 32
GER
   (gastroesophageal reflux) 302
GERD *see* gastroesophageal
   reflux disease
"Getting Diagnosed"
   (Office on Women's Health) 456n
"Giant Cell Arteritis" (American
   College of Rheumatology) 355n
giant cell arteritis (GCA),
   described 91, 355–57
"Glossary" (Beth Israel
   Medical Center) 597n
"Glossary" (Office on
   Women's Health) 597n
glossopharyngeal neuralgia 371
"Glossopharyngeal Neuralgia
   Information Page"
   (NINDS) 371n
glutamate 4–5
golfer's elbow, described 202

gonadotropin-releasing
   hormone agonists (GnRHa)
   endometriosis 330
   uterine fibroids 333
gout, described 91, 107–9
granulomas, midline 412
growing pains 161–63
"Growing pains"
   (Nemours Foundation) 161n
guarding, appendicitis 289
guided imagery
   cancer pain 252
   described 479, 505
   surgical pain 429
"Guide to Safe Use of Pain
   Medicine" (FDA) 509n

H

Haglund's deformity,
   described 156
hallux valgus
   described 148
   surgery 149
"Halt the Hurt! Dealing
   with Chronic Pain" (NIH) 52n
hammertoes, described 150–51
hamstring muscle stretch 187
"Handout on Health: Back Pain"
   (NIAMS) 114n
"Handout on Health:
   Osteoarthritis" (NIAMS) 98n
"Handout on Health:
   Rheumatoid Arthritis"
   (NIAMS) 94n
"Handout on Health:
   Sports Injuries" (NIAMS) 223n
harm avoidance,
   pain experience 29, 30
"Headache: Hope Through
   Research" (NINDS) 340n
headaches
   CAM therapies 490, 494, 506
   coping 352
   diagnosis 342–43
   introduction 340–41
   lost productivity time 13
   medication overuse 345–46, 354
   primary 340, 343–49
   requiring medical care 341–42

headaches, *continued*
secondary 340, 349–51
sleep disorders 351
types 22
see also migraine
head and facial pain,
described 22
Health Resources and
Services Administration,
Lower Extremity Amputation
Prevention Program,
contact information 614
"Healthy Woman: Pain"
(Office on Women's Health) 456n
hearing
described 279–80
difficulties 281
heart attack
incidence 11
neck pain 192
signs and symptoms 254–55
heartburn, described 302
"Heartburn, Gastroesophageal
Reflux (GER), and
Gastroesophageal Reflux
Disease (GERD)"
(NDDIC) 302n
heat, computers 82
heat therapy
back pain 116
cancer pain 251
described 478
neck pain 191
osteoarthritis 101
post-stroke pain 420
rehabilitation 485, 486
sports injuries 231
surgical pain 430
heel pain, types 154–59
heel spur syndrome,
described 156–59
Helpguide.org, stress
management publication 57n
hematocrit, rheumatic diseases 93
hemicrania continua,
described 348–49
hemorrhoids, defined 602
herbal supplements,
described 497, 498

herpesviruses, types 376
hindfoot pain, described 146
Hippocrates 501
hip replacement surgery 585
Hip Society,
contact information 614
histamine type 2
(H2) receptor blockers
described 521, 522
GERD 303, 304
hormonal therapies
chronic pelvic pain 318
endometriosis 330
migraine 353
uterine fibroids 332–33
hormones
migraine 352–53
pain response 5, 6, 27
"Hormones and Migraine"
(National Headache
Foundation) 352n
hospice
defined 602
versus palliative care 590–91
hospice home care, defined 602
Human Factors and Ergonomics
Society, contact information 83
Hunner's ulcers, interstitial
cystitis 438, 441, 442
hyaluronic acid substitutes,
osteoarthritis 102, 563–64
hydrocodone 533
hydromorphone 534
hydroxyurea, sickle cell
pain 404
hyperalgesia, defined 602
hyperpathia, defined 602
hyperuricemia, gout 107, 108
hypnic headache, described 349
hypnosis
burn pain 241
cancer pain 252
defined 602
described 505
irritable bowel syndrome 308
hysterectomy
chronic pelvic pain 319, 320
endometriosis 330
uterine fibroids 333–34

I

IBS *see* irritable bowel
 syndrome
ibuprofen
 defined 602
 described 523
 intravenous 521
 opioids containing 533, 534
ice cream headache, described 349
IDET (intradiscal
 electrothermal treatment) 577
iliotibial band syndrome
 knee pain 172
 sports injury 224
imagery *see* guided imagery
immobilization,
 sports injuries 229–30
immunosuppressive drugs
 peripheral neuropathy 387
 reactive arthritis 106
impingement syndrome,
 shoulder 202–3, 218
implanted intrathecal drug
 delivery systems 566–68
infants, pain scales 458–61
infectious arthritis,
 described 90–91
inflammation
 back pain 124–25
 defined 602
 depression 35
 reactive arthritis 104
 rheumatoid arthritis 95, 96–97
inflammatory bowel disease
 defined 602
 types 291–92
informed consent, defined 602
ingrown toenails,
 described 151–52
Institute of Medicine,
 pain statistics 9, 15–16
interdisciplinary pain
 management programs 451–54
International RadioSurgery
 Association,
 contact information 614
International Research
 Foundation for RDS/CRPS,
 contact information 614

interstitial cystitis
 chronic pelvic pain 318
 defined 602–3
 described 438–43
Interstitial Cystitis Association,
 contact information 614
"Interstitial Cystitis/Painful
 Bladder Syndrome" (National
 Kidney and Urologic Diseases
 Information Clearinghouse) 438n
intestinal obstruction,
 abdominal adhesions 286–87
intradiscal electrothermal
 treatment (IDET) 577
intrathecal drug
 delivery systems 566–68
irritable bowel syndrome (IBS)
 chronic pelvic pain 318
 described 305–8
 gas 300
 relaxation techniques 506
"Irritable Bowel Syndrome"
 (NDDIC) 305n
"Is Post-Surgery Codeine a
 Risk for Kids?" (FDA) 434n

J, K

Jabbari, Bahman 554–55
Jarrett, Christian 25n
jaw, osteonecrosis 136
joint care, arthritis 96, 100
joint replacement surgery
 described 583–87
 knee 173–74
 osteonecrosis 138
 rheumatoid arthritis 97
 shoulder 222
 TMJ disorders 274
"Joint Replacement Surgery:
 Information for Multicultural
 Communities" (NIAMS) 583n
jumper's knee, described 171, 203
juvenile arthritis, described 90
Juvenile Diabetes
 Research Foundation,
 contact information 614
kappa-opioids 6
Keefe, Francis 27
Kelly, Brendan P. 399n

Keppra (levetiracetam) 549
ketoprofen 524
kidney stones
  defined 603
  described 444–46
"Kidney Stones in Adults"
  (National Kidney and
  Urologic Diseases Information
  Clearinghouse) 444n
Killen, John 52, 53
Klonopin (clonazepam) 548, 552
knee
  structures 165–67, *166*
  tendinitis 170–71, 203, 224
knee injuries, common 167–73, 224
knee pain
  acupuncture 495
  injuries and problems 167–73
  joint replacement 173–74, 585
knee-to-chest exercises *69*
Komiyama, Osamu 28
kyphoplasty, percutaneous 576

L

labor and delivery, pain 314–17
laboratory tests,
  rheumatic diseases 92–93
lacosamide 548
lactase tablets or drops 301
Lamaze
  defined 603
  described 315
laminectomy
  defined 603
  described 574
  spinal stenosis 130
lamotrigine 548
laparoscopic surgery
  abdominal adhesions 287
  appendicitis 290
  chronic pelvic pain 319–20
  endometriosis 330
laparotomy
  appendicitis 290
  endometriosis 330
laxatives
  constipation 538–39
  irritable bowel syndrome 307
leiomyoma, uterine 331–34

leuprolide
  chronic pelvic pain 318
  uterine fibroids 333
levetiracetam 549
Levine, Fredric 26
levorphanol 534
lidocaine
  intravenous 549
  topical 379, 514–16, 517
lifestyle changes
  angina 261, 262
  anxiety disorders 39
  GERD 303
  migraine 346
  peripheral neuropathy 387
  rheumatoid arthritis 95–96
  stress management 63–64
ligaments
  injuries 120–21, 224
  knee *166*, 166–67, 169–70
  repair 150
Lioresal (baclofen) 553
lithotripsy, kidney
  stones 445–46
living will, defined 603
L.M.X.4 cream 515, 516
loperamide, irritable
  bowel syndrome 307
low back pain *see* back pain
lower esophageal sphincter (LES)
  function 302
  surgery 304–5
Lower Extremity Amputation
  Prevention Program, Health
  Resources and Services
  Administration,
  contact information 614
lubiprostone, irritable
  bowel syndrome 308
lumbar degenerative
  joint disease, back pain 123
lumbar radiculopathy,
  electrodiagnostic tests 470–71
lumbar strain, back pain 120–21
Lunesta (eszopiclone) 551
Lupron (leuprolide)
  chronic pelvic pain 318
  uterine fibroids 333
Lyme disease, described 90–91

Lyrica (pregabalin)
  described 547–48
  diabetic neuropathy 392
  fibromyalgia 141

M

Mackey, Sean 53–54
magnetic fields, computers 82
magnetic resonance imaging (MRI)
  defined 603
  described 8
  neck, back, or radicular
    pain 115, 464–68
  shoulder pain 216
  whiplash 196
*Magnetic Resonance
  Imaging* (NASS) 464n
Maloni, Heidi 359n
"Managing Pain after Burn
  Injury" (MSKTC) 238
MAOIs (monoamine oxidase
  inhibitors) 546–47
marijuana, medicinal 47–48
massage therapy
  cancer pain 252
  described 482–83, 501–3
  osteoarthritis 101
  sports injuries 231
"Massage Therapy: An
  Introduction" (NCCAM) 501n
maxillary sinuses,
  location 407, *407*, 411
Mayo Clinic, website address 398
medial branch block (MBB)
  described 569
  whiplash 195, 196
"Medication Guide" (FDA) 529
medication overuse
  headache (MOH),
  described 345–46, 354
meditation
  cancer pain 252
  described 480
melanoma, paranasal sinus
  and nasal cavity 412
meloxicam 520, 524
men, pain perception 5–6, 26–27
meningitis, neck pain 192
meniscal injuries, knee 168

menstrual cycle
  described 322, 329
  migraine 344, 352–53
meperidine
  described 534
  sickle cell pain 403
meralgia paresthetica 372
"Meralgia Paresthetica
  Information Page"
  (NINDS) 372n
mesalamine,
  Crohn disease 292–93
metaxalone 553
methadone 534
methocarbamol 552
mexiletine, neuropathic
  pain 387, 549–50
microdiscectomy
  defined 600
  described 573
microvascular decompression,
  trigeminal neuralgia 278
"Middle Ear Infections"
  (Nemours Foundation) 279n
middle ear infections,
  about 280–84
migraine
  anxiety disorders 37
  defined 603
  described 22, 343–46
  hormones 352–53
  treatment 494, 556–57
milnacipran, fibromyalgia 141
mindfulness training,
  irritable bowel syndrome 308
"Minimally Invasive Spine
  Surgery (MIS)" (AANS) 577n
Mirena, uterine fibroids 333
misoprostol 521, 522
Mobic (meloxicam) 520, 524
Model Systems Knowledge
  Translation Center (MSKTC)
  burn pain publication 238n
  contact information 614
MOH (medication
  overuse headache),
  described 345–46, 354
monoamine oxidase
  inhibitors (MAOIs) 546–47

morphine
  codeine metabolism 435
  described 534
  intrathecal infusion 567–68
  palliative care 593
Morton's neuroma,
  described 152–53
motor neuropathy,
  described 385
motor vehicle accident,
  whiplash 193–94
Motrin (ibuprofen) 523–24
MRI *see* magnetic
  resonance imaging
MSKTC *see* Model Systems
  Knowledge Translation
  Center
multiple sclerosis pain 359–61
"Multiple Sclerosis Pain"
  (Maloni) 359n
"Muscle Cramp" (AAOS) 184n
muscle cramps 184–87
muscle injuries,
  back pain 120–21
muscle pain
  described 22
  versus nerve pain 366
  polymyalgia rheumatica 111
muscle relaxants
  back pain 118
  described 552–53
muscle strain, neck pain 195
Muscular Dystrophy Association,
  contact information 614
MyDr, contact information 615
Myers, Cynthia 26–27
Mylanta Gas (simethicone) 301
myofascial pain
  acupuncture 494
  defined 603
  temporomandibular joint 271
myofascial pain syndrome,
  described 22, 176–79
myolysis, uterine fibroids 334
myoma, uterine 331–34
myomectomy,
  uterine fibroids 333
myopathy,
  electrodiagnostic tests 471

N

nalbuphine 6, 537
naproxen and sumatriptan,
  migraine 557
naproxen sodium 524
narcotics
  back pain 117
  migraine 345
  osteoarthritis 102
  see also opioids
nasal cavity
  cancer 412–13
  structure and function 411
nasal sprays, sinusitis 409
NASS *see* North
  American Spine Society
National Amputation Foundation,
  website address 398
National Athletic Trainers
  Association,
  contact information 615
National Cancer Institute
  contact information 615
  publications
    bone cancer 132n
    cancer pain 243n
    paranasal sinus and nasal
      cavity cancer 411n
National Center for
  Chronic Disease Prevention
  and Health Promotion,
  contact information 615
National Center for
  Complementary and
  Alternative Medicine (NCCAM)
  contact information 615
  publications
    acupuncture 492n
    chronic pain and CAM 488n
    dietary supplements 496n
    massage therapy 501n
    relaxation techniques 504n
    spinal manipulation 499n
    yoga 507n
National Center for Health
  Statistics, pain data 12, 16
National Diabetes Education
  Program, contact
  information 394, 615

National Diabetes Information
  Clearinghouse
  contact information 394, 615
  diabetic neuropathy
    publication 389n
National Digestive Diseases
  Information Clearinghouse
  (NDDIC)
  contact information 615
  publications
    abdominal adhesions 286n
    appendicitis 288n
    Crohn disease 291n
    diverticulosis and
      diverticulitis 294n
    gallstones 297n
    gas 299n
    heartburn 302n
    irritable bowel syndrome 305n
    pancreatitis 309n
National Fibromyalgia Association,
  contact information 616
National Fibromyalgia Partnership,
  Inc., contact information 616
National Headache Foundation
  contact information 616
  publications
    analgesic rebound 354n
    hormones and migraine 352n
National Health and Nutrition
  Examination Survey (NHANES),
  pain data 16
National Health
  Interview Survey (DHHS)
  acupuncture 492
  health statistics 16–17
National Heart, Lung,
  and Blood Institute (NHLBI)
  contact information 616
  publications
    angina 256n
    heart attack 254n
National Institute for Occupational
  Safety and Health, contact
  information 83, 616
National Institute of Allergy and
  Infectious Diseases (NIAID)
  contact information 616
  sinusitis publication 406n

National Institute of Arthritis
  and Musculoskeletal and Skin
  Diseases (NIAMS)
  contact information 616
  publications
    arthritis and rheumatic
      diseases 88n
    back pain 114n
    bursitis and tendinitis 201n
    gout 107n
    joint replacement surgery 583n
    knee pain 165n
    osteoarthritis 98n
    osteonecrosis 136n
    Paget's disease 134n
    reactive arthritis 104n
    rheumatoid arthritis 94n
    shoulder pain 213n
    spinal stenosis 126n
    sports injuries 223n
National Institute of
  Child Health and Human
  Development (NICHD)
  contact information 617
  vulvodynia publication 335n
National Institute of Dental and
  Craniofacial Research (NIDCR)
  contact information 617
  TMJ disorders publication 270n
National Institute of General Medical
  Sciences, burns publication 236n
National Institute of
  Mental Health (NIMH)
  contact information 617
  depression and chronic
    pain publication 34n
National Institute of Neurological
  Disorders and Stroke (NINDS)
  contact information 617
  publications
    arachnoiditis 367n
    carpal tunnel syndrome 206n
    central pain syndrome 368n
    complex regional pain
      syndrome 370n
    glossary 597n
    glossopharyngeal
      neuralgia 371n
    headaches 340n

National Institute of Neurological
Disorders and Stroke (NINDS)
publications, *continued*
  meralgia paresthetica 372n
  pain 3n
  pain types 20n
  paresthesia 373n
  peripheral neuropathy 384n
  pinched nerve 374n
  piriformis syndrome 375n
  repetitive motion
    disorders 200n
  shingles and postherpetic
    neuralgia 376n
  tabes dorsalis 380n
  Tarlov cysts 381n
  trigeminal neuralgia 274n
National Institute of Nursing
Research (NINR)
contact information 617
palliative care publication 589n
National Institute on Aging,
contact information 617
National Institutes of Health (NIH)
contact information
  Osteoporosis and Related
    Bone Diseases—National
    Resource Center 618
  Pain Consortium 618
publications
  chronic pain control 52n
  pain intensity scales 456n
RePORTER website 587
National Kidney and Urologic
Diseases Information
Clearinghouse
contact information 617
publications
  interstitial cystitis 438n
  kidney stones 444n
National Osteonecrosis Foundation,
contact information 618
National Women's
Health Information Center,
contact information 618
NCCAM *see* National Center
for Complementary and
Alternative Medicine
NCS *see* nerve conduction studies

NDDIC *see* National Digestive
Diseases Information
Clearinghouse
neck, anatomy 194
neck pain
  CAM therapies 490, 494
  causes 190–93
  ergonomics 80–81
  magnetic resonance
    imaging 465–67
  whiplash 194–95
"Neck Pain"
  (A.D.A.M., Inc.) 190n
Nemours Foundation,
  publications
  childbirth and pain 314n
  costochondritis 264n
  ear pain 279n
  growing pains 161n
nephrolithiasis, defined 444
  see also kidney stones
nephrolithotomy,
  percutaneous 446
nerve blocks
  back pain 119
  cancer pain 250
  defined 603
  described 483, 569, 580–82
  spinal stenosis 128
  surgical pain 427–28
"Nerve Blocks" (Regents
  of the University
  of California) 580n
nerve conduction studies (NCS)
  described 7–8, 469–72
  whiplash 197
nerve pain
  see neuropathic pain
nerves
  defined 603–4
  pinched 374–75
nerve stimulation,
  invasive 484
neurectomy,
  trigeminal neuralgia 277
neurological examinations,
  described 8
neuroma, interdigital 152–53
Neurontin (gabapentin) 547–48

neuropathic pain
  burns 239
  cancer therapy 246
  described 22–23, 364–66
  incidence 10
  multiple sclerosis 359–60
  peripheral neuropathy 386,
    387–88
Neuropathy Association,
  contact information 618
neurostimulatory procedures,
  types 475
neurosurgery, cancer pain 250
neuroticism, pain experience 29, 31
neurotransmitters 4–5
new daily persistent
  headache, described 349
New Zealand Dermatological Society
  dyspareunia publication 324n
  website address 618
NHANES (National Health and
  Nutrition Examination Survey),
  pain data 16
NHLBI *see* National Heart,
  Lung, and Blood Institute
NIAID *see* National Institute of
  Allergy and Infectious Diseases
NIAMS *see* National Institute of
  Arthritis and Musculoskeletal
  and Skin Diseases
NICHD *see* National Institute
  of Child Health and Human
  Development
nicotine 45
nicotine replacement therapy 44
NIDCR *see* National Institute of
  Dental and Craniofacial Research
NIH *see* National Institutes of
  Health
"NIH Research Plan on
  Vulvodynia" (NICHD) 335n
NIMH *see* National Institute
  of Mental Health
NINDS *see* National Institute of
  Neurological Disorders and Stroke
NINR *see* National Institute
  of Nursing Research
Nissen fundoplication, GERD 304
nitrates, angina 262

nociceptors, described 5
nonsteroidal anti-inflammatory
  drugs (NSAIDs)
  adverse/side effects 520–21
  back pain 117–18
  burn pain 240
  cancer pain 247–48
  carpal tunnel syndrome 209
  chronic pain 53
  cytoprotective
    medications 521–22
  defined 604
  described 519, 522–25
  foot injury 160
  gout 108–9
  intravenous 521
  migraine 345, 353
  older adults and children 7
  osteoarthritis 102–3
  osteonecrosis 137
  over-the-counter 510–12
  plantar fasciitis 157
  polymyalgia rheumatica 112
  reactive arthritis 105
  spinal stenosis 128
  sports injuries 229
  surgical pain 429
  topical 514, 520–21
norepinephrine 5, 45
Norflex (orphenadrine) 553
North American
  Spine Society (NASS)
  contact information 618
  publications
    electromyograms and nerve
      conduction studies 469n
    exercise and spinal pain 65n
    magnetic resonance
      imaging 464n
    whiplash 193n
    x-rays 462n
NSAIDs *see* nonsteroidal anti-
  inflammatory drugs
Nubain (nalbuphine) 6, 537
Nucynta (tapentadol) 535
Numeric Rating Scale 457–58
Numorphan (oxymorphone) 535
nutrition/hydration, defined 604
  see also diet and nutrition

O

obturator sign, appendicitis 290

Occupational Safety and Health Administration (OSHA), contact information 84, 618

Office of National Drug Control Policy (ONDCP), prescription drug abuse facts 14–15

Office on Women's Health (DHHS), publications
  chronic pain diagnosis 456n
  endometriosis 328n
  fibromyalgia 139n
  glossary 597n
  uterine fibroids 331n

Ofirmev (acetaminophen) 521

older adults
  pain experience 6–7
  treatment plans 475

ONSOLIS (fentanyl) 533

Opana (oxymorphone) 535

"Opiate Use for Chronic Non-Terminal Pain is Controversial" (Cooke) 541n

opioid agonists
  described 530
  examples 532–36
  short- and long-acting 531–32
  slow-release tablets 532, 536

opioid mixed agonists/antagonists
  described 530–31
  examples 536–37

opioids
  adverse/side effects 538–41
  burn pain 240
  cancer pain 248–49
  chronic pain 53, 528–29, 541–42
  classification 530–31
  defined 604
  delivery 531–32
  diabetic neuropathy 392
  endogenous 5, 27, 529, 530
  history 4
  intrathecal infusion 567–68
  kappa- 6
  older adults and children 7
  overdose deaths 17–18, 529, 541
  palliative care 593
  postherpetic neuralgia 379

opioids, *continue*
  receptors 5
  sickle cell pain 402, 403
  surgical pain 428–29
  tolerance and addiction 250

orphenadrine 553

orthopaedic surgeon 228

orthotics, heel pain 158

Orudis, Oruvail (ketoprofen) 524

Osgood-Schlatter disease 171–72

OSHA (Occupational Safety and Health Administration), contact information 84, 618

osteoarthritis
  acupuncture 495
  defined 604
  described 88–89, *89*, 98–99, *99*
  lumbar, back pain 123
  treatment 99–103, 563–64
  see also arthritis

osteochondritis dissecans 172–73

osteolysis, joint replacement 586

osteonecrosis 136–38

osteoporosis
  back pain 125
  defined 604

osteosarcoma, described 132

osteotomy
  osteonecrosis 138
  toe 149

otitis media, described 280–84

Oucher pain scale 401

"Ouch! The different ways people experience pain" (Jarrett) 25n

overdose deaths, prescription opioid 17–18, 529, 541

over-the-counter pain relievers 509–12, 519

oxcarbazepine 549

oxycodone 534–35

oxymorphone 535

P

packed cell volume (PCV), rheumatic diseases 93

Paget Foundation, contact information 619

Paget's disease of bone 134–36

pain
  defined 20, 604
  history 3–4
  types 20–25
  see also acute pain; chronic pain
"Pain" (Beth Israel
  Medical Center) 476n
"Pain: Hope Through Research"
  (NINDS) 3n, 20n, 597n
"Pain after Stroke"
  (US Department of
  Veterans Affairs) 419n
"Pain and Paget's Disease
  of Bone" (NIAMS) 134n
pain conditions, common
  lost productivity time 13
  types 11–12, 20–25
"Pain Control: Support
  for People with Cancer"
  (National Cancer
  Institute) 243n
pain due to nerve injury,
  defined 604
Paine, Peter 30–31
painful bladder syndrome
  see interstitial cystitis
"Painful Periods (Dysmenorrhea)"
  (Regents of the University
  of California) 321n
"Painful sex in women
  (dyspareunia)" (New Zealand
  Dermatological Society) 324n
pain history 7
"Pain in Sickle Cell Disease
  (Sickle Cell Anemia)"
  (Boyse and Kelly) 399n
pain intensity scales
  cancer pain 246, 247–50
  children 401–2, 458–61
  post-stroke pain 421
  surgical pain 425
  types 457–61
"Pain Intensity Scales"
  (NIH Pain Consortium) 456n
painkillers *see* analgesics
pain management
  methods 8, 474–75
  plans 474–76
  programs 451–54

pain management, *continued*
  therapies 476–84
    advances 4
    anesthesiologic 483–84
    complementary/
      alternative 482–83
    invasive and
      implanted 563–70
    non-pharmacological 477
    pharmacological 476–77
    physiatrist 477–78
    psychoeducational 479–82
    stimulatory 479, 484
"Pain Management Programs"
  (ACPA) 451n
pain medicine, defined 450
pain pathway, described 3
pain perception
  differences 25–32, 53–54
    ethnicity 27–29
    gender 6, 26–27
    personality 29–31
  theories 3
pain pumps 566–68
palliative care
  cancer pain 243
  defined 604
  described 589–93
"Palliative Care: The Relief You
  Need When You're Experiencing
  the Symptoms of Serious Illness"
  (NINR) 589n
Palmer, Ben 28–29
pancreatitis
  described 309–12
  gallstone 297
"Pancreatitis" (NDDIC) 309n
papilloma, paranasal sinus
  and nasal cavity 412
Parafon Forte DSC
  (chlorzoxazone) 553
"Paranasal Sinus and
  Nasal Cavity Cancer
  Treatment (PDQ): Patient
  version" (National
  Cancer Institute) 411n
paranasal sinuses
  cancer 412–13
  names 406–7, *407*, 411

paresthesia
  described 373
  peripheral neuropathy 384
"Paresthesia Information Page"
  (NINDS) 373n
Partners Against Pain,
  contact information 619
passing gas, described 300
patella, described 166, *166*
patient-controlled analgesia (PCA)
  defined 604
  surgical pain 426–27
Paulson, Pamela 26
PCV (packed cell volume),
  rheumatic diseases 93
"PDQ Cancer Information Summary"
  (National Cancer Institute) 411n
pediatric population *see* children
Pedorthotic Footwear Association,
  contact information 619
pelvic pain, chronic 318–20
pentazocine and pentazocine/
  naloxone 537
pentosan polysulfate sodium,
  interstitial cystitis 440
peptides 5
peripheral nervous system,
  defined 605
peripheral neuropathy
  defined 605
  described 384–88
  diabetic 390
  electrodiagnostic tests 471
"Peripheral Neuropathy
  Fact Sheet" (NINDS) 384n
personality, pain experience 29–31
Phalen test, carpal
  tunnel syndrome 209
"Phantom and Stump Pain"
  (Beth Israel Medical Center) 395n
phantom pain
  cancer surgery 246
  defined 605
  described 395–97
  websites 397–98
pharmacotherapy
  defined 605
  types 476–77
phenytoin 548

PHN *see* postherpetic neuralgia
Phoenix Society for Burn Survivors
  contact information 619
  website address 242
physiatric approaches, types 477–78
physical activity
  burn pain 241
  program 179–80
  readiness questionnaire 183–84
  see also exercise(s)
physical therapy
  cancer pain 252
  described 485
  interstitial cystitis 442
  spinal stenosis 128
  sports injuries 228–29
physician assisted suicide,
  defined 605
pinched nerve 374–75
"Pinched Nerve Information Page"
  (NINDS) 374n
piriformis syndrome,
  described 121, 375
"Piriformis Syndrome
  Information Page" (NINDS) 375n
placebos
  acupuncture 493
  defined 605
plantar fasciitis, described 156–59
plasmapheresis, peripheral
  neuropathy 387
plica syndrome 173
PLO (Pluronic Lecithin
  Organogel) 517
polymethylmethacrylate
  bone cement, FDA warning 576
"Polymyalgia Rheumatica"
  (American College of
  Rheumatology) 110n
polymyalgia rheumatica (PMR)
  described 91, 110–12
  giant cell arteritis 355, 356
polymyositis, described 22, 91
posterior calcaneal exostosis,
  described 156
postherpetic itch 379
postherpetic neuralgia (PHN)
  defined 605
  described 23, 378–79

post-nasal drip, sinusitis 407
posture
  ergonomics 76, 77, 79–80
  standing and seated 68, *68*
PPIs *see* proton pump inhibitors
pregabalin
  described 547–48
  diabetic neuropathy 392
  fibromyalgia 141
press-ups exercise 66–67, *67*
Prialt (ziconotide),
  intrathecal 568
primary exertional/stabbing
  headaches, described 349
probiotics, irritable
  bowel syndrome 308
progestins, endometriosis 330
progressive muscle relaxation,
  described 479, 505
prokinetics, GERD 304
pronation, excessive foot 155
propoxyphene 537–38
prostaglandins
  drugs inhibiting 323
  dysmenorrhea 322
proton pump inhibitors (PPIs)
  GERD 304
  types 522
psoas sign, appendicitis 289–90
psoriatic arthritis
  back pain 125
  described 91
psychological approaches
  back pain 118
  burn pain 240–41
  defined 605
  fibromyalgia 142
  irritable bowel syndrome 308
  types 475, 479–82
psychotherapy, described 481–82
Pud, Dorit 29

Q

quadriceps muscle stretch 187
quality of life
  chronic pain 12–13
  measurement 55–56
  palliative care 589
"Quality of Life Scale" (ACPA) 55n

"Questions and Answers about
  Arthritis and Rheumatic
  Diseases" (NIAMS) 88n
"Questions and Answers about
  Bursitis and Tendinitis"
  (NIAMS) 201n
"Questions and Answers
  about Gout" (NIAMS) 107n
"Questions and Answers about
  Knee Problems" (NIAMS) 165n
"Questions and Answers about
  Osteonecrosis" (NIAMS) 136n
"Questions and Answers about
  Reactive Arthritis"
  (NIAMS) 104n
"Questions and Answers
  about Shoulder Problems"
  (NIAMS) 213n
"Questions and Answers about
  Spinal Stenosis" (NIAMS) 126n
Qutenza (capsaicin) 515

R

radiation therapy
  bone cancer 133
  cancer pain 250
radiculopathy
  electrodiagnostic tests 470–71
  magnetic resonance
    imaging 465–67
radiofrequency ablation,
  described 569–70
*Radiographic Assessment
  for Back Pain* (NASS) 462n
Rahim-Williams, F. Bridgett 28
raloxifene 318
ramelteon 551
Rappaport, Bob 434, 435, 436
reactive arthritis
  back pain 124–25
  described 90, 104–7
rebound headache,
  described 345–46, 354
rebound tenderness,
  appendicitis 289
receptors, neurotransmitter 4–5
referred pain
  polymyalgia rheumatica 111
  whiplash 195–96

reflex sympathetic dystrophy
    defined 605–6
    described 23
    see also complex regional
        pain syndrome
Reflex Sympathetic Dystrophy
    Syndrome Association,
    contact information 619
reframing, described 480–81
Regents of the University of
    California, publications
    dysmenorrhea 321n
    nerve blocks 580n
rehabilitation
    approaches 475, 485–86
    cardiac 263
    defined 606
    sports injuries 230–31
"Rehabilitation Approaches"
    (Beth Israel Medical Center) 485n
Reiki, cancer pain 252
Reiter syndrome, back pain 124–25
relaxation response 504, 505–6
relaxation techniques
    anxiety disorders 38
    burn pain 241
    cancer pain 252
    described 504–7
    stress management 62–63
    surgical pain 429
"Relaxation Techniques for Health:
    An Introduction" (NCCAM) 504n
*Relieving Pain in America:
    A Blueprint for Transforming
    Prevention, Care, Education, and
    Research* (Institute of Medicine) 9,
    15–16
repeated actions, ergonomics 76, 81
repetitive motion disorders (RMDs)
    described 23, 74–75, 200–201
    fibromyalgia 140
    risk factors 76–77
"Repetitive Motion Disorders
    Information Page" (NINDS) 200n
Research! America, pain survey 13–14
resting pain, burns 239
rheumatic diseases,
    questions and answers 88–94
    see also arthritis

rheumatoid arthritis
    defined 606
    described *89*, 90, 94–98
    see also arthritis
rheumatoid factor 93
rheumatologists 112, 357
rhinosinusitis, chronic,
    treatment 408–9
rhizotomy
    defined 606
    described 569–70
    trigeminal neuralgia 277–78
RICE (rest, ice, compression,
    and elevation)
    bursitis and tendinitis 204–5
    defined 606
    foot injury 160
    sports injuries 228, 229
rifaximin, irritable
    bowel syndrome 308
Rimso-50 (dimethyl sulfoxide) 439–40
RMDs *see* repetitive motion disorders
Robaxin (methocarbamol) 553
Rolfing, back pain 120
Roman chair extension exercise 70, *70*
rotator cuff
    structure 214, *215*
    tendinitis and bursitis 202–3, 218
    torn 219–20
Rovsing's sign, appendicitis 289
Roxicodone (oxycodone) 534–35
Rozerem (ramelteon) 551

S

SAFER mnemonic,
    medication safety 512
salicylates
    described 523
    topical 513
Salonpas Pain Relief Patch 514
sarcoma, paranasal sinus
    and nasal cavity 412
Savella (milnacipran),
    fibromyalgia 141
Schmahl, Christian 30
sciatica
    described 21, 23, 121
    piriformis syndrome 375
scleroderma, described 90

SCS *see* spinal cord stimulation
seated posture 68, *68*
seating, ergonomic 80–81
sedatives, described 550–51
Segal, Robert 57n
selective serotonin and
    norepinephrine
    reuptake inhibitors (SNRIs)
    depression 36
    pain control 546
selective serotonin
    reuptake inhibitors (SSRIs)
    depression 36
    pain control 544, 545–46
self-efficacy, pain experience 30
self-hypnosis *see* hypnosis
sensory neuropathy,
    described 385–86
separation, shoulder 217–18
serotonin 5, 557
sesamoiditis 153
sex, painful, described 324–27
sexual problems,
    diabetic neuropathy 393
Sforzo, Gary 179n
shingles
    defined 606
    described 23, 376–78
"Shingles: Hope through
    Research" (NINDS) 376n
shin splints, sports injuries 225
shock wave lithotripsy,
    kidney stones 445–46
shoes
    bunion relief 148–49
    heel pain 158
shoulder
    structure and function 213–14, *215*
    tendinitis, bursitis, and
        impingement syndrome 202–3
shoulder pain
    common problems 213, 216–22
    diagnosis 215–16
    ergonomics 80–81
sickle cell anemia, defined 606
Sickle Cell Disease
    Association of America,
    contact information 619
sickle cell pain 399–404

simethicone 301
sinusitis 406–10
    see also paranasal sinuses
"Sinusitis" (NIAID) 406n
Skelaxin (metaxalone) 553
skin disorders, painful 23–24
skin grafting, burns 236–37
skull fracture 225–26
SLE (systemic lupus
    erythematosus), described 90
sleep
    anxiety disorders 39
    fibromyalgia 141–43
    headache 351
    medications 240, 550–52
    pain and 40–42
    stress management 64
"Sleep and Pain" (Sleep
    HealthCenters) 40n
"Sleep Deprivation"
    (Sleep HealthCenters) 40n
sleep deprivation, described 40–41
Sleep HealthCenters
    contact information 619
    pain and sleep publication 40n
slings, sports injuries 230
Smith, Melinda 57n
smoking
    effects on pain 44–45
    interstitial cystitis 441
    sickle cell disease 400
    stress management 64
SNRIs *see* selective serotonin
    and norepinephrine
    reuptake inhibitors
Social Security Administration,
    disability benefits 144
social support
    chronic pain 51
    described 481–82
sodium channel blocking 549–50
Soma (carisoprodol) 552
somatoform pain disorder 415–17
"Somatoform Pain Disorder"
    (A.D.A.M., Inc.) 415n
sphenoid sinuses,
    location 407, *407*, 411
sphincterotomy,
    pancreatic or bile ducts 312

spinal cord
  compression 244–45
  pain transmission 3, 4
  traumatic injuries 225–26
spinal cord stimulation (SCS)
  defined 606
  described 484, 564–66
spinal fusion
  defined 606–7
  described 574–76
spinal infusion, described 483
spinal injections, whiplash 197–98
spinal manipulation
  back pain 119, 499–500
  whiplash 198
"Spinal Manipulation for
  Low-Back Pain" (NCCAM) 499n
spinal pain *see* back pain
spinal stenosis
  back pain 123
  described 24, 126–30, *127*
  magnetic resonance imaging 466
spine
  minimally invasive
    surgery 577–79
  structures *127*
Spine Care Treatment Centers,
  website address 619
splints
  heel pain 158
  osteoarthritis 100
  sports injuries 230
  surgical pain 430
  TMJ disorders 273
Spondylitis Association of America,
  contact information 619
spondyloarthropathies
  described 90
  seronegative 104, 124–25
spondylolisthesis
  back pain 124
  described 21
sports injuries
  acute *versus* chronic 227
  treatment 227–32
  types 24, 223–27
sprains, sports injuries 224
squamous cell carcinoma,
  paranasal sinus and nasal cavity 412

SSRIs *see* selective serotonin
  reuptake inhibitors
Stadol (butorphanol) 6, 537
standing backbends 66–67, *67*
standing posture 68, *68*
stent placement,
  pancreatic or bile ducts 312
steroids, types 559
  see also corticosteroid injections
stimulatory therapies
  invasive 484
  non-invasive 479
strains
  back pain 120–21
  neck pain 195
  sports injuries 224
strength training *see* exercise(s)
stress
  responses 59–62, 505
  sources 57–58
  workplace 82–83
stress fracture
  forefoot 153–54
  sports injuries 226–27
stress management
  chronic pain 50, 57–64
  healthy strategies 59–64
  rheumatoid arthritis 96
  unhealthy strategies 58–59
"Stress Management"
  (Smith and Segal) 57n
stress testing, angina 260
stretching *see* exercise(s)
stroke
  headache 350
  incidence 11
  pain after 419–22
struvite stones, described 445
stump pain, described 395–97
  see also phantom pain
Suboxone
  (buprenorphine/naloxone) 537
Subutex (buprenorphine) 536
sucralfate 521, 522
sulfasalazine, Crohn disease 292–93
sumatriptan and naproxen,
  migraine 557
supine ball extension exercise *71*
surgical approaches, pain control 484

surgical pain
  control
    codeine for children 7, 434–36
    frequently asked
      questions 431–32
    home 430–31
    importance 424
    options 426–30
    patient role 432–33
  described 24
Swiss ball exercises 70, *70, 71, 72*
Synalgos-DC (dihydrocodeine
  bitartrate, aspirin, caffeine) 533
synovectomy,
  rheumatoid arthritis 97
synovial fluid examination,
  rheumatic diseases 93
systemic lupus erythematosus
  (SLE), described 90

T

tabes dorsalis 380
"Tabes Dorsalis Information
  Page" (NINDS) 380n
tai chi
  cancer pain 252
  fibromyalgia 53
Talwin (pentazocine) 537
Tambocor (flecainide) 549–50
tapentadol 535
tardive dyskinesia,
  anti-psychotic drugs 554
Tarlov cysts 381–82
"Tarlov Cysts Information Page"
  (NINDS) 381n
tarsal tunnel syndrome,
  described 159
TCAs *see* tricyclic
  antidepressants
Tegretol
  (carbamazepine) 547, 548
temporal arteritis
  see giant cell arteritis
temporomandibular joint
  (TMJ) 270–71, *271*
temporomandibular joint
  (TMJ) disorders
  described 24, 270–74
  relaxation techniques 506

tendinitis
  Achilles 154–55, 203–4
  described 23, 91, 201–6
  knee 170–71, 203, 224
  shoulder 202–3, 218
tendons
  defined 201
  injuries 170–71, 224
  knee 166, *166*
  repair 97, 150
tennis elbow
  acupuncture 495
  described 202
TENS *see* transcutaneous
electrical nerve stimulation
tension headaches,
  described 22, 346–47
testosterone, pain response 5, 6
thalamus, function 4, 341
thermotherapy *see* cold therapy;
  heat therapy
tiagabine 548
tic douloureux
  see trigeminal neuralgia
Tinel test, carpal
  tunnel syndrome 209
tissue engineering,
  sports injuries 232
tizanidine 553
TMJ
  see temporomandibular joint
"TMJ Disorders" (NIDCR) 270n
TNA—Facial Pain Association,
  contact information 620
TNF inhibitors,
  reactive arthritis 106
toenails, ingrown 151–52
toe problems, types 146–52
tolerance, pain medication 250
tooth pain
  acupuncture 495
  described 268–69
"Tooth Pain" (American
  Association of Endodontists) 268n
Topamax (topiramate) 549
topical pain relievers
  described 513–17
  NSAID 520–21
topiramate 549

traction, back pain 118
tramadol 102, 536
tranquilizers
  described 550–52
  labor pain 316
transcutaneous electrical
  nerve stimulation (TENS)
  back pain 119
  cancer pain 251
  defined 607
  described 479
  interstitial cystitis 441
  osteoarthritis 101
  post-stroke pain 421
transdermal drugs 513
trauma, pain conditions 24–25
  see also sports injuries
traumatic brain injury,
  described 225–26
trazodone 546
"Treating Chronic Pelvic Pain:
  A Review of the Research for
  Women" (AHRQ) 318n
treatment withdrawal, defined 607
Treximet (naproxen
  and sumatriptan) 557
tricyclic antidepressants (TCAs)
  chronic pain 544–45
  diabetic neuropathy 392
  interstitial cystitis 440
  postherpetic neuralgia 378–79
  trigeminal neuralgia 276
trigeminal autonomic cephalgias,
  described 347–48
trigeminal nerve, branches 275, 341
trigeminal neuralgia
  defined 607
  described 22, 274–78
  headache 351
Trigeminal Neuralgia Association,
  contact information 620
"Trigeminal Neuralgia
  Fact Sheet" (NINDS) 274n
trigger point injections
  back pain 119
  described 484
trigger points,
  myofascial 176, 177, 501
Trileptal (oxcarbazepine) 549

Trilisate (choline magnesium
  trisalicylate) 523
triptan drugs,
  migraine 345, 353, 556
tumor necrosis factor (TNF)
  inhibitors, reactive arthritis 106
Tylenol *see* acetaminophen
tympanostomy tubes,
  ear infections 283–84

U

Ultram (tramadol) 536
ultrasound
  heat therapy 486
  shoulder pain 216
  sports injuries 231
"Understanding Nerve
  Pain" (ACPA) 364n
University of California, San Diego
  contact information 620
  dysmenorrhea publication 321n
University of California, San
  Francisco
  contact information 620
  nerve blocks publication 580n
University of Michigan
  Health System
  contact information 620
  sickle cell pain publication 399n
University of Washington
  Model Systems Knowledge
  Translation Center, burn
  pain publication 238n
ureteroscopy, kidney stones 446
uric acid, defined 607
uric acid stones, described 445
urinalysis, rheumatic diseases 93
urinary problems, diabetic
  neuropathy 393
urolithiasis or ureterolithiasis,
  defined 444
  see also kidney stones
Urology Care Foundation,
  contact information 620
urostomy, interstitial cystitis 443
US Department of Health
  and Human Services (DHHS),
  health survey 16–17, 492
  see also Office on Women's Health

US Department of Veterans Affairs
   contact information 620
   publications
      multiple sclerosis pain 359n
      stroke and pain 419n
   website address 397
US Food and Drug
   Administration (FDA)
   botulinum toxin 555–56
   contact information 620
   dietary supplements 497
   MedWatch program 274, 436, 498
   opioid safety 529
   publications
      codeine for children 434n
      over-the-counter
         pain relievers 509n
"Using Dietary Supplements
   Wisely" (NCCAM) 496n
uterine fibroid embolization
   (UFE) or uterine artery
   embolization (UAE) 334
uterine fibroids
   defined 607
   described 331–34
"Uterine Fibroids Fact Sheet"
   (Office on Women's Health) 331n

V

Valium (diazepam) 552, 553
valproic acid 548
varenicline 45
varicella zoster virus (VZV)
   shingles 376
   vaccine 378
vascular disease, pain 25
vertebroplasty, percutaneous 576
vibration, ergonomics 77
Vimpat (lacosamide) 548
viscosupplementation,
   osteoarthritis 102, 563–64
vision correction, workplace 79
Voltaren 1% Gel (diclofenac) 520–21
Vossen, Helen 29
vulvodynia 335–37

W

walking, back pain 66–67, *67*
warm-up activities 182, 187

weight control, osteoarthritis 100
"What Are the Signs and
   Symptoms of a Heart Attack"
   (NHLBI) 254n
"What Is a Cortisone Shot?"
   (Cluett) 559n
"What Is Angina?" (NHLBI) 256n
"What Is Pain Medicine?"
   (American Board of
   Pain Medicine) 450n
"What Is Sleep and
   Why Is It Important?"
   (Sleep HealthCenters) 40n
"What You Need to
   Know About Pain
   Control after Surgery"
   (Cleveland Clinic) 424n
whiplash 193–98
*Whiplash and Whiplash-Associated
   Disorders* (NASS) 193n
women
   hormones and migraine 352–53
   pain perception 5–6, 26–27
Wong-Baker FACES
   Pain Rating Scale 401, 458
work/workplace
   carpal tunnel syndrome 208, 311
   costs of pain 9, 11, 13
   ergonomics 73–84
   fibromyalgia 143, 144
writer's cramp, described 23, 208

X, Y, Z

x-rays
   angina 260
   back pain 115, 462–64
   described 8
   whiplash 196
yoga
   cancer pain 252
   described 507–8
"Yoga for Health" (NCCAM) 507n
Zanaflex (tizanidine) 553
ziconotide, intrathecal 568
zolpidem tartrate 550–51
zonisamide 549
Zostavax (VZV vaccine) 378
Zubieta, Jon-Kar 27
Zyban (bupropion) 45

Health Reference Series

Adolescent Health Sourcebook, 3rd Edition

Adult Health Concerns Sourcebook

AIDS Sourcebook, 5th Edition

Alcoholism Sourcebook, 3rd Edition

Allergies Sourcebook, 4th Edition

Alzheimer Disease Sourcebook, 5th Edition

Arthritis Sourcebook, 3rd Edition

Asthma Sourcebook, 3rd Edition

Attention Deficit Disorder Sourcebook

Autism & Pervasive Developmental Disorders
Sourcebook, 2nd Edition

Back & Neck Sourcebook, 2nd Edition

Blood & Circulatory Disorders Sourcebook,
3rd Edition

Brain Disorders Sourcebook, 3rd Edition

Breast Cancer Sourcebook, 4th Edition

Breastfeeding Sourcebook

Burns Sourcebook

Cancer Sourcebook for Women, 4th Edition

Cancer Sourcebook, 6th Edition

Cancer Survivorship Sourcebook

Cardiovascular Disorders Sourcebook,
5th Edition

Caregiving Sourcebook

Child Abuse Sourcebook, 3rd Edition

Childhood Diseases & Disorders Sourcebook,
3rd Edition

Colds, Flu & Other Common Ailments
Sourcebook

Communication Disorders Sourcebook

Complementary & Alternative Medicine
Sourcebook, 4th Edition

Congenital Disorders Sourcebook, 3rd Edition

Contagious Diseases Sourcebook, 2nd Edition

Cosmetic & Reconstructive Surgery Sourcebook,
2nd Edition

Death & Dying Sourcebook, 2nd Edition

Dental Care & Oral Health Sourcebook,
4th Edition

Depression Sourcebook, 3rd Edition

Dermatological Disorders Sourcebook,
2nd Edition

Diabetes Sourcebook, 5th Edition

Diet & Nutrition Sourcebook, 4th Edition

Digestive Diseases & Disorder Sourcebook

Disabilities Sourcebook, 2nd Edition

Disease Management Sourcebook

Domestic Violence Sourcebook, 4th Edition

Drug Abuse Sourcebook, 4th Edition

Ear, Nose & Throat Disorders Sourcebook,
2nd Edition

Eating Disorders Sourcebook, 3rd Edition

Emergency Medical Services Sourcebook

Endocrine & Metabolic Disorders Sourcebook,
2nd Edition

Environmental Health Sourcebook, 3rd Edition

Ethnic Diseases Sourcebook

Eye Care Sourcebook, 4th Edition

Family Planning Sourcebook

Fitness & Exercise Sourcebook, 4th Edition

Food Safety Sourcebook

Forensic Medicine Sourcebook

Gastrointestinal Diseases & Disorders
Sourcebook, 2nd Edition

Genetic Disorders Sourcebook, 5th Edition

Head Trauma Sourcebook

Headache Sourcebook

Health Insurance Sourcebook

Healthy Aging Sourcebook

Healthy Children Sourcebook

Healthy Heart Sourcebook for Women

Hepatitis Sourcebook

Household Safety Sourcebook

Hypertension Sourcebook

Immune System Disorders Sourcebook,
2nd Edition

Infant & Toddler Health Sourcebook

Infectious Diseases Sourcebook